Ethics and Professionalism
A Guide for the Physician Assistant

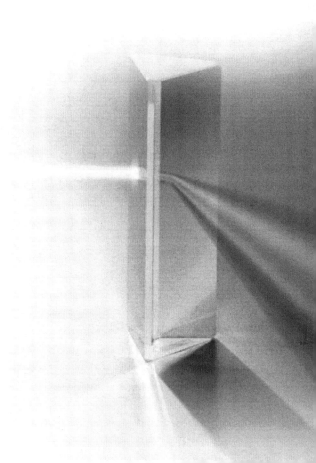

Ethics and Professionalism
A Guide for the Physician Assistant

Barry A. Cassidy, PhD, PA-C

Senior Vice-President Professional Services
NEXTCARE Urgent Care
Mesa, Arizona
Former Executive Director
Arizona Medical Board and Arizona Regulatory
    Board of Physician Assistants
Former Professor, Associate Dean and Director
    Physician Assistant Program
Midwestern University
Glendale, Arizona

J. Dennis Blessing, PhD, PA-C

Associate Dean for South Texas Programs
School of Allied Health Sciences
Professor and Chair
Department of Physician Assistant Studies
The University of Texas Health Science Center at
    San Antonio
San Antonio, Texas

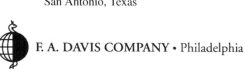 F. A. DAVIS COMPANY • Philadelphia

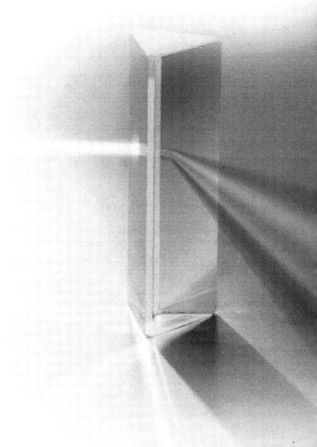

F.A. Davis Company
1915 Arch Street
Philadelphia, PA 19103
www. fadavis.com

Printed in the United States of America

Last digit indicates print number: 10 9 8 7 6

Publisher: Margaret M. Biblis
Acquisitions Editor: Andy McPhee
Manager, Content Development: Deborah J. Thorp
Developmental Editor: Jennifer A. Pine
Manager Art and Design: Carolyn O'Brien

As new scientific information becomes available through basic and clinical research, recommended treatments and drug therapies undergo changes. The author(s) and publisher have done everything possible to make this book accurate, up to date, and in accord with accepted standards at the time of publication. The authors, editors, and publisher are not responsible for errors or omissions or for consequences from application of the book, and make no warranty, expressed or implied, in regard to the contents of the book. Any practice described in this book should be applied by the reader in accordance with professional standards of care used in regard to the unique circumstances that may apply in each situation. The reader is advised always to check product information (package inserts) for changes and new information regarding dose and contraindications before administering any drug. Caution is especially urged when using new or infrequently ordered drugs.

Library of Congress Cataloging-in-Publication Data

Ethics and professionalism : a guide for the physician assistant /
[edited by] Barry A. Cassidy, J. Dennis Blessing.
    p. ; cm.

  Includes bibliographical references and index.
  ISBN-13: 978-0-8036-1338-6 (pbk. : alk. paper)
  ISBN-10: 0-8036-1338-5 (pbk. : alk. paper)
  1. Physicians assistants—Professional ethics. 2. Physicians assistants—Training of—Moral and ethical aspects. 3. Medical ethics. I. Cassidy, Barry A. II. Blessing, J. Dennis.
  [DNLM: 1. Physician Assistants—ethics. 2. Clinical Competence. 3. Decision Making. 4. Ethics, Clinical. W 21.5 E84 2008]
  R697.P45E84 2008
  174.2—dc22
                                        2007002960

Dedication

My efforts for this book are dedicated to the memory of Eugene A. Stead, Jr., MD, founding father of the PA concept; and James R. Pluth, MD, retired thoracic and cardiovascular surgeon. Both men were mentors, friends, and ethical role models for me. I also dedicate this book to my wife Barbie Cassidy, who keeps me grounded and helps me live an ethical life with love.

—BAC

My efforts for this book are dedicated to Richard R. Rahr, EdD, PA-C, colleague, mentor, friend. A role model and example of ethical behavior for us all.

—JDB

Preface

This book was conceived more than 5 years ago. Its production was a labor of love and a program of persistence. In our roles as educators of physician assistant students, we recognized that a textbook discussing ethics and professionalism focused specifically for PA students would be helpful to both them and their educators.

Physician assistants are unique health-care professionals in many ways. During the beginning years of the profession, typical PA students had a significant amount of health-care experience; many of them were military corpsmen and medics. This experience allowed these early PAs the opportunity to see other health-care professionals in action and to appreciate not only the culture of the physician-patient relationship but also the interdependent professional interactions of all members of the health-care team.

Today's PA students have far more academic preparation and less health-care experience than their older colleagues. The PA medical education curriculum is academically intense and accomplished quickly. The clinical curriculum is also intense and attempts to provide PA students with clinical exposure across a wide range of medical experiences and specialties. The standards for PA education require curricula to include education in ethics and professionalism. A component of becoming a critical thinker involves understanding the ethics of decision making that affects others.

Ethics and professionalism are usually included in the academic portion of the PA curriculum. Faculty need to lead and encourage discussion and analysis of issues that involve professional behavior and ethical conflicts to help students prepare for approaching clinical dilemmas. This text was designed to help PA educators and students accomplish this important task.

In putting this book together, we looked across the nation for experts in physician assistant education and ethical training who also had a clear understanding of the challenges facing PAs in today's practice environment. While many excellent books and treatises are available concerning issues in medical ethics, none have been written from the perspective of a dependent practitioner who shares in one of the most intimate of life's experiences, the physician-patient relationship. For PAs and their supervisors and patients, this has evolved to the physician assistant–patient–physician relationship. It is not a lesser relationship; it includes all the same ethical and professional issues.

This book has been designed not only for today's PAs but also for PAs in the future. Cases are presented to help illustrate ethical principles and provide insight into the ethics and professionalism considerations of being a PA student. All chapters are designed to stimulate discussion and blend theory and practice.

Although the process of completing this work has been long, we hope you'll agree that the wait has been worthwhile.

Barry A. Cassidy, PhD, PA-C

J. Dennis Blessing, PhD, PA-C

Contributors

Barry A. Cassidy, PhD, PA-C
Senior Vice-President Professional Services
NEXTCARE Urgent Care
Mesa, Arizona
Former Executive Director
Arizona Medical Board and Arizona Regulatory Board of
    Physician Assistants
Former Professor, Associate Dean and Director
    Physician Assistant Program
Midwestern University
Glendale, Arizona

Randy D. Danielsen, PhD, PA-C
Arizona School of Health Sciences
Associate Professor and Chair
Physician Assistant Studies
Mesa, Arizona

Ann Davis, MS, PA-C
Director of State Government Affairs
American Academy of Physician Assistants
Alexandria, Virginia

Moira Fordyce, MD, MB, ChB, FRCP Edin, AGSF
Laguna Niguel, California

Danny L. Franke, PhD
Alderson-Broaddus College
Philippi, West Virginia

FJ Gianola, PA-C
Faculty
MEDEX Northwest Physician Assistant Program
School of Medicine and Center for Health Sciences
    Interprofessional Education and Research
University of Washington
Seattle, Washington

Therese Jones, PhD
Associate Professor
Department of Internal Medicine,
    Division of Medical Ethics and
    Humanities
University of Utah Health Sciences Center
Editor, *Journal of Medical Humanities*

James E. Meyer, MD
Midwestern University
Glendale, Arizona

Elin Armeau, PhD, PA-C
Eastern Virginia Medical School PA Program
Norfolk, Virginia

Michael Potts, PhD
Department of Philosophy and Religion
Methodist College
Fayetteville, North Carolina

Peter M. Stanford, MPH, PA-C
Academic Coordinator
Clinical Assistant Professor
Physician Assistant Department
University of Maryland Eastern Shore
Princess Anne, Maryland

Reviewers

Gilbert A. Boissonneault, PhD, PA-C
Professor
Division of Physician Assistant
   Studies
University of Kentucky
Lexington, Kentucky

Courtney Cribbs
Graduate
Physician Assistant Program
University of Findlay
Findlay, Ohio

Katherine M. Erdman, MPAS, PA-C
Assistant Director and Instructor
Physician Assistant Program
Baylor College of Medicine
Houston, Texas

Carl Fasser, BA, PA-C
Director and Associate Professor
Physician Assistant Program
Baylor College of Medicine
Houston, Texas

James Hammond, MA, PA-C
Director
Physician Assistant Program
James Madison University
Harrisonburg, Virginia

Wanda Hancock, MHSA, RT(R)(T), PA-C
Professor Emeritus
Physician Assistant Program
Medical University of South Carolina
Charleston, South Carolina

Julie B. Keena, MMSc, PA-C
Chair and Associate Professor
Physician Assistant Program
Nova Southeastern University
Naples, Florida

Pat Kenney-Moore, MS, PA-C
Associate Director and Academic
   Coordinator
Physician Assistant Program
Oregon Health and Science University
Portland, Oregon

Deborah E. Kortyna, MMS, PA-C
Assistant Professor
Physician Assistant Program
Chatham College
Chatham, Pennsylvania

Clara LaBoy, MS, PA-C
Assistant Professor
School of Physician Assistant Studies
Pacific University
Forest Grove, Oregon

Mary Ann Laxen, MAB, PA-C
Director and Associate Professor
Physician Assistant Program
University of North Dakota
Grand Forks, North Dakota

Anthony A. Miller, MEd, PA-C
Director
Division of Physician Assistant
   Studies
Shenandoah University
Winchester, Virginia

Rena N. Mitchell, MS, CHES, RPA-C
Acting Chairperson and Clinical
   Assistant Professor
Physician Assistant Program
SUNY Downstate Medical Center
Brooklyn, New York

John M. Schroeder, JD, PA-C
Director
Physician Assistant Program
Idaho State University
Pocatello, Idaho

Victoria Scott, MHS, PA-C
Director and Senior Physician
   Assistant
Breast Wellness Clinic
Duke University Medical Center
Durham, North Carolina

Robert J. Spears, MPAS, PA-C
Former Assistant Professor
Physician Assistant Program
University of Findlay
Findlay, Ohio

Erica Young
Student
Physician Assistant Program
Baylor College of Medicine
Houston, Texas

Acknowledgments

In modern times, no book is the result of the efforts of one person. Even the best writer needs help with research, development, proofing, review, critique, and so forth. This effort is no different.

First, the contributors deserve the most praise for their work. Their efforts have resulted in a body of work new to physician assistant literature. They are a truly dedicated group of people, and we are lucky to be able to share in their expertise.

Our world presents a set of challenges at every level, and the professional and ethical development of our students is one key to our survival and growth. Life, much less the practice of medicine, presents us with ethical challenges every day. Every decision in medicine has an ethical component, some with huge components that affect provider, patient, family, and society as a whole. Helping students master and understand these ethics is a challenge. The needs of those students drive what we do in education. So we must acknowledge our students—we are certain our contributors will agree— as the primary source of our efforts to help define and clarify ethical challenges.

Equal thanks must go to the people who work "behind the scenes" at F.A. Davis. We know working with editors and authors is like herding cats, but the people at F.A. Davis are special, with high levels of tolerance and patience. Our initial contact was Carl Holm, who directed us to Jennifer Pine and Andy McPhee. Jennifer and Andy certainly went way beyond the call to duty to make this effort succeed. Their guidance has been invaluable because this book took a lot of effort at every level and more time than we ever imagined. We are sure that our stops, starts, turnabouts, and changes of minds on this book would have driven other people crazy. Fortunately, they stayed sane (even when we were not), and we are eternally grateful for that.

We also want to acknowledge our colleagues who inspire us to make such efforts and those who support us while we do. Of course, we can never forget our families and friends. They are the ones who keeps us grounded, which we often need.

Contents

Ethics and the Physician Assistant Student

James E. Meyer, MD

CASE STUDIES

Ethical Violations and Their Significance

Case 1.1
During the third week of class of a new group of physician assistant (PA) students, one of the students makes a derogatory comment to this instructor. The instructor is offended and retaliates with a demeaning verbal put-down. Several other students hear the exchange and report the faculty member's behavior to the program director.

Case 1.2
Later in the year, a faculty member learns that a student was allowed to copy another student's SOAP note and submitted the copy as her own. The faculty member decides to confront both students to discuss their unethical, unprofessional behavior.

Case 1.3
A professor creates an instructional CD for use as a teaching aid in a course that she teaches. She publishes the CD and makes it a required learning tool for the course. Rather than purchasing the CD, several of the class members decide to "burn" copies and sell them to their classmates. Their rationale: "We learned in an undergraduate ethics class that there may be an 'ethical conflict' if a professor requires students to purchase a teaching tool from which the professor may benefit financially."

Case 1.4
While on his Women's Health rotation, a male student asks one of the female patients to go out on a date with him. His preceptor is quite upset and wants to know how the PA Program would like to handle this situation.

Case 1.5
About 2 weeks into a new clinical rotation, a second-year PA student calls to inform the PA program that her preceptor has been introducing her as a medical student rather than as a PA student. At first, the student was reluctant to object, for fear of upsetting her preceptor, but she is now feeling more uncomfortable about being introduced this way. She calls to ask for advice.

Case 1.6
The office manager from a family practice site discovers that a PA student has been taking samples of antibiotics and Viagra from the sample closet. The office manager is trying to decide whether to dismiss the student from the rotation and wants to discuss the situation with the PA program.

A ll of the preceding scenarios are, with minor variations, real events that this author has heard about in the past few years while working with PA students. Unethical behavior of PA students is something that all PA programs must confront sooner or later. Breaches of ethical behavior occur during both the didactic year and the clinical year. Although most PA students, like most students enrolled in other professional fields, demonstrate good moral character, there are always a few students who exhibit inappropriate, unethical, uncivil, or unprofessional behavior. Similar types of behaviors are seen in most clinical training programs, whether the trainees are medical students or students in pharmacy, nursing. or other programs.

The examples cited at the beginning of this chapter may seem relatively mild compared with some of the more serious cases of clinician misbehavior handled by state boards. However, these milder forms of unethical behavior may be early indicators of future problems and should be viewed as "teaching moments" for professionals-in-training. They are some of the "stuff" that must be addressed by the training institution if students are to learn what it means to be an ethical professional. As Wayne Sotile, Ph.D. (a psychotherapist who works with physicians), put it, "Problem medical students can grow up to be problem physicians....You either learn [professionalism] in medical school or you're going to be forced to learn it later."[1] This applies to PA students as well.

Papadakis et al found that physicians who had engaged in unethical or unprofessional behavior as students were more than twice as likely eventually to be disciplined by their state medical board than physicians who had a clean student record.[2] In addition, these researchers assert that "we can now advocate from an evidence-based position that professionalism is an essential competency that must be demonstrated for a student to graduate from medical school."[2] Traditional forms of academic evaluation were much less likely to be predictive of future disciplinary action. The authors make a plea for the development of better tools to evaluate personal attributes of student applicants and better training in professionalism, with testing for competency.

d'Oronzio describes his work with physicians who have had their licenses suspended for inappropriate behavior related to "transgressions of professional ethics."[3] He observes that the most common types of professional misbehavior fit into one of the following three general categories: (1) boundary violations, (2) misrepresentation, and (3) financial infractions. Each of the examples given at the beginning of this chapter could fit into one of these three categories.

Students in PA training programs are less likely to get into difficulty with unethical financial behavior than with boundary violations or misrepresentation. Financial fraud is more likely to develop after graduation, in a practice setting. Because of the dependent nature of the PA's practice, the supervising physician may be more likely to be the culprit in financially unethical practices. However, stealing samples from a preceptor's office would fit into a student category. Up-coding for services rendered, submitting false claims, and similar financial indiscretions may be committed by any practicing clinician. PAs are not immune and certainly need to be aware of these types of unethical behavior and the need to avoid them. Added to this is the consideration of PAs' guilt if they know their services are being up-coded.

In Search of Common Meaning: Ethical Integrity Versus Professionalism Versus Civility

Much of the literature dealing with problematic behavior among clinicians and clinicians-in-training discusses "professionalism" and its characteristics, with lapses described as "unprofessional behavior." Other articles talk about "civility" and "incivility,"[4] "moral integrity," or "professional integrity."[5] References to "ethical behavior" and the nature of ethics and its role in clinician behavior appear more commonly in the bioethics literature than in literature geared primarily for clinicians. There are considerably fewer articles dealing with the ethical behavior of PAs than ones dealing with medical student and resident behavior. For all practical purposes, the principles are the same, with medical students and residents facing the same challenges as those faced by PA students and practicing PAs. Issues related to conflicts between a student and faculty member or student and clinical preceptor are also similar. All trainees are in a dependent relationship with their preceptor or attending physician.

The terminology used in discussions of ethics and professionalism can be confusing. In spite of the extensive literature on the subject (or because of it?), there is still no common understanding of how best to define professionalism.[6] Doukas remarks that "the concept of professionalism has been bandied about in whatever context the user intends. The current discussion of professionalism is like the fable of six men assessing an elephant: you believe what you perceive."[7] Numerous professional groups have recently produced or revised their statements on professionalism. The American Board of Internal Medicine's (ABIM) Project Professionalism outlines "the six elements of professionalism" (altruism, accountability, excellence, duty, honor and integrity, and respect for others) and the challenges to those elements (abuse of power, arrogance, greed, misrepresentation, impairment, lack of conscientiousness, and conflict of interest)[8] (Box 1-1 and 1-2). Robins et al suggest using these elements as the basis for teaching ethics to medical students.[9] In 2002, European and American internal medicine organizations published "The Charter on Medical Professionalism," which presented a list of standards for professionalism that the authors think should be universally accepted.[10] (Box 1-3)

In May 2000, the American Academy of Physician Assistants (AAPA) adopted its Guidelines for Ethical Conduct for the Physician Assistant, which discusses the four main bioethical principles (autonomy, beneficence, nonmaleficence, and justice) and reviews a statement of values of the PA profession[11] (Box 1-4). These principles and values are used as the basis for the guidelines for a PA's work as a professional engaged with patients, other professionals, the health-care system, and society. The American Medical Association recently published similar Principles of Medical Ethics[12] (Box 1-5).

Box 1-1   **Six Elements of Professionalism**
1. Altruism 2. Accountability 3. Excellence 4. Duty 5. Honor and Integrity 6. Respect for Others

From Project Professionalism. American Board of Internal Medicine, 1995.

Box 1-2	Seven Challenges to Elements of Professionalism

1. Abuse of power
2. Arrogance
3. Greed
4. Misrepresentation
5. Impairment
6. Lack of conscientiousness
7. Conflict of interest

From Project Professionalism. American Board of Internal Medicine, 1995.

Is Ethics (Ethical Integrity) the Same as Professionalism?

Dr. Peter Singer, Professor of Medicine and Director of the University of Toronto Joint Centre for Bioethics, in his article "Strengthening the Role of Ethics in Medical Education" states that professionalism and the role of ethics in medical education are so similar that there is no real benefit in distinguishing between the two. He believes that the most important issue for the professional is to create a "shared medical experience with the patient."[13] Dr. Singer believes that a "Flexner-like commission" needs to be created to strengthen the role of ethics in medical education, much like what Abraham Flexner did nearly 100 years ago to standardize and improve the quality of general medical education.

Wear and Kuczewski, in their discussion of the professionalism movement, seem to differ with Dr. Singer by stating that "Perhaps the greatest potential danger is that we educators will simply rename what has been called 'medical ethics' as 'professionalism' in the curriculum and consider ourselves done."[14] The authors take issue with the "seemingly immutable...group of attitudes, values, and behaviors subsumed under the label of 'professionalism.'" They note that the typical features of professionalism have been developed "by and for male physicians who traditionally have few domestic obligations." The excessive work schedules demanded of clinicians in training and other forms of mistreatment of students, along with the "traditional focus on limitless ideals," creates an *environment* that "deprofessionalizes" students and is more likely to damage a student's character than to enrich it.

As an example of the limitless ideals, Wear and Kuczewski quote from the ABIM Project Professionalism's definition of duty, one of the so-called "immutable" features of professionalism: "the free acceptance of a commitment to service. This commit-

Box 1-3	The Charter on Medical Professionalism

Preamble
Professionalism is the basis of medicine's contract with society.

Fundamental Principles
1. *Principle of primacy of patient welfare*
2. *Principle of patient autonomy*
3. *Principle of social justice*

A Set of Professional Responsibilities
1. *Commitment to professional competence*
2. *Commitment to honesty with patients*
3. *Commitment to patient confidentiality*
4. *Commitment to maintaining appropriate relations with patients*
5. *Commitment to improving quality of care*
6. *Commitment to improving access to care*
7. *Commitment to a just distribution of finite resources*
8. *Commitment to scientific knowledge*
9. *Commitment to maintaining trust by managing conflicts of interest*
10. *Commitment to professional responsibilities*

Summary
To maintain the fidelity of medicine's social contract during this turbulent time, we believe that physicians must reaffirm their active dedication to the principles of professionalism, which entails not only their personal commitment to the welfare of their patients but also collective efforts to improve the health care system for the welfare of society. This Charter on Medical Professionalism is intended to encourage such dedication and to promote an action agenda for the profession of medicine that is universal in scope and purpose.

Adapted from Annals of Internal Medicine, 5 Feb 2002, 136:3, pp. 243-246.

ment entails being available and responsive when 'on call,' accepting inconvenience to meet the needs of one's patients, enduring unavoidable risks to oneself when a patient's welfare is at stake, advocating the best possible care regardless of ability to pay, seeking active roles in professional organizations, and volunteering one's skills and expertise for the welfare of the community."[14] They also express concern that the emphasis on objective measurements of professionalism might make us "attempt to test for the untestable."[14] There is more to ethics than professionalism,

Box 1-4	Statement of Values of the Physician Assistant Profession

- Physician assistants hold as their primary responsibility the health, safety, welfare, and dignity of all human beings.
- Physician assistants uphold the tenets of patient autonomy, beneficence, nonmaleficence, and justice.
- Physician assistants recognize and promote the value of diversity.
- Physician assistants treat equally all persons who seek their care.
- Physician assistants hold in confidence the information shared in the course of practicing medicine.
- Physician assistants assess their personal capabilities and limitations, striving always to improve their medical practice.
- Physician assistants actively seek to expand their knowledge and skills, keeping abreast of advances in medicine.
- Physician assistants work with other members of the health care team to provide compassionate and effective care of patients.
- Physician assistants use their knowledge and experience to contribute to an improved community.
- Physician assistants respect their professional relationship with physicians.
- Physician assistants share and expand knowledge within the profession.

Courtesy of American Academy of Physician Assistants: JAAPA, 2001;14:10-20, 2001. Policy of the AAPA, adopted May 2000.

and professionalism does not necessarily guarantee ethical behavior.

So how are the two different? Dudzinski relates a story from the book *My Own Country* [by Verghese, 1994] in which an AIDS patient went to see a new doctor: "The doctor said to the patient, 'I don't approve of your lifestyle and what it represents. It is ungodly in my view. But that doesn't mean I won't continue to take good care of you....' To which the patient replied, 'Oh yes it does!' Whether uttered aloud or kept secret, the values, attitudes, and experiences physicians bring with them deeply impact their practice. I fear that professionalism divorced from medical ethics would advise this physician to keep quiet. But when ethics takes precedence, he might realize that it is disrespectful to reduce a person to his sexual orientation and disease. He might

Box 1-5	The American Medical Association Principles of Medical Ethics

Preamble:
The medical profession has long subscribed to a body of ethical statements developed primarily for the benefit of the patient. As a member of this profession, a physician must recognize responsibility to patients first and foremost, as well as to society, to other health professionals, and to self. The following Principles adopted by the American Medical Association are not laws, but standards of conduct which define the essentials of honorable behavior for the physician.

I. A physician shall be dedicated to providing competent medical care, with compassion and respect for human dignity and rights.
II. A physician shall uphold the standards of professionalism, be honest in all professional interactions, and strive to report physicians deficient in character or competence, or engaging in fraud or deception, to appropriate entities.
III. A physician shall respect the law and also recognize a responsibility to seek changes in those requirements which are contrary to the best interests of the patient.
IV. A physician shall respect the rights of patients, colleagues, and other health professionals, and shall safeguard patient confidences and privacy within the constraints of the law.
V. A physician shall continue to study, apply, and advance scientific knowledge, maintain a commitment to medical education, make relevant information available to patients, colleagues, and the public, obtain consultation, and use the talents of other health professionals when indicated.
VI. A physician shall, in the provision of appropriate patient care, except in emergencies, be free to choose whom to serve, with whom to associate, and the environment in which to provide medical care.
VII. A physician shall recognize a responsibility to participate in activities contributing

Accessed from http://www.ama-assn.org/ama/pub/category/8600.html

(box continues on page 6)

Box 1-5   The American Medical Association
Principles of Medical Ethics (continued)

to the improvement of the community and
the betterment of public health.

VIII. A physician shall, while caring for a
patient, regard responsibility to the
patient as paramount.

IX. A physician shall support access to
medical care for all people.

learn to be more compassionate with his patients,
neighbors, and colleagues. Then, and only then, does
professionalism have integrity."[15] Dudzinski's explanation seems to indicate that a professional would
simply not verbalize his personal beliefs, whereas a
physician with ethical integrity would be aware of his
own values and work to deal with the patient in a nonjudgmental way.

In his example, Dudzinski seems to be equating
"professionalism" with competent application of clinical guidelines for treatment of disease rather than
with the more complete elements of professionalism
as proposed by the ABIM. This more limited view of
professionalism lacks compassion, and it also appears
to lack civility (respect for others) and "justice"
(equal treatment for all). Treating patients with beneficence and nonmaleficence and allowing them the
autonomy of their own lifestyle choices are all consistent with basic bioethical principles. Treating them
justly, without bias or prejudice, conforms to the
fourth principle of bioethics. Is the concept of professionalism lacking, or is the real problem "professionals" who allow their own incivilities and arrogance to
get in the way of proper behavior?

Shirley and Padgett from the University of
Washington School of Nursing argue that "professionalism is no longer helpful as an organizing
ethical framework....it is too deeply entangled
with physician privilege and power, too limited in
its concept of normative responsibilities, and too
diffuse in the ways it has been deployed within
the healthcare system."[16] They contend that professionalism operates differently, depending on the professional group to which one belongs. "For nurses
and social workers, for example [could PAs be
added?] the power and privileges of professionalism
are far more tenuous than for physicians." Shirley
and Padgett may be referring to the "social prestige"
of physicians, one of the structural attributes of
professionalism alluded to by Hammer.[17] Nurses
and PAs may view physicians as taking advantage
of their prestige in a way that borders on *abuse of*

power and *arrogance*, characteristics that the ABIM
lists as challenges to the elements of professionalism (see Box 1-2).

Anyone who has worked in the medical field
knows clinicians who are viewed as "professionals"
in the popular sense of the term but who do not
behave with civility and ethical integrity, demonstrating the six elements of professionalism (see Box 1-1).
Coulehan and Williams cite the following examples
that seem to illustrate this: "He's an extremely good
doctor, but he sure is nasty with patients." "Her bedside manner is terrible, but she's the best gastroen-
terologist in...the city."[18] Their comments suggest
that certain forms of unethical, or at least "uncivil,"
behavior do not prevent someone from being viewed
as a "good professional." What is the value system
that is being used to define these physicians as
"good" professionals? Characteristics such as empathy, communication skills, patience, and kindness do
not seem to count as much as technical, and perhaps
diagnostic, competence.

Civility as the Behavioral Expression of Ethical Integrity and Professionalism

Descriptions of arrogant, impatient, unkind clinicians
as "good" are further evidence that the term "professionalism" has different meanings to different people.
It is laudable that professional organizations are
attempting to incorporate ethics and civility into the
definition of professionalism, but common usage of
the term may not always include those components.
Perhaps this is where some of the confusion and dis-
taste for the term as expressed by Dudzinski and
Shirley and Padget comes from.

Is there a way to conceptualize the various aspects
of professionalism and ethical behavior so that confusion is minimized? Bruce Berger, Ph.D., R.Ph., uses
the term "civility" to describe appropriate behavior.[4]
He conceptualizes civility as a foundational value for
professionalism. A basic definition of an *incivility*
may be "a speech or action that is disrespectful or
rude."[4] Should the physicians mentioned above be
described as "uncivil" but "good professionals," or
does their incivility provide proof that they are not
truly "good" professionals? Should clinicians be
referred to simply as good "technicians" rather than
"professionals" if they do not exhibit the full range of
desirable character traits listed in the proposed "Six
Elements of Professionalism"? Or should those who
are exhibiting unprofessional behavior be called professionals?

Berger has edited an excellent text for pharmacy
students and faculty titled *Promoting Civility in
Pharmacy Education*. The text is a very practical

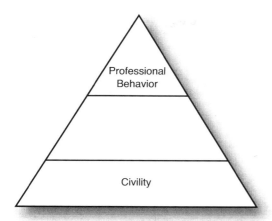

Figure 1.1 Civility as the foundation for professional behavior.

approach to dealing with some of the typical behavioral problems exhibited by students and faculty in *any* professional training program. The authors state that civility is the foundation for professionalism, and they illustrate this with a diagram of a triangle, with civility at the base and professional behavior at the peak, representing a specialized and more refined type of behavior, but behavior that has civility as its foundation[17] (Fig. 1.1).

Following a review of pertinent social science literature, Hammer concludes that "professionalism is a complex composite of structural, attitudinal, and behavioral attributes."[17] The *structural* attributes include:

• Specialized body of knowledge and skills
• Unique socialization of student members
• Licensure/certification
• Professional associations
• Governance by peers
• Social prestige
• Vital service to society
• Code of ethics
• Autonomy
• Equivalence of members
• Special relationship with clients

Attitudinal attributes of professionals are described as:

• Use of the professional organization as a major reference
• Belief in service to the public
• Belief in self-regulation
• Sense of calling to the field
• Autonomy[17]

Civility is viewed as the *behavioral* component of professionalism, and its features are described as:

• Tolerance
• Respect
• Proper conduct
• Diplomacy[19,20]

Civility is, therefore, viewed as the behavioral expression of, and foundation for, professionalism; the minimum behavioral standard.

It can be argued that moral or ethical principles are the basis for appropriate thoughts and behavior. It is reasonable to propose a modified diagram, with ethics or "ethical integrity" at the base, civility at the midpoint, with professionalism at the top (Fig. 1.2).

Civility is the behavioral expression of underlying ethical integrity. Professionalism is the more specialized development of ethical and civil behavior, above and beyond what is expected from the nonprofessional. Professionalism's structural and attitudinal features also further define its specialized nature and will vary depending on the specific professional field represented. A medical professional will be expected to demonstrate behavioral characteristics, attitudes, and structural attributes (body of knowledge and skills, licensure, etc) that are different from those of a "professional" engineer, hockey player, or lawyer.

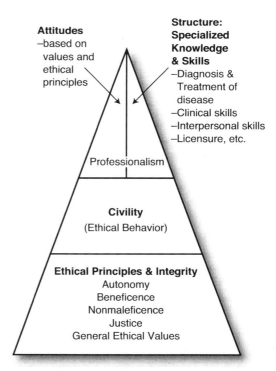

Figure 1.2 Modified diagram with civility as a support for professional behavior.

Ethics and the
Traditional Curriculum

Current medical training programs seem to have a pretty good grasp of what it takes to teach students the foundational principles of the basic sciences and clinical sciences, which some have simply called "bioscience." "Medical education has traditionally placed the highest value on scientific (rationalistic) knowledge, which may have little to do with the critical thinking about oneself, the medical profession, and society, all of which are basic to professional development."[21] So what does all this scientific knowledge "have to do with educating doctors [and PAs] to be compassionate, communicative, and socially responsible?" Wear and Castellani worry that the overwhelming immersion in bioscience may cause students to believe that the principles of science are also the key to relationships with patients and colleagues,[21] when in fact this is not the case.

Robert Coles, MD, of Harvard Medical School writes that "Medical education barrages students with information, fosters sometimes ruthless competition, and perpetuates rote memorization and an obsession with test scores—all of which stifle moral reflection."[22] He wonders how we can teach students to really know what it means to be a "good doctor"—and, one might add, a good PA.

Where do students learn moral values, ethical integrity, and civility? What are the unique characteristics [or "character"] of a professional such as a physician or PA, or for that matter anyone working in one of the "helping professions?" Where in our curriculum do students learn compassion, empathy, respect, tolerance, diplomacy—characteristics that have been traditionally exemplified by the medical professional? As Goleman states in his excellent book *Emotional Intelligence*,[23] "Academic intelligence offers virtually no preparation for the turmoil—or opportunity—life's vicissitudes bring....our schools and our culture fixate on academic abilities, ignoring emotional intelligence, a set of traits—*some might call it character*—that also matters immensely for our personal destiny."[23]

Kenny et al raise an important issue in their discussion of the attempt by medical training institutions to teach medical ethics: ethics seems to be taught primarily with an interest in learning how to solve ethical dilemmas, and in so doing, "the *ethics of character* has been lost. The Hippocratic tradition is rooted in virtue ethics where the moral agent, rather than principles for problem solving, is central."[24] And Singer states that "Moral reasoning is a precondition for ethical behaviour in medicine."[13] Where in the medical curriculum is moral reasoning taught? Do we assume that students have this capability fully developed when they matriculate?

Glick encourages teachers of ethics in medical training programs to "help create an academic environment in which well motivated students have reinforcement of their inherent good qualities."[25] This must be done actively, and with awareness of the potential consequences of leaving this teaching to chance. Is the current academic environment in PA programs one that promotes the reinforcement and further development of "character"—of ethical behavior? Can we, in our pluralistic society, promote key ethical values in a medical culture that is increasingly controlled by financial and time constraints determined by nonclinicians and by excessive work (and study) demands?

Some reports on the physician training process are rather disturbing. There are numerous articles about the negative impact that medical training has on the moral and emotional development of medical students and residents. Coulehan and Williams, in their article "Vanquishing Virtue: The Impact of Medical Education," state that American medical education "favors an *explicit* commitment to traditional values of doctoring—empathy, compassion, and altruism among them—and a *tacit* commitment to behaviors grounded in an ethic of detachment, self-interest, and objectivity."[18] These disparate values provide one good explanation for the confusion generated by the term "professionalism." When confronted with this dichotomy, students seem to respond in one of three ways. They (1) give up the traditional values and become technicians, (2) they give lip service to the traditional values but remain coolly objective and "scientific," or (3) they manage to hold-on to the traditional values, resist the tacit values, and "internalize and develop professional virtue."[18] For this latter group of trainees, something about their deeply ingrained character has "immunized" them against the tacit values.

The so-called *tacit values* are referred to elsewhere as the "hidden curriculum"[26] or the "informal curriculum"[27] of medical training. In spite of the formal teaching regarding the desirable features of professionalism and medical ethics, the truth of the matter is that trainees are exposed to environmental influences that have been shown to damage or erode the moral values and commitment to the ideals of medicine that they originally held.[18,28,29] These influences are not discussed openly; rather, they are experienced in the day-to-day activities of the developing clinician. Feudtner et al studied 665 third- and fourth-year medical students in six Pennsylvania medical schools; 62% believed that at least some of their ethical principles had been eroded or lost as a direct result of their medical training.[30] Dr. Coles reminds us that during the medical training process "many of us...forsake certain ideals or principles—not in one grand gesture, but in moment-to-moment decisions, in day-to-day rationalizations and self-deceptions, until we find ourselves caught in lives whose implications we have long ago stopped examining, never mind judging."[22]

"Tacit learning...stresses objectivity, detachment, wariness, and distrust of emotions, patients, insurance companies, administrators, and the state."[18] Long hours of work, which have now been generously limited to no more than the equivalent of two full-time jobs (80 hours per week), create a "self-care deficit"[31] including physical and emotional exhaustion and sleep deprivation. The ability to truly care becomes impaired, empathy suffers, and a degree of self-protective *detachment* develops. Placing others first and relegating one's own health and contact with one's family to after-thoughts eventually create a sense of *entitlement*.[18] Physicians come to believe that they deserve respect and ample income and become intolerant when their expectations are not fulfilled. The stresses of the training process eventually wear down even the most committed and idealistic trainee. It is only with great inner courage and commitment that those "immunized" students and residents are able to retain and consistently exhibit the high standards of an ethical medical professional. As one fourth-year medical student put it, "my personal challenge was to maintain this humanism and idealism throughout the years of medical school, to resist the desensitization and disillusionment that were probably natural. I know that many of my classmates felt the same way. And many of them felt as if they have lost too much through the process. It is ironic that the system itself squelches so much of the idealism and the spark of professionalism that educators are, in the classroom at least, trying to teach, preserve, and foster."[28] So how does all of this relate to ethics for the PA student?

PA Training Versus Physician Training: Impact on Ethical Development

PA training is a *fast track* to medical practice. It is also a fast track to the development of professionalism and ethically appropriate medical behavior. There are advantages and disadvantages to this fast track approach.

The most obvious *disadvantage* is its short duration. PAs have less time to learn the complex body of medical knowledge and less time to develop their clinical skills. They have only 1 year of exposure to the necessary didactic material, including formal instruction in ethical and professional behavior. In addition,

they have less exposure to experienced clinicians and observe fewer encounters of skilled clinicians interacting with patients, families, and professionals. Medical training has been referred to as a "transformative process of socialization,"[32] and this process for the PA student is necessarily truncated. PAs make up the difference in their initial years of clinical practice.

The most obvious *advantage* to the fast-track PA training is also its short duration. The average PA program is 26 months. The didactic year is usually only 12 months. The training is all-consuming and intense, and students are typically exhausted by the end of the first year. However, the total duration of training program stress is considerably shorter than the 7-plus years of heavy demands on time and energy that is characteristic of the average medical school and residency process. PAs are spared the extra years of the chronic daily stress of an extremely long, arduous, and at times downright abusive training process. Exposure to a potentially morally erosive environment is considerably shorter. By the end of their training program, PA students are more likely to retain their enthusiasm, idealism, and moral values. Principles taught in their didactic year may be more likely to "stick," with less exposure to the *tacit values* and *hidden curriculum* discussed above.

One of the dilemmas faced by PA faculty members is the desire to be humane and reasonable in their expectations for students, yet at the same time to prepare their students for the demands and challenges in the clinical environment that await them after graduation. Students routinely imply that they have to put their "normal life" on hold for 2 years in order to meet the obligations of the program successfully. If the curriculum is lightened to allow for more personal and family time, will the students learn enough to pass their certification examination? Will they be adequately prepared for the realities of practice?

Many programs pride themselves on their academic rigor. How rigorous is too rigorous? Are the demands too extreme? Is it ethical to require so much time and energy from students? Are students treated with respect and compassion, or do programs tacitly allow emotionally abusive treatment to exist? Does the PA training process contribute to the "ethical erosion" mentioned in the earlier discussion, or does this happen only in physician training programs? How many PA faculty personnel were trained during an era, not too long ago, when "intimidation and abusive behavior were viewed as ways to harden future doctors [and PAs?] so that they would not flinch when faced with difficult medical challenges."[33] Do some faculty members still exhibit those attitudes in their interactions with students? How can a balance be achieved between academic rigor and humane expectations and treatment of students?

Today's PA Students

Selection and Evaluation

One of the major issues facing every PA program is the selection of worthy applicants. The application process includes evaluation of a student's academic ability based on undergraduate grade point average, perhaps the Graduate Record Examination and/or other standardized tests of bioscientific knowledge, and perhaps general information. A written personal statement provides more information, which may highlight certain aspects of a student's personality. Evaluating a student's moral character is an entirely different matter. The interview process is certainly the most commonly used procedure for getting a sense of an applicant's values. Questions geared to an applicant's method of handling a variety of hypothetical scenarios are often quite informative. However, it is unlikely that a 20- to 30-minute interview and a review of a student's personal statement are adequate indicators of a student's moral character.

Some clinical training programs use standardized tests designed to evaluate cognitive moral development. One of these is the Defining Issues Test (DIT), which is thought to be helpful in screening out "amoral" students.[34] Carrothers et al administered a 34-item test for "emotional intelligence" to medical school applicants, which seemed to be helpful in measuring desirable personal attributes.[35] Obviously, there is no perfect test for assessing an applicant's moral character and his or her future likelihood of behaving in a professional manner.

Experience and Expectations

Students admitted to PA programs have had varying amounts of clinical experience. Some are already well grounded in the tenets of ethical medical behavior; others have had more limited experience and are familiar with professional expectations only in a rather superficial way. Compared with students from previous generations, Generation X students entering PA programs today have different backgrounds and different social and educational expectations. Berger indicates that "Students of today prefer self-directed learning, dislike close supervision, are cynical, tend to be less respectful or in awe of authority figures/faculty, desire immediate feedback, and like faculty who get to the point."[4] They also like lots of visuals and activities; they get bored easily—they are part of the media generation. These personality traits and expectations may present challenges for those involved in their training program.

Moral Values

What types of values do today's students possess? The "moral absolutes" of 50 to 75 years ago have undergone change, with an increasing amount of moral relativism in our culture. How has this affected the values of our entering students? There seem to be fewer "black or white" moral issues, and many more of them with shades of gray. What effect could this have on teaching today's students the principles of professionalism and ethical medical behavior? In spite of Kenny's concern that the *ethics of character* has been lost and that current ethical training is focused on solving ethical dilemmas,[24] it may be more politically correct to deal with ethical dilemmas than with underlying moral/ethical values.

Unethical Behavior as "Incivilities"

In view of today's ambiguous moral and ethical climate, it may be more expedient and accepted to use the terms "civility" and "incivilities" when discussing ethical and unethical behavior. As Berger notes, "in the past, rules of civility were instilled during childhood…[I]n addition to a decreased emphasis in teaching children rules of civility, other factors, such as the introduction of technology, have contributed to an overall decline in civility in our society."[4] The average young adult has seen thousands of hours of television and film interactions where the "put-down" of one person by another is the primary means of generating "humor." Disrespectful, intolerant, and emotionally abusive behavior is glamorized on a regular basis. Attempts by parents and teachers to instill respect, tolerance, and courteous behavior in children have certainly been hindered by media influences.

Incivilities in PA education may occur during the didactic year and the clinical year. Incivilities can be categorized as passive and active.[4] During the didactic year, being late for class, reading a newspaper, or sleeping during class are all impolite, disrespectful behaviors. Active incivilities include more overt behavior such as talking back to instructors, vulgar language, sexual harassment, cheating on tests, or copying a fellow student's write-up. Faculty may also be guilty of incivilities. Being consistently late for lectures, ignoring student requests, lack of follow-through on promises, and verbal attacks on students are all examples of unprofessional faculty behavior, i.e. "incivilities."

Clinical-year incivilities include inappropriate dress while on rotations, talking negatively about preceptors or fellow students, taking medication samples from the preceptor's office, challenging one's preceptor in front of patients, tardiness, and failing to introduce oneself as a PA student. These uncivil behaviors have their roots in a student's underlying value system and may also be influenced by ignorance of appropriate protocols in medical settings (such as challenging a preceptor in front of a patient; inappropriate dress). Some PA programs attempt to "immunize" students prior to the start of their clinical year with presentations on the "Do's and Don'ts of the Clinical Year," or a "Top Ten List of What Not to Do on Your Clinical Rotations!" In this way students learn about the common examples of unethical and unprofessional behavior that are known to occur on clinical rotations. Most students seem to benefit from this, but mere lectures on the topic may not be sufficient for those students who most need to learn the principles.

Preventing and Responding to Incivilities

It may not be entirely appropriate to expect to admit students whose character and qualities of professionalism are fully developed at the time of admission.[24] Although there are programs that rather aggressively weed out students who exhibit unethical and/or unprofessional behavior during the course of their training, the majority of programs try to work with students in ways that use these breaches of propriety as "teaching moments." The underlying assumption is that what needs to be taught is both bioscientific facts and how to *be a professional* and behave in an ethically appropriate manner in the midst of a complex medical-legal-social environment.

Basic principles for preventing and/or confronting incivilities include making expectations known, communicating effectively, modeling civil behavior, maintaining appropriate boundaries, holding people responsible for transgressions, and having an effective grievance process.[36] The course syllabus is an excellent source for clarifying the instructor's expectations with regard to behavior as well as academic issues. Some programs have developed an honor code along with an honor board, which investigates incivilities (unethical behavior). Berger suggests that instructors also reexamine their course to determine if it is boring, if the material that is being covered is really necessary, and if the instructor is aloof, defensive, complacent about disruptive behavior, or whether he or she allows and seeks adequate feedback from students.[4]

The same basic principles are important during the student's clinical year. With a program that is primarily preceptor-based, communication must be optimized between preceptors, students, and the PA program. The expectations of each must be clearly understood. Preceptors and students must be willing to contact the PA program promptly when problems arise, and programs must have protocols in place for handling these problems.

Role modeling by preceptors is the most important means of teaching ethical behavior. Professionalism can best be learned by observing and interacting with skilled clinicians who are articulate, enjoy teaching, demonstrate healthy boundaries, and model competent, compassionate care.[24,37] Exemplary clinicians abound in the field of medicine. Hard-working, selfless clinicians continue to be an inspiration to anyone who is in training. Fourth-year medical student Jennifer Fesher relates that she best learned what professionalism is by observing the behavior of other doctors in clinical settings. She describes her experience with a resident who was caring for a woman with terminal breast cancer. "Despite the fact that my resident was being paged relentlessly, a sign of the dozens of other responsibilities he held that night, he chose to sit and listen to the dying patient's husband for nearly an hour, letting him cry and listening to his many stories about this wife. I was in awe of this compassionate, empathetic, and humanistic approach, especially when he began to prepare this man for the fact that his wife might not live through the night. He handled the situation with such compassion—with such professionalism, in the truest sense of the word—that I learned volumes....Thus, while I was formally taught in the classroom the framework within which to consider and understand the concept of professionalism, it was largely through observation, mentoring and role modeling that the concepts were finally solidified and internalized."[28]

Uncivil behavior by students should be dealt with promptly and in a civil and professional manner. Extreme cases of unethical/unprofessional behavior may need to be dealt with by dismissal from the program. Less extreme situations should be dealt with in a way that provides an important learning experience for the offender. This process, when done respectfully and consistently, can be a highly effective teaching modality. Ideally, it would seem desirable for other students to learn from the offender's behavior. Student privacy issues are a concern, of course, but there is good evidence from the literature that students learn best from case scenarios that hit close to home.[7] For example, in one PA program a class officer was asked to step down because it was learned that she deliberately misrepresented some facts on a class sign-up sheet that would have given her an unfair advantage over other classmates. Although no general announcement was made about this issue, the class eventually learned what happened. The overall impact on the class seemed to be positive. The class as a whole learned that a "white lie" can have serious consequences.

Many cases of unprofessional behavior by students are have a "low profile," and class members do not become aware of them. Confidentiality requirements mandate private handling of the offense. As a consequence, other students do not learn valuable lessons related to unprofessional behavior. One way to highlight these types of issues is to have "ethics or professionalism grand rounds" to discuss issues that have occurred, either in one's own program or in other programs, as a means of case-based instruction in ethics. Students might also benefit from attending a session of the state PA board to observe the process of dealing with problem behaviors.

d'Oronzio believes that discussions of case material from actual ethical or professional breaches is more valuable for teaching ethics than heady discussions of abstract principles and theories. This belief is based on feedback from professionals undergoing treatment for unethical behavior or "professional lapses." They wondered why they had not had a course in their professional training that dealt with the common types of unprofessional behavior.[3]

In addition to the above teaching methods, medical student Jennifer Fesher recommends including the following components in an ethics and professionalism curriculum:

1. "Teach us more of the historical context of professionalism in America.
2. Teach us about the noble tradition of doctors here and their long history of obligation to society, so that we can truly understand where medicine has been and where it is going.
3. Teach us that…the autonomy which the field of medicine has enjoyed historically was granted in exchange for a stated commitment to altruism and public service.
4. Also teach us about lapses in professionalism that occurred in the past so that we can learn to recognize them and to prevent them effectively.
5. Acknowledge the inherent conflict between professionalism and a doctor's own financial security and how these issues have been dealt with in the past and how they will be addressed in the future.
6. Teach us about how professionalism as we know it is threatened by forces such as managed care and how the field of medicine must adapt. How can we be humanistic and compassionate when we have only 10 minutes to see the patient? How can we truly care for our patients if insurance companies are telling us which tests to run, which medicines to prescribe, and how much time we will be allocated to do it? Give us the knowledge

and the tools so that we can maintain the principles of professionalism as health care reform continues—so that we, the next generation of doctors, can lead the reform ourselves."[28]

These suggestions apply to PA students as well. They need to know the history of their own profession—the challenges it has faced in the past and those it must face in the present and future.

Emotional Intelligence as an Important Prerequisite for Civility

An issue of great importance for developing clinicians is the ability to deal with the emotionality they will encounter in the course of clinical training. Student experiences with patients generate the whole range of emotions. "Positive emotions," such as happiness, compassion, and pride, as well as "difficult emotions," such as guilt, grief, anxiety, anger, and shame, are experienced during clinical interactions with patients and other clinicians. The way in which students and their supervisors deal with these emotions can determine to what extent students become more "emotionally intelligent" or more emotionally repressed or damaged.[37] Training programs would do well to evaluate the emotional learning, as well as the cognitive learning, by their students.

Ethical integrity is the foundation for civility and professionalism (see Fig 1.2). Moral values are taught to children by parents and other early caregivers. Values are further developed during adolescence and early adulthood. Emotional development follows a similar process.

The term "emotional intelligence" was first discussed by Salovey and Mayer as the ability to monitor one's own emotions and to guide one's thoughts and actions in a healthy manner.[38] Goleman popularized the term in his best-selling book *Emotional Intelligence*,[23] in which he indicates that "There is growing evidence that fundamental ethical stances in life stem from underlying emotional capacities. For one, impulse is the medium of emotions; the seed of all impulse is a feeling bursting to express itself in action. Those who are at the mercy of impulse—who lack self-control—suffer a moral deficiency: The ability to control impulse is the base of will and character. By the same token, the root of altruism lies in empathy, the ability to read emotions in others; lacking a sense of another's need or despair, there is no caring. And if there are any two moral stances that our times call for, they are precisely these, self-restraint and compassion."[23]

The five domains of emotional intelligence described by Goleman are (1) knowing one's own emotions, (2) managing one's own emotions, (3) motivating oneself, (4) recognizing emotions in others, and (5) handling relationships. Understanding and mastering one's emotions greatly improves one's ability to achieve a healthy degree of self-restraint and compassion. Emotional distress can have a "devastating effect" on mental clarity, with the "emotional brain [able] to overpower, even paralyze, the thinking brain."[23]

Knowing One's Own Emotions

Socrates' injunction "know thyself" is the keystone of emotional intelligence. It is a well-established psychological principle that the *inability* to notice our true feelings leaves us at their mercy. Childhood experiences play a significant role in an individual's self-awareness. Children raised with love and caring and with permission to feel the whole range of normal human emotions come into adulthood with an ability to feel their own happiness, sadness, fear, anger, shame, and sexual feelings. On the other hand, children who were punished or shamed for one or more of their emotions, for instance expressing sadness ("big boys don't cry—stop that crying or I'll give you something to cry about"), come into adulthood with part of their emotional potential repressed—out of their conscious awareness. This boy, as many males in our culture can attest, will have difficulty expressing sadness (especially with tears) without at the same time feeling ashamed of his sadness. For many whose emotions have been shamed ("shame-bound"), it is easier to simply "not feel" those emotions than to feel both the emotion and the distress of the accompanying shame. Being unable to feel an emotion in oneself certainly makes it equally difficult to feel it for another person—to empathize with a patient or family member who is experiencing profound sadness, for instance.

As James S. Gordon, MD, puts it in his intriguing book, *Manifesto for a New Medicine*, "Most of us spend much of our lives in ...psychological sleep.... Waking up, self-awareness, is the beginning of wisdom and the prerequisite for self-care."[39] It is this self-awareness and self-care that allow students and teachers to better deal with the stresses of life and to be more effectively attuned to their patients, so they can understand them and help them, and to their colleagues, so they can work harmoniously with them.

Managing One's Own Emotions

Managing emotions in oneself is the second key component of emotional intelligence. Children who have developed a secure sense of attachment to loving parents are more successful in learning how to modulate their emotions. Bowlby and Winnicott have postulated that "emotionally sound infants learn to soothe themselves by treating themselves as their caretakers have treated them, leaving them less vulnerable to the upheavals of the emotional brain."[23] This ability to "self-soothe" carries over into adulthood when emotions such as anger and fear are triggered. Individuals with the ability to calm themselves are more successful in exercising self-restraint.

Students and faculty who are unable to self-soothe may have a more difficult time dealing with intense emotional experiences. They may be more vulnerable to the "upheavals of the emotional brain" and more likely to overreact to stressors. Because of this, they have greater difficulty managing their emotions and are more likely to react in unprofessional ways.

In addition to the inability to self-soothe, another factor limiting the ability to manage one's emotions is the presence of unresolved, residual feelings from the past. When an event in the present triggers highly emotionally charged feelings from the past, these feelings may resurface with a vengeance.[23] These feelings from the past have been called "carried feelings." The affected individual is frequently not consciously aware of the past experience that is adding emotional fuel to the present experience. The most dramatic example of the impact of these carried feelings is in the post-traumatic stress disorder (PTSD).

Motivating Oneself

Motivating oneself is Goleman's third domain of emotional intelligence. Students and teachers who learn positive self-talk are more likely to feel optimistic and hopeful about the future.[23] These attributes enable them to be self-motivated, self-assured, and proactive. Optimism allows individuals to face adversity with the underlying expectation that things will ultimately turn out well. One might say that such individuals have learned to implement Covey's first three Habits of Highly Effective People, namely to (1) be proactive, (2) begin with the end in mind, and (3) put first things first.[40]

Recognizing Emotions in Others

Goleman's fourth domain, recognizing emotions in others, is closely related to awareness of one's own emotions. Without self-awareness, "other awareness" is difficult, if not impossible. Effectiveness as a skilled medical professional in the full sense of the term—not just the "bioscientist" sense of the term—requires empathy and the ability to connect with other people. Communication training is most effective if it is coupled with training in how to accurately recognize emotions in oneself and in others.

Handling Relationships

The art of handling relationships is, in large part, skill in managing our reactions to the emotions in others. This fifth domain is of crucial importance for any clinician. One of the greatest challenges facing any clinician is dealing with a patient whose emotions are "out of control." People who are overwhelmed with emotion are said to be "flooded." They do not hear clearly, can not think rationally, and resort to primitive emotional reactions. The ability to listen actively, validate, and empathize if possible, all the while maintaining one's own sense of control and self-restraint, is one of the most difficult tests of one's emotional intelligence.[23]

When an irate surgeon in the operating room throws his instruments across the room, he is regressing to behavior characteristic of a 2-year-old throwing a temper tantrum. The student who angrily confronts her professor in a blaming manner when she gets a failing grade on a test is probably reacting with primitive, childhood emotions while flooded with feelings of shame and inadequacy masquerading as anger. Instructors must be able to soothe their own defensive or fearful feelings and set boundaries with firmness and respect in order to handle such situations with professionalism. Dealing with the surgeon in the operating room may be more of a challenge. Students observing this type of behavior will be influenced by the behavior itself and by the way the behavior is handled. Is it an example of the "tacit value system"—the hidden curriculum—and therefore to be tolerated? Whatever the response to this behavior, it will provide powerful instruction to students.

Student Disagreements With Preceptors/ Attending Physicians

Another area where relationship skills are very important is in the interaction between a PA student and the preceptor. The ability to communicate clearly, avoid emotional flooding, and discuss disagreements in a healthy manner are of crucial importance if one wishes to maintain a professional, respectful, and trusting relationship. These skills become even more important following graduation when a PA must work closely when a supervising physician.

What ethical principles should be followed when a student disagrees with a preceptor? How is the student to know when it is appropriate to simply follow the directives of the preceptor or to follow the dictates of his/her conscience? The student's underlying ethical value system will play an important role in this decision. Those with strongly held values, which are in conflict with those of their preceptor, will probably find that it is harder to simply "follow their leader" than those with less clearly defined values. When these situations arise, an excellent resource is the Guidelines for Ethical Conduct for the Physician Assistant.[11]

J. Van Rhee, MS, PA-C, describes an interesting case in which a PA thought that his supervising physician was "incompetent" to provide appropriate medical care and supervisory expertise.[41] Guidelines for Ethical Conduct for the Physician Assistant adhere to the dictum to "do no harm" (nonmaleficence), and the statement of values includes the promotion of the health, safety, and welfare of all human beings. The values also include "respect [for] their professional relationship with physicians."[11] The Guidelines state that "Physician assistants have an ethical responsibility to protect patients and the public by identifying and assisting impaired colleagues."[11] The best ethical approach in this case was to report the physician to the appropriate hospital committee. In so doing, the PA placed himself in a difficult political and employment position, but ultimately the physician relinquished his hospital privileges. The ethical principles involved in protecting patients from an impaired physician won out over any attempt to use the PA's dependent relationship to the physician as an argument for ignoring the PA's concerns.

The above case involved a physician with hospital privileges who was answerable to a hospital committee. Many PAs work exclusively in office settings where hospital committees have no authority and are unable to play a disciplinary role. These situations are more difficult for PAs to handle, particularly if there is only one physician in the office. In these cases, the PA ultimately needs to decide on the severity of the problem. The two decisions faced by the PA are whether to remain as an employee of that physician and whether the problem is serious enough to report to the state licensing board. Confidential consultation with another professional or possibly an attorney or confidential anonymous consultations with the state medical board are reasonable options.

Shreves and Moss report on "Residents' Ethical Disagreements With Attending Physicians: An Unrecognized Problem."[42] In their study, a survey was conducted of 42 internal medicine house staff members and 51 faculty members who were attending at the West Virginia University Hospitals. They found that house staff reported 127 ethical disagreements but that the faculty were aware of only 19 of these disagreements. The conclusion of the study was that the faculty were not aware of most of the disagreements because the house staff did not voice their concerns to the attendings.

The dependent relationship of the house staff to the faculty attendings is very similar to the dependent relationship of PAs and PA students to their supervising physicians and preceptors. One of the goals of PA training is to teach students how to develop collegial relationships with physicians and how to communicate their own viewpoints clearly and with "professionalism." It might be informative to do a study similar to the one by Shreves and Moss on PA disagreements with their supervising physicians.

Application of Principles of Ethical Professionalism to Case Studies

How should the six case scenarios at the beginning of this chapter be dealt with? The principles discussed in this chapter can be applied to these cases.

CASE STUDY DISCUSSION

● **Case 1.1:** The behavioral components of professionalism that were described earlier as "civility" are: *tolerance, respect, proper conduct,* and *diplomacy.* The ABIM's six elements of professionalism (see Box 1-1) include *respect for others* and *accountability* as two of the important elements. In this case, the student violated the principles of civility by lack of respect for his instructor; the instructor also behaved in a disrespectful way toward the student by his verbal put-down of the student in front of the student's classmates. The classmates who reported the faculty member's behavior to the program director probably had the right idea. As in the clinical arena where the clinician has the responsibility for retaining composure and taking the "high road" when dealing with irate patients, the instructor also has the responsibility for behaving in a controlled manner. Such control includes appropriate restraint with proper management of a student's inappropriate outburst. It takes emotional intelligence to be able to manage one's own emotions when confronted by a disrespectful student. Some options for proper management of this situation by the instructor include the following: (1) after class she could ask the student to meet with her to discuss his behavior; (2) during class she could state, "I hear your concerns—let's discuss it after class" and educate the student on appropriate professional conduct, or (3) respond in some other nondemeaning way. Any of these responses would be more appropriate than a verbal put-down and more in keeping with the principles of ethical professionalism. It is the duty of the program director to discuss these types of issues with any faculty member who responds in an unprofessional manner with students or others. Left unchecked, persistence of this behavior will create tension in the classroom and poor modeling of professionalism.

Regardless of the instructor's reaction, the disrespectful student should be informed about inappropriate behavior. In the above situation, this would best be carried out by another faculty member or the program director.

● **Case 1.2:** This is an obvious case of dishonesty. *Honor and integrity, excellence,* and *respect for others* are three of the six elements of professionalism. By using another student's work and benefiting from it, the student who copied the other's work violated these three elements. This student also exhibited two of the "Seven Challenges to the Elements of Professionalism," namely *misrepresentation* and *lack of conscientiousness.* The student who allowed the other student to copy the SOAP note is also participating in a deceptive practice. Students who continue these breaches of ethics and professionalism are in danger of repeating similar deceptive practices when they graduate. They will become the clinicians who falsify medical records, record data that they have not actually obtained, and take advantage of professional colleagues because of their own lack of conscientiousness. The ethical principles that are violated here need to be confronted.

Accountability is a fourth element of professionalism. It is the duty of faculty to confront students who exhibit these unethical behaviors and hold them accountable. In the above case, both students who participated in the copied SOAP note met with the faculty member to discuss the reasons why their behavior was inappropriate. Neither student was given credit for the SOAP note. Both students apologized to the instructor. The student who copied the SOAP note felt remorseful about causing a friend to lose credit for the note. The process was performed in a manner that did not demean either student yet very clearly identified their behavior as completely unacceptable and not in keeping with professional behavior.

● **Case 1.3:** This is a very interesting case. The professor became aware of the CD duplication and mentioned her concerns to the class as a whole. One of the students asked the professor, in front of the rest of the class, if it is ethical to require that a class purchase an educational item from which the professor stands to profit. In a sense, the questioner attempted to deflect attention away from the illegal CD duplication and toward the ethics of making a profit from the product. The professor responded by merely stating that in her experience as a medical professional she had been required to purchase many books and other educational materials that had been authored by her professors. In addition, she stated that she did not think it was inappropriate for those who expend their time and creative energies on an educational product to benefit financially from their efforts. No attempt was made to identify the student "entrepreneur(s)" who duplicated and sold the CDs or those who purchased them. One could debate whether the students should have been identified or whether the class could have benefited from a more open discussion of the ethical principles involved. This situation might have been an opportunity to discuss the professionalism elements of *honor and integrity, respect for others*, and the challenge to professionalism, *greed*.

● Case 1.4: This case brings up the issue of professional boundaries, an issue that could use further discussion and was mentioned by d'Oronzio as one of the three main categories of professional misbehavior that he has observed in his work with physicians who have had their licenses suspended.[3] Unclear sexual boundaries may result in inappropriate sexualized comments, inappropriate sexual touch, and romanticized relationships with patients. Students need to be made aware of the dangers inherent in crossing sexual boundaries. Two of the seven challenges to professionalism are *abuse of power* and *conflict of interest*. A student who asks a patient for a date is acting on his romantic interest in the patient rather than his professional interest in her well-being. Health-care professionals are viewed by regulatory boards and by general principles of medical ethics as individuals with a power advantage over their patients. Using this advantage to get a date or become involved romantically is seen as an *abuse of power*. In addition, such a relationship can be viewed as a *conflict of interest*—having both a professional relationship as a treating clinician whose primary interest is for the patient's health and well-being and a romantic relationship where personal gratification is the goal.

● Case 1.5: *Honor and integrity* are key elements of professionalism, and one of the challenges to professionalism is *misrepresentation*. The ABIM's Charter on Medical Professionalism lists *Commitment to honesty with patients* as a professional responsibility (see Box 1-3). In addition, honesty is a foundational ethical principle at the base of the pyramid described in Figure 1.2. Whatever the rationale of the physician who preferred to describe the student as a medical student rather than a PA student, the rationale is not sufficient to

condone that type of misrepresentation. The PA student's concern was justified. In all states, PAs are required by law to identify themselves as such; any failure to do so is considered to be unprofessional conduct and is subject to disciplinary action.

During their didactic year, students must learn about the need to properly identify themselves while on rotations and when they are graduate PAs. In this case, the student must be supported in correcting the error of the preceptor. Several approaches are possible. One approach would be to have the student remind the preceptor that PA students must be introduced as PA students. In many cases this is sufficient to get the preceptor to comply. If the student is reluctant to confront the preceptor, or if the preceptor does not comply with the student's request, then it is the responsibility of the PA program to call or meet with the preceptor to discuss and clarify this issue.

● Case 1.6: This case illustrates both *boundary violations* and *financial infractions*, two of the three most common categories of misbehavior for which physicians have had their licenses suspended.[3] Although the severity of this student's misbehavior may be viewed as relatively minor, these types of "minor indiscretions" may lead to more serious forms of misbehavior later, if they are not confronted. Any type of stealing is, by definition, a boundary violation—going beyond the limits, taking something that does not belong to you. Although the medical office may have received the samples at no cost, the samples are still the property of the office, regardless of their monetary value. Samples are there for patients and should not be taken without permission.

Students need to be told about boundary violations, with practical examples of what they might look like in real life. When these violations occur, students need to be confronted, and a forceful message must be conveyed. There are a variety of options for dealing with this type of situation, ranging from a verbal warning meeting with the PA Academic Review Committee and being placed on probation for unprofessional behavior to failing the rotation.

SUMMARY

PA students have much to learn in a short time. In addition to learning a large volume of bioscientific knowledge, they must also learn how to behave in a complex medical-legal-social climate. PA programs have an obligation to teach the principles of medical professionalism, which are based on foundational ethical principles. Students must develop greater awareness of their own values and how these may influence their attitudes about the whole range of issues that they will be dealing with as medical professionals. In addition, they must become more aware of their own emotional inner life—they must become more emotionally intelligent—in order to immunize themselves against ethical lapses.

References

1. Adams D. (2004, March 15). Professionalism starts in med school: Students who don't get it are likely to become physicians who spend time before state medical boards. AMNews.
2. Papadakis MA, Hodgson CS, Teherani A, et al. Unprofessional behavior in medical school is associated with subsequent disciplinary action by a state medical board. Academic Medicine, 2004;79:244-249.
3. d'Oronzio JC. Avoiding fallacies of misplaced concreteness in medical professionalism. The American Journal of Bioethics, 2004;4:31-33.
4. Berger BA, ed. Promoting Civility in Pharmacy Education. New York: Pharmaceutical Products Press, 2003.
5. Wear D, Castellani B. The development of professionalism: Curriculum matters. Academic Medicine 2000;75:602-611.
6. Swick HM. Toward a normative definition of medical professionalism. Academic Medicine, 2000;75: 612-616.
7. Doukas DJ. Returning to professionalism: The re-emergence of medicine's art. The American Journal of Bioethics, 2004;4:18-19.
8. American Board of Internal Medicine, 1995. Project professionalism. Retrieved June 20, 2004, from http://www.abim.org/pubs/p2/index.htm
9. Robins LS, Braddock CH, Fryer-Edwards KA. Using the American Board of Internal Medicine's "elements of professionalism" for undergraduate ethics education. Academic Medicine, 2002;77:523-531.
10. Medical professionalism in the new millennium: A physician charter. Annals of Internal Medicine, 2002;136:243-246.
11. Guidelines for the ethical conduct for the physician assistant. JAAPA, 2001;14:10-20 [policy of the AAPA, adopted May 2000].
12. American Medical Association. Principles of medical ethics. Retrieved July 6, 2004, from http://www.ama-assn.org/ama/pub/category/8600.html
13. Singer PA. Strengthening the role of ethics in medical education. Canadian Medical Association Journal, 2003;168:854-855.
14. Wear D, Kuczewski MG. The professionalism movement: Can we pause? The American Journal of Bioethics, 2004;4:1-10.
15. Dudzinski DM. Integrity in the relationship between medical ethics and professionalism. The American Journal of Bioethics, 2004;4:26-27.
16. Shirley JL, Padgett SM. Professionalism and discourse: But wait, there's more! The American Journal of Bioethics, 2004;4:36-37.
17. Hammer DP. Civility and professionalism. In Berger BA, ed. Promoting Civility in Pharmacy Education. New York: Pharmaceutical Products Press, 2003.
18. Coulehan J, Willams PC. Vanquishing virtue: The impact of medical education. Academic Medicine, 2001;76:598-605.
19. Carter SL. Civility. New York: Basic Books, 1998.
20. Beck DE, Krueger JL, Byrd DC. Experiential learning: Transitioning students from civility to professionalism. In Berger BA, ed. Promoting Civility in Pharmacy Education. New York: Pharmaceutical Products Press, 2003.
21. Wear D, Castellani B. The development of professionalism: Curriculum matters. Academic Medicine 2000;75:602-611.
22. Coles R. The moral education of medical students. Academic Medicine, 1998;73:55-57.
23. Goleman D. Emotional Intelligence: Why It Can Matter More Than IQ. New York: Bantam Books, 1995.
24. Kenny NP, Mann KV, MacLeon H. Role modeling in physicians' professional formation: Reconsidering an essential but untapped educational strategy. Academic Medicine, 2003;78:1203-1210.

25. Glick SM. The teaching of medical ethics to medical students. Journal of Medical Ethics, 1994;20:239-243.

26. Hafferty FW. What medical students know about professionalism. The Mount Sinai Journal of Medicine, 2002;69:385-397.

27. Hundert EM, Hafferty F, Christakis D. Characteristics of the informal curriculum and trainees' ethical choices. Academic Medicine, 1996;71:624-642.

28. Fesher J. Teaching professionalism: A student's perspective. The Mount Sinai Journal of Medicine 2002;69:412-414.

29. Patenaude J, Niyonsenga T, Fafard D. Changes in students' moral development during medical school: A cohort study. Canadian Medical Association Journal, 2003;168:840-844.

30. Feudtner C, Christakis DA, Christakis NA. Do clinical clerks suffer ethical erosion? Students' perceptions of their ethical environment and personal development. Academic Medicine, 1994;69:670-679.

31. Skelly FJ. (1990, July 6/13). Permission granted. AMNews.

32. Hensel WA, Dickey NW. Teaching professionalism: Passing the torch. Academic Medicine, 1998;73: 865-870.

33. Whitcomb ME. Fostering and evaluating professionalism in medical education. Academic Medicine, 2002;77:473-474.

34. Fleisher WP, Kristjanson C, Bourgeois-Law G, et al. Pilot study of the defining issues test. Canadian Medical Association Journal, 2003;169:1145-1146.

35. Carrothers RM, Gregory SW, Gallagher TJ. Measuring emotional intelligence of medical school applicants. Academic Medicine, 2000;75:456-463.

36. Mason HL. Promoting civility in graduate student education. In Berger BA, ed. Promoting Civility in Pharmacy Education. New York: Pharmaceutical Products Press, 2003.

37. Kasman DL, Fryer-Edwards K, Braddock CH. Educating for professionalism: Trainees' emotional experiences on IM and pediatrics inpatient wards. Academic Medicine, 2003;78:730-741.

38. Salovey P, Mayer JD. Emotional intelligence. Imagination, Cognition and Personality. 1990; 9:185-211.

39. Gordon JS. Manifesto for a New Medicine. New York: Addison-Wesley, 1996.

40. Covey SR. The 7 Habits of Highly Effective People: Restoring the Character Ethic. New York: Simon and Schuster, 1989.

41. Van Rhee J. Dealing with the incompetent supervising physician: An ethical dilemma. JAAPA, 2003;16: 31-33.

42. Shreves JG, Moss AH. Residents' ethical disagreements with attending physicians: An unrecognized problem. Academic Medicine, 1996;71:1103-1105.

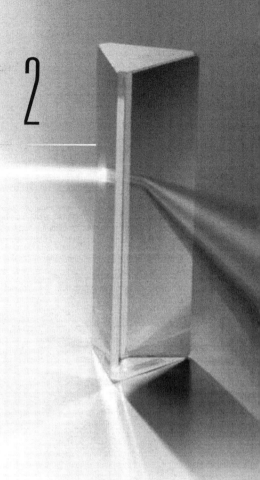

Ethical Decision Making and Ethical Principles

Therese Jones, PhD

"It appears to me that in Ethics, difficulties and disagreements are due to a very simple cause: namely, to the attempt to answer questions, without first discovering precisely what question it is which you desire to answer."

George Edward Moore, *Principia Ethica*

Ethical Decision Making

Several years ago, a journalist who regularly writes on religion and culture titled his column, "Everyday Ethics," and opened with the following: "Many people treat ethics like the good set of dishes, something to be saved for special occasions."[1] When we think and talk about ethical issues in health care, we typically focus on the big issues such as embryonic stem cell research, physician-assisted suicide, technology at the end of life, and the allocation of organs. Like the good set of dishes, these are the topics we often bring out for public debate in legislatures, courtrooms, classrooms, congregations, living rooms, research facilities, and ethics conferences.

Most people, as this journalist notes, recognize the moral and ethical components of these dramatic and polarizing issues, but ethical questions permeate many less dramatic and more ambiguous everyday situations. Thomas Shanks, an ethicist at the Markkula Center for Applied Ethics, spent several years talking with hundreds of people, including students, teachers, lawyers, physicians, and allied health providers, about the commonplace moral questions, the "everyday ethics," that they encounter in their daily lives.[2] Some of those questions are:

- "Is it right to keep my mouth shut when a colleague or classmate is getting into real trouble?"
- "Do I laugh at a sexist, racist, or homophobic joke?"
- "Is it right to be chronically late for class, work, or meetings because I am so busy?"

Shanks notes that not only do many of us share such everyday questions, but many of us also share a hunger for ethical approaches to such questions. He cites a recent survey conducted by the *Times Mirror* that showed ethics, or rather a decline in ethics, as one of the most important concerns of Americans.[2] Perhaps such widespread concern is what prompted the *New York Times Magazine* in 1999 to create a weekly column, "The Ethicist," which is widely syndicated in newspapers and regularly broadcast. For Randy Cohen, the man behind "The Ethicist," the objective of the column is to bring about an honorable society and to make visible the assumptions that underpin our individual decisions and the workings of

the society in which we live. Cohen, himself an avowed flawed and busy human being, knows that it would be impossible for us to pause and question the propriety of each and every one of our actions: "we'd never get out of the house, stuck by the closet door as we pondered the acceptability of leather shoes."[3] However, he also knows that individual ethical behavior is far likelier to flourish within a just society, and he responds to the quandaries of those who write to "The Ethicist" with that end in mind. What is most encouraging, he says, is how seriously people think about the ethical questions of daily life.[4]

Waiting for a big dramatic event, such as cloning, before tackling ethical considerations is like playing a sport only on the weekend, according to Elizabeth Bounds, a Christian ethicist at Emory University: "Just as a weekend warrior often ends up with pulled muscles and poor performance, people who seldom consider the moral implications of daily activities won't have the coordination to work through the more difficult times in their lives."[1]

Thus, making moral decisions, like other decisions in daily life and in health care, is not a precise art but a learned skill, promising a degree of proficiency and confidence to those willing to take the time and effort to practice. And how such ethical decisions are best made has long been an object of intense interest and extensive scholarship.

In this chapter, you will have the opportunity to become more familiar with the major ethical principles that frame the moral context of health care and with the essential features of ethical decision making as well as with some of the more prominent ethical theories that have been developed to guide that decision making. Acquiring this familiarity will help foster responsible ethical decision making.

Principles of Health-Care Ethics

The *American Heritage Dictionary* defines a principle as a "basic truth," "law," "assumption," or "source." The principles of health-care ethics are meant to inform, guide, and shape the behaviors and decisions of those involved. Since its emergence as a discipline in the 1960s, contemporary health-care ethics has relied on four principles:

- Respect for autonomy
- Beneficence
- Nonmaleficence
- Justice

From these principles are derived particular rules of conduct, such as informed consent, confidentiality, and negligence. In their influential book, *Principles of Biomedical Ethics,* Beauchamp and Childress codified these "four clusters of principles," but they were quick to point out that these principles provide only a framework for identifying and reflecting on moral problems and that they do not constitute a general moral theory.[5] Below is a brief description of each principle; a more detailed discussion will follow in the second part of this chapter, including several landmark cases that exemplify the principles.

Respect for Autonomy

The principle of respect for autonomy is no less important in health care than it is in every other aspect of our lives. As members of a moral community that values individuals and their personal freedom, we believe we can best flourish when others treat us with dignity and permit us the opportunity to make our own decisions in our own ways. Even though patients, because of illness or accident, may lose some measure of their independence, they still deserve to be treated with respect and to remain in control of their lives.

Health-care professionals have specific professional responsibilities that help ensure that patients are treated with respect and are given the opportunity to retain control over their bodies and their lives. These responsibilities include respecting patient confidences, communicating with patients honestly, and obtaining patients' informed consent or refusal as treatment plans develop.

Beneficence and Nonmaleficence

The principle of beneficence instructs us to promote the well-being of others. Its complement, nonmaleficence, instructs us not to harm others deliberately. Beneficence arguably captures the true moral essence of the professional responsibilities of health-care providers. It is the guiding purpose of health care to help those who suffer from illness either by treating that illness, by making them more comfortable, or by providing them with information about how to cope and adjust to their situation. Being of help to patients is what being a health-care professional is all about. Examples of responsibilities that flow from the principle of beneficence are competency, discernment, and service.

Justice

The principle of justice, often equated with fairness, speaks to our belief that we each be treated equally, that we all share the good and the bad alike. Justice is important to health care in a variety of ways, especially given its cost in our society. There is very often an excess of demand on public services coupled with a shortage of the goods used to meet those demands. As an example, consider all the possible ways the wealth of the government could be used to benefit the population, such as providing health care, education, military defense, or public transportation. We can not

do all these things to the extent we would like; we have to choose. Justice helps guide our choices. As citizens, we expect that health professionals, who are entrusted with society's resources to provide health care, will be responsible in their actions and will not waste resources.

Conflicting Principles

At times, these principles may conflict with one another. For example, a patient may suffer a life-threatening injury that can be treated successfully with surgery and blood transfusions. However, the patient may believe that it is wrong, based on religious principles, to receive the blood of another human being. In this instance, respect for autonomy and beneficence are in irreconcilable conflict. One principle must be judged as having priority over the other.

At other times, principles will complement one another in providing ethical guidance. For example, someone may be diagnosed with a terminal illness that can not be cured but may be treated so as to control symptoms and possibly extend that patient's life. However, that treatment may have serious and uncomfortable side effects. Treating someone to extend her life is apparently helping her, whereas treating someone so that he is caused pain is apparently harming him. On the surface, it is hard to know which is more important. Does benefiting take precedence over not harming?

We can answer this question only to the extent that we truly know what constitutes benefit and what constitutes harm. By consulting the patient and learning that person's preferences and values, we can then, and only then, have sufficient information to determine what counts as benefit and harm and what constitutes the proper course of action. Here the principle of respect for autonomy has complemented and clarified the guidance offered by the principles of beneficence and nonmaleficence.

Features of Ethical Decision Making

Whenever we are faced with an ethical choice, there are four constant and essential components:

- Agent
- Choices
- Consequences
- Context

Agent

The person, or moral agent, who is faced with making a choice serves as the focus for responsibility. As moral agents, we have the responsibility to make an appropriate decision. Our capacity to make these decisions is heavily influenced by our character: the set of personal characteristics, beliefs, and values that predispose us to act in certain ways and seek certain outcomes. As you become a health-care professional, your profession will inform your character to the extent that, when joined with your own personal values and beliefs, it influences and shapes the tendencies that guide your actions when you act in your professional role.

Choices

In making ethical decisions, moral agents always have choices that they can select from as they make their decisions. We typically discriminate among these choices because we perceive some to be generally right, such as telling the truth, or generally wrong, such as deliberately hurting people.

Consequences

It is also the case that we usually anticipate that certain consequences will occur if certain choices are made. Again, we tend to understand that some consequences are better than others. For example, one state of affairs that works to the benefit of those involved in the situation is valued more highly than another state of affairs that works to their detriment.

Context

Finally, there is always a setting, or context, that influences the ethical decisions we make. The salient feature of the context, which situates the ethical decisions of health-care professionals, is that your decisions involve and affect patients. Patients are made vulnerable by their illness; not only is their ability to function typically diminished but so also is their capacity to act as full agents in their community. They are dependent on the support and assistance of others, and they are struggling to give meaning to their illness within the context of their own lives framed by family, race, gender, and culture.

Ethical Theories

Ethical theories serve as frameworks or perspectives that individual moral agents can bring to bear on the situations confronting them. Just as is the case with science, art, and other areas of applied knowledge, there are competing theories constructed to facilitate the making of ethically responsible decisions. What follows is a very concise overview of predominant theoretical and methodological approaches to ethical decision making.

These different theories tend to view one of the essential features of ethical decision making as having greater importance over the others. For example, one theory may place a greater emphasis on achieving certain outcomes, whereas another may place a greater emphasis on the characteristics of the moral agent who is making the decision.

Virtue Ethics

Virtue ethics is characterized by an emphasis on the moral character of the **agent** because it is presumed that morally appropriate decisions occur as a result of being decided by morally sensitive and skilled people. Accordingly, virtue theorists focus principally on the education and development of the agent making the decision. By cultivating certain skills or certain virtues, people will make appropriate decisions. The task is to ensure that people, first of all, want to do that which is right and best. However, desire, on its own, is not sufficient—good intentions alone do not make for good decisions. There must also be in place the knowledge of how to accomplish that which we see as being good. And this knowledge comes only from practice.

Virtue ethics has been criticized for treating moral virtue as a sufficient rather than necessary condition for ethical decisions being made. In other words, joining proper motivation with knowledge and practice is not enough to guarantee good decisions on all occasions. To illustrate, consider what happened when people began to ask whether withdrawing a feeding tube was the moral equivalent of starving someone to death. Critics contend that no matter how much skill and practice a health-care professional may have had making ethical decisions, this was a choice that required more than experienced thinkers to make the right decision.

Deontology or Formalism

In contrast to virtue ethics, deontological or formalist theories begin with the assumption that what makes an action primarily right or wrong is some intrinsic property not of the moral agent but of the **action** itself. According to legend, George Washington confessed to chopping down the cherry tree; he did the right thing because his action had the feature of honesty attached to it, and honesty can be shown to be good on a variety of accounts. From a Judeo-Christian perspective, for instance, it con*forms* (hence, the term *form*alism) with one of the Ten Commandments: "Thou shalt not bear false witness." From another point of view, it conforms to the golden rule: "Treat others as you would wish to be treated yourself."

There is the assumption in all deontological or formalist theories that a guide to truth exists, that there is a moral litmus test. And if you subject an action to this moral test and it passes, then it is the right thing to do; if it fails the test, then it is the wrong thing to do.

The major drawback to deontological or formalist theories is that they leave us hanging in the lurch far too often. If we apply any of the tests for generating knowledge of right and wrong actions, we will generate a list of duties: tell the truth, do not steal, do not harm innocent people, keep your promises, help those in need. However, what do we do when telling the truth will harm innocent people? Which duty is more important? Sometimes honesty will triumph, and sometimes not hurting others will.

The most common example used to illustrate such a conflict is that of the Gestapo during the Nazi regime in Germany who come pounding on your front door behind which you have hidden your Jewish friends and neighbors. Do you lie to protect your friends from harm? Or do you tell the truth and send your friends to certain torture and death? It is not clear that we can know which one triumphs just by applying the test that generated our list of duties in the first place. In other words, there is not a litmus test after all.

Consequentialism and Utilitarianism

Consequentialist theories, on the other hand, think the trap of conflicting duties that ensnares deontology can be avoided if we evaluate the moral worth of actions focusing not on the agent or on the action but on what we seek to accomplish with an action. Actions that are thought to most likely produce **good consequences** are good actions; actions that are thought to most likely produce **bad consequences** are bad actions.

The most prevalent form of a consequentialist theory is utilitarianism, the theory that instructs us to act so as to cause the greatest net amount of pleasure for the greatest number of people. Thus, when we are faced with making an ethical decision, utilitarians claim there is a very straightforward approach that, if followed correctly, will tell us what to do.

First, we must examine the consequences, both short-term and long-term, that will likely result from the decisions that might conceivably be made. Second, those consequences must be compared in terms of how many people will be helped and to what degree and how many people will be harmed and to what degree. The decision that will produce the greatest amount of benefit for the most people or produce the least amount of harm emerges as the proper course of action.

Not surprising, utilitarianism has its critics, too. Because the theory tells us to make decisions based on consequences, we need to be able to know what consequences to pursue. Critics argue that the theory can not tell us exactly which consequences to seek. Complicating the picture even more is the fact that some actions benefit some and harm others to differing degrees. Critics point out that knowing whether the harm to the few is offset by the benefit to the many is like comparing apples with oranges; they can not be compared. The final major criticism centers on our ability to predict consequences. Even if we knew which consequence is the one we should attempt to achieve, there is the fact that very frequently we are in no position to predict accurately what the conse-

quence of our actions will be. Critics conclude that for these reasons utilitarianism is just not workable in practice.

Casuistry

Casuistry employs analogical reasoning to resolve difficult cases and proceeds on the basis of comparing one case with other, similar paradigm cases in which the right course of action is known. On the basis of these comparisons, such as degrees of similarity or dissimilarity between the paradigm case and the present case, we can infer a course of action. Paradigm cases are often dramatic and involve court decisions, such as the Karen Ann Quinlan and Nancy Cruzan decisions (described below). However, there are dilemmas that arise more frequently and that are resolved in less dramatic ways than petitioning the courts. For instance, what should you do about the patient who demands penicillin for a viral infection? This case involves nonmaleficence, truth-telling, justice, and patient autonomy. How have experienced health-care professionals decided what to do? What reasoning led them to their decisions? Is the present case similar in relevant ways?

Casuists argue that determinations can be made only by paying strict attention to the salient features of the current situation and then making a decision, one that is based upon experience, judgment, and skills. Proponents of casuistry say that its strength lies in its attention to the context, to the concrete situations of real patients and real caregivers.

Narrative

One method of understanding these concrete situations is with narrative that views medical knowledge as storytelling knowledge. The patient's illness is the telling of a story that requires empathy and compassion and that is introduced into the patient-professional relationship through the use of language. Narrative ethics is considered a methodology that increases sensitivity to detail and to the particulars of cases. How can we deliberate responsibly about moral choices if we fail to understand the nuance and subtlety intrinsic to human dilemmas, whose features can get easily lost when trying to impose some absolute standard on a situation, such as "doing one's duty" or "promoting the greatest good for the greatest number"?

Narrative ethics, according to its proponents, is a tool that allows for deeper penetration and deeper insight into the human moral drama that is involved in illness. Through understanding of the context and illumination of the experiences, values, beliefs, and cultural practices within illness, the narrative or story approach permits us to peer closer—a kind of interpretive stethoscope. As a methodology, it helps people hear and see in heightened ways and improves their perception of the moral dilemma and its complexity. Narrative theorists see this as essential if we are to remain interested and focused on the moral and existential elements involved in patient care.

The prevalent criticisms of narrative ethics are with the inherent difficulties of knowing both how to interpret and how to complete a narrative. What or whose point of view should be adopted for interpretation? Moreover, knowing the story in the present does not guarantee that we can know how the story will or must end.

Conclusion

In summary, the most prominent ethical theories and methods can be connected to the essential elements of ethical decision making:

- Agent: virtue theory
- Action: deontological or formalist theory
- Outcome: consequentialist and utilitarian theory
- Context: casuistry and narrative theories

The dispute over approach and method can only be introduced and certainly not resolved here. Some approaches to ethics assume there is an approach from "on high," even though there is disagreement exactly where this "on high" is. Other approaches encourage decision makers to get as deep "in the trenches" as possible. The tensions among these approaches produce insight into the situations and tasks of those who have to make ethical decisions. However, even though these approaches are not perfect does not mean they are not useful. The limitations of the various approaches to decision making can guide our actions. The greater care we show in our thinking, the greater our chances of making better rather than worse decisions.

An Ethical Decision-Making Framework

The following ethical decision-making framework, an amalgam of several similar frameworks and matrices used by health-care professionals, identifies the key steps in making such decisions[6]:

I. Gather relevant information
  A. Clinical indications
    1. Is the problem acute? chronic? emergent? reversible?
    2. What is the usual or customary treatment?
    3. What will relieve suffering and provide comfort?
  B. Patient preferences
    1. Has the patient been informed of risks and benefits? understood? given consent?
    2. Is the patient mentally capable? If not, is there a surrogate?
  C. Quality of life
    1. What is the patient's judgment?
    2. What is the health professional's judgment?
    3. Is there a future plan?
  D. Context
    1. What are the patient's values? religious beliefs? cultural traditions?
    2. Are there financial concerns?
    3. Are there institutional policies? legal issues?
II. State the nature of the ethical dilemma
  A. Ethical principles
  B. Professional virtues
  C. Projected outcomes
  D. Paradigm cases
  E. Particular features
III. Explore the options
IV. Select and justify a resolution

Ethical Principles

This section includes a more detailed discussion of the four principles of health-care ethics and introduces several landmark legal and ethical cases in the United States.

Respect for Autonomy

"One's own free unfettered choice, one's own caprice—however wild it may be….What one wants is simply independent choice, whatever that independence may cost and wherever it may lead."

Dostoyevsky, The Brothers Karamazov

In their groundbreaking work, *Clinical Ethics: A Practical Approach to Ethical Decisions in Clinical Medicine*, Jonsen and Siegler begin by discussing the significance of those actions required by the principle of respect for autonomy: "When there are medical indications for treatment or care, a [health professional] normally proposes a plan that a competent patient may either accept or refuse. An informed, competent patient's preference to accept or to refuse medically indicated treatment is of great clinical, legal, psychological and ethical significance."[7]

The authors emphasize how patient preferences are the ethical and legal nucleus of the patient-professional relationship and how the "knowledge of those preferences is essential to good care, since the patient's cooperation and satisfaction reflect the degree to which intervention and therapy fulfill the patient's choices, values and needs" (p. 37). The following discussion presents a brief summary of both the consequences of and the requirements for identifying and respecting patient preferences as outlined by Jonsen and Siegler.

Clinical Significance: Better Outcomes
Patient preferences are clinically significant because patients who interact actively with health professionals to reach a shared decision have greater trust and loyalty in the patient-professional relationship, cooperate more completely to implement the shared decision, express greater satisfaction with their health care and, most important, have been shown to have better clinical outcomes.

Legal Significance: Self-Determination
As Jonsen and Siegler note, patient preferences are "legally significant because the American legal system recognizes that each person has a fundamental right to control his or her own body and the right to be protected from unwanted intrusions or 'unconsented touchings'"(p. 38). One of the earliest judicial opinions on this matter was in 1914, *Schloendorff v New York Hospital:* "Every human being of adult years and of sound mind has a right to determine what shall be done with his body." This legal requirement of explicit consent prior to specific treatment "protects patients' legal right to control what is done to their own bodies," and the documentation of that patient's consent "serves as a defense for the [health professional] against a claim that the patient was coerced" (p. 38).

Moreover, Jonsen and Siegler discuss the now quite common legal distinction of the fiduciary nature of the patient-professional relationship. The fiduciary, in this case the health professional, "has an obligation to promote the best interests of persons who have entrusted themselves" to that professional's care, and the patient's consent both "initiates this relationship and sustains it by accepting recommendations" (p 39).

Psychological Significance: Control
Common sense tells us that when patients have both the freedom to express their preferences and the belief that those preferences are respected, their sense of self-worth is nurtured and reinforced. As Jonsen and Siegler write, patients "already threatened by illness or accident may have a vital need for some sense of control," and if they believe their preferences are denied or devalued, they are likely to distrust and disregard the recommendations of a health professional, however clinically sound and medically necessary those recommendations might be (p. 39). Moreover, the open and honest expression of a patient's preferences offers the opportunity for the revelation and the

discussion of other important factors such as his or her fears, fantasies, beliefs, and values (p. 39).

Ethical Significance: Autonomy
Patient preferences are ethically significant because they make explicit the value of personal autonomy that is deeply rooted in the ethics of our culture. As discussed above, moral philosophers emphasize the principle of autonomy, the right to choose and follow one's own plan of life and action, and Jonsen and Siegler concur, describing respect for autonomy as "the moral attitude that disposes one to refrain from interference with others' autonomous beliefs and actions in the pursuit of their goals" (p. 38).

The word *autonomy* is derived from the Greek, *autos* ("self") and *nomos* ("rule," "governance," or "law") and originally referred to the self-rule or self-governance of independent city-states. Autonomy has since been extended to individuals and has acquired meanings as diverse as self-governance, liberty, rights, privacy, individual choice, freedom of will, and being one's own person.

Defined by Beauchamp and Childress, personal autonomy is, at a minimum, "self-rule that is free from both controlling interference by others and from limitations, such as inadequate understanding, that prevent meaningful choice" (p. 58). The autonomous individual acts freely in accordance with a self-chosen plan. Virtually all theories of autonomy agree that two conditions are essential: "liberty (independence from controlling influences) and agency (capacity for intentional action)" (p. 58).

Thus, respect for autonomy is not simply an ideal in health care; it is a professional obligation. And autonomous choice is a right, not a duty, of patients. To respect an autonomous person is to acknowledge that person's right to hold views, to make choices, and to take actions based on personal values and beliefs. Such respect involves respectful action, not merely a respectful attitude. For health professionals, it not only requires noninterference in their patients' personal affairs but also includes the obligation to strengthen or restore their patients' capacity for free choice while helping to allay any fears or other conditions that might hamper or prevent that free choice. Finally, respect involves acknowledging decision-making rights and enabling persons to act autonomously, whereas disrespect for autonomy involves attitudes and actions that ignore, insult, or demean others' rights of autonomy.

Beauchamp and Childress make the further distinction in their exploration of the principle of respect for autonomy as both a negative and a positive obligation: "As a *negative* obligation: *Autonomous actions should not be subjected to controlling con-*

straints by others. As a positive obligation: this principle requires respectful treatment in disclosing information and fostering autonomous decision making" (p 64).

Consequently, respect for autonomy "obligates professionals in health care and research involving human subjects to disclose information, to probe for and ensure understanding and voluntariness, and to foster adequate decision making" (p. 64). Because of various ways in which the negative and positive sides of respect for autonomy function in the moral life, they are capable of supporting many specific moral rules, such as these enumerated by Beauchamp and Childress (p. 65):

• Tell the truth to patients.
• Respect the privacy of patients.
• Protect confidential information.
• Obtain consent from patients.
• Help patients make important decisions at their request.

Paternalism

As Jonsen and Siegler point out, one of the most common ethical issues raised by the principle of respect for autonomy is that of paternalism. Paternalism in health care refers to "the practice of overriding or ignoring preferences of patients in order to benefit them or enhance their welfare" (p. 39). Such a practice is usually justified by a health professional when he or she judges that the principle of beneficence trumps, or takes priority over, the principle of respect for autonomy. Although paternalism has been endorsed by health-care professionals historically, it is now considered to be ethically suspect.

Informed Consent and Refusal

Patient preferences are typically expressed by informed consent. It is the practical application of respect for the patient's autonomy and is defined by Jonsen and Siegler as the willing acceptance of a medical intervention by a patient after adequate disclosure by a health professional about the nature of an intervention with its risks and benefits and alternatives with their risks and benefits (p. 40). Thus, as the ethical basis for the patient-professional relationship, informed consent refers to an encounter that is characterized by mutual participation, respect, and shared decision making.

By the 1970s, most jurisdictions in the United States had adopted the doctrine of informed consent as an essential aspect of professional responsibility in the care of patients. The states divided evenly, however, on standards of disclosure. A very slight majority adopted a "professional standard" of disclosure, according to which a health-care professional may disclose information to a patient that a reasonable

professional under the same or similar circumstances would disclose. A significant minority of states adopted a "reasonable patient standard," according to which the health-care professional must disclose information to a patient that a reasonable person in a similar situation would wish to know in deciding whether or not to consent. Over time, however, the reasonable patient standard has increasingly replaced the professional standard. A third standard, the "subjective standard," is patient-specific, providing information that is specifically tailored to a particular patient's need for information and understanding.

Essential Elements of a Fully Informed Consent

Informed consent should represent a dialogue between patient and professional, establishing a reciprocal relationship or therapeutic alliance and leading to agreement about the course of treatment or care. A properly negotiated informed consent benefits both the health professional and the patient. The following information must be conveyed to the patient in comprehensible language rather than clinical or scientific jargon:

• Diagnosis and recommendation for procedure/treatment
• Nature of the recommended procedure/treatment
• Risks and benefits of the procedure/treatment (excluding those that are extremely remote unless extremely significant such as paralysis or death)
• Alternatives to the recommended procedure/treatment (including doing nothing) and their risks and benefits
• Likelihood that the anticipated risks or benefits will be realized
• Identity, credentials, and experience of those performing the procedure or providing the treatment
• Cost of the procedure/treatment

Informed consent is an ongoing process rather than a single event. The consent is only as informed and as effective as the discussion that preceded it. The ultimate goal is the patient's understanding, not the patient's agreement with the professional's recommendation and not the patient's signature on a form. The consent form signed by the patient is the best documentary evidence that a consent process has taken place.

Decisional Capacity

As Jonsen and Siegler point out, consent to treatment is complicated by the difficulties of disclosure for health professionals, such as the uncertainty intrinsic to all medical information, the worry about harming or alarming a patient, and the burden of a tight and complicated schedule (p. 44). Patients may be limited in understanding; they may be inattentive and distracted; and they may be overcome by fear and anxiety. Moreover, some patients lack the mental capacity to understand or to make choices. The law often uses the terms competence and incompetence to designate whether people have the legal authority to make personal choices, such as managing their finances or making health-care decisions. Judges alone have the right to rule that a person is legally incompetent.

However, health professionals may encounter legally competent patients who appear to have their mental capacities compromised by illness, anxiety, pain, or hospitalization. Such a situation is referred to as decisional capacity or incapacity in order to distinguish it from the legal determination of competency. It is necessary to assess decisional capacity as an essential part of the informed consent process.

Determining Patient Competency

The following are some of the factors to be remembered about patient competency in making health-care decisions:

- The capacity to make a rational decision rather than the decision itself is what is sought in determining competency.
- This capacity is not a continuous, 24-hour capacity but is rather the mental capacity to make a particular medical decision at the time the decision is required.
- A patient may be incompetent in some areas of life, such as inability to make financial decisions, yet be competent in other areas.
- Determining capacity is not an expert medical diagnosis.

Equally important are some of the elements in determining patient competency in making health-care decisions:

- The patient possesses a set of personal goals and values.
- The patient is able to give and receive information and to appreciate the meaning of potential medical alternatives.
- The patient is able to compare the impact of alternative outcomes on his or her personal goals and life plans.

Landmark Case: Dax Cowart

In the summer of 1973, after graduating from college and serving 3 years as a jet pilot in the Air Force, Donald "Dax" Cowart was critically injured in a propane gas explosion that killed his father, who was also his partner in a successful real estate venture. Dax sustained primarily third-degree burns over 68% of his body; both eyes were blinded by corneal damage, both ears were mostly destroyed, both hands were so badly burned that the distal parts of the fin-

gers required amputation, and the hands were so badly deformed that they appeared as useless, unsightly stubs. Within minutes after the accident and throughout the days and weeks and months of excruciatingly painful treatment, such as repeated skin grafts and daily immersions in the household bleach and water mixture of a Hubbard tank for infection control, Dax consistently and coherently stated that he did not want medical care, that he did not want to live.

In April 1974, Dax was admitted to the University of Texas Medical Branch in Galveston (the third care facility since the accident), where he adamantly refused to give consent for corrective surgery on his hands and persistently demanded to leave the hospital and return home to die. Despite his protests, the tankings were continued. Eventually, Dr. Robert B. White was called in as a psychiatric consultant to determine the patient's competency.

Finding Dax to be mentally able to make a rational and informed decision but feeling deeply troubled about the circumstances, White first conferred with a colleague, who agreed with the initial evaluation, and next obtained permission from Dax and his mother, Ada Cowart, to do a videotaped interview for educational purposes. That interview functions as the structural centerpiece of a 30-minute documentary *Please Let Me Die*. Although viewers of this documentary are stunned by the total helplessness of a bedridden and bandaged patient without eyes or fingers, they are also persuaded by the clear and cogent argument he makes for his own free choice: "What gives any physician the right to keep alive a patient who wants to die?"[8] Dax's ordeal became what one scholar describes as a "celebrated case study in medical ethics and human meaning...a classic among professionals concerned with the treatment and care of the hopelessly ill and helplessly deformed."[9] Dax became a cause célèbre in the growing "right to die" movement of the 1970s. A second documentary, *Dax's Case,* followed in 1985, along with hundreds of television and print interviews, countless panel discussions, many articles, and at least six books.

Dax's story raises a fundamental moral issue in health care: how can a professional respect a patient's autonomy while looking out for his or her best interests? According to bioethicist H. Tristram Englehardt, Jr., that issue foregrounds the "bounds and legitimacy of paternalism."[10] The options in Dax's case were to force treatment, to stop treatment, or try to convince Dax to continue to treatment. This third alternative would respect both the freedom of the patient as well as the commitment of the health-care professionals to preserve the patient's life. However, as Englehardt writes, "in the end, individuals, when able, must be allowed to decide their own destiny, even that of death."[11]

After earning a law degree from Texas Tech University, Dax Cowart went on to specialize in patients' rights. While he affirms that his life is happy and fulfilled, he insists that he should have been allowed to die. To this day, he still maintains that health-care professionals violated his right to choose not to be treated and still resents the powerlessness of patients who are forced to live when they beg to die.

Summary of Respect for Autonomy

What follows is an illustrative but selective list of actions derived from the principle of respect for autonomy[12]:

- Respect the ability of competent patients to hold views, make choices, and take actions based on their personal values and beliefs.
- Respect the choice of competent patients to refuse treatment or care.
- It is impermissible to lie to patients or to withhold information necessary for them to understand adequately.
- It is impermissible to treat competent patients without their informed consent.
- Respect and protect patient privacy and confidentiality.

Beneficence and Nonmaleficence

"If I can stop one Heart from breaking/I shall not live in vain/If I can ease one Life the Aching/Or cool one Pain/Or help one fainting Robin/Unto his Nest again/I shall not live in Vain."

Emily Dickinson, No. 919

Beauchamp and Childress are direct in their admonition that morality requires not only that we treat persons autonomously but that we also contribute to their welfare and refrain from harming them (p. 165). Nursing ethicist Rose Mary Volbrecht is equally clear in her own discussion of beneficence: "The provision of health care is fundamentally tied to beneficence....Health-care professionals commit themselves to the care of the sick and to the promotion of health. Our duty of universalized respect for persons implies that we all have duties to promote the well-being of others as well as our own well-being."[13]

Because human beings have intrinsic value and dignity, health professionals demonstrate respect for this value by taking care not to harm people. The category of nonmaleficence includes rules that prohibit killing, physical and emotional harm, negligence, stealing, sexual exploitation, and breaking promises or contract.

Beneficence

The principle of beneficence, the obligation to benefit others or to seek their good, potentially demands more than the principle of nonmaleficence because agents must take positive steps to help others, not merely refrain from harmful acts. The *Oxford English Dictionary* defines beneficence as "doing good, the manifestation of benevolence or kindly feeling." And as Beauchamp and Childress demonstrate, beneficence supports an array of specific moral rules (p. 167):

- Protect and defend the rights of persons.
- Prevent harm from occurring to persons.
- Remove conditions that will cause harm to persons.
- Help persons with disabilities.
- Rescue persons in danger.

While beneficence is important to many philosophical and religious systems of ethics, it is central to the health professions. However, if beneficent duties are not really optional for health professionals, a persistent issue is how to discern their proper scope. Where do obligations to benefit others end? Are health professionals obligated never to say "no" to patients as long as there is any hope for improvement? Would beneficence require acceptance of higher taxes to fund universal health coverage, or does acting for the good of one's fellow citizens require that those who can afford it must forgo very expensive and highly technological interventions and treatments?

Beneficent duties may be limited in two ways. The first limit is duty to oneself. Self-respect and personal well-being will necessarily restrict activities for the good of others. A second limit involves the health professional's psychological capacity for identification of and sympathy with those who need their help. To attempt to respond to a seemingly inexhaustible world of suffering would be debilitating. Thus, limits to the duty of promoting good restrict health professionals but also orient and direct their finite capacities.

Distinguishing Beneficence From Nonmaleficence

The principle and rules of beneficence differ in several ways from those of nonmaleficence. The rules of nonmaleficence (as stated below) are negative prohibitions of actions that must be followed impartially and that provide moral reasons for legal prohibitions of certain forms of conduct. By contrast, the rules of beneficence present positive requirements for action that need not be followed impartially and rarely, if ever, provide reasons for legal punishment when persons fail to abide by the rules.

Beneficence and Respect for Autonomy

Throughout the history of health care, the professional's obligations and virtues have been interpreted as commitments of beneficence. As Beauchamp and Childress note, health professionals were traditionally able to rely almost exclusively on their own judgments about their patients' needs for treatment and information (p. 176). However, in recent years, patients have asserted their rights to make independent judgments about their health care, and as assertions of autonomy have increased, the problem of paternalism has loomed larger.

Beauchamp and Childress also note that the question of whether respect for the autonomy of patients should have priority over professional beneficence directed at those patients is a central problem in health-care ethics (p. 176). For some, the health professional's primary obligation to the patient (disclosure, informed consent, and confidentiality) is established by the principle of respect for autonomy. For others, the health professional's primary obligation is to act for the patient's benefit, not to encourage autonomous decision making.

Confusion has often marked the debate between proponents of one model over another. Sometimes beneficence is viewed as competing with a principle of respect for autonomy, and sometimes beneficence is viewed as incorporating the patient's autonomous choices in the sense that the patient's preferences help to determine what counts as a benefit. Beauchamp and Childress argue that rather than defending one principle against another or making one principle absolute, beneficence can provide the primary goal and rationale of health care, whereas respect for autonomy (along with nonmaleficence and justice) can set moral limits on the health professional's actions in pursuit of this goal (p. 177).

Nonmaleficence

The principle of nonmaleficence asserts an obligation not to inflict harm on others. In health-care ethics, it has been closely associated with the maxim, *Primum non nocere*—"Above all, do no harm." Obligations not to harm others are distinct from obligations to help others and are generally more stringent. The principle of nonmaleficence supports many moral rules, such as these specified by Beauchamp and Childress (p. 117):

• Do not kill.
• Do not cause pain or suffering.
• Do not incapacitate.
• Do not offend.
• Do not deprive others of the goods of life.

Due Care and Negligence

The principle of nonmaleficence obligates health professionals neither to inflict harm nor to impose risks of harm. For instance, a person can harm or risk harming another person without malicious or harmful intent. In cases of risk imposition, law and morality recognize a standard of due care, a standard that is a specification of the principle of nonmaleficence. As

defined by Beauchamp and Childress: "Due care is taking sufficient and appropriate care to avoid causing harm to a patient given what the circumstances would demand of a reasonable and prudent health professional. The standard requires that the goals pursued justify the risks that must be imposed to achieve those goals" (p. 118).

Negligence, then, is the absence of due care. In the health professions, it involves a departure from the professional standards that determine due care in certain circumstances. The term negligence covers two types of situations, according to Beauchamp and Childress (p. 118):

• Intentionally imposing risks of harm that are unreasonable
• Unintentionally but carelessly imposing risks of harm

Too often in our society, it is left to our courts of law to determine responsibility and liability for harm when a patient is seeking compensation. However, as Beauchamp and Childress recommend, the legal model of responsibility for harmful action provides a framework that can and should be adapted for health-care professionals (pp. 118-119):

• The health professional must have a duty to the affected person.
• The health professional must breach that duty.
• The affected person must experience a harm.
• The harm must be caused by the breach of duty.

Distinguishing Nonmaleficence From Beneficence

As already mentioned, obligations of nonmaleficence are more stringent than those of beneficence. Beauchamp and Childress group the principles of both as follows (p. 115):

Nonmaleficence
• One ought not to inflict evil or harm.
  Beneficence
• One ought to prevent evil or harm.
• One ought to remove evil or harm.
• One ought to do or promote good.

Thus, each of the three forms of beneficence requires taking an action by helping someone, whereas nonmaleficence requires intentionally refraining from an action that will harm someone.

As a society, we continue to confront the risks and benefits, the moral dilemmas, and the ethical questions regarding new and emergent medical technologies and scientific discoveries. In the past, we developed some guidelines and some distinctions that derive from religious traditions, philosophical discourses, professional codes, and laws to specify requirements of beneficence and nonmaleficence in health care, particularly with regard to treatment and nontreatment decisions.

Withholding and Withdrawing Life-Sustaining Treatment

As Beauchamp and Childress write, much debate about the principle of nonmaleficence and foregoing life-sustaining treatments has centered on the distinction between withholding and withdrawing treatments: "Many professionals and family members feel justified in withholding treatments they never started but not in withdrawing treatments already initiated. They sense that decisions to stop treatments are more momentous and consequential than decisions not to start them. Stopping a respirator, for example, seems to cause a person's death, whereas not starting the respirator does not seem to have this direct causal role" (p. 120).

Certainly, moral uneasiness and emotional conflict around the withdrawal of treatment are understandable, but ethicists maintain that the distinction between withdrawing and withholding is both irrelevant and dangerous. Beauchamp and Childress articulate any number of potential situations and potential consequences that arise from this unclear distinction. For instance, what of the possibility of withdrawing treatment through an omission (withholding) such as neglecting to recharge the batteries that power a respirator or neglecting to put the infusion in a feeding tube? Moreover, giving a priority to withholding over withdrawing treatment can lead to over-treatment in some cases, such as continuing a treatment that is no longer beneficial or desirable for the patient, and under-treatment in others, such as not authorizing a potentially beneficial technology because of the fear of being trapped by it (pp. 121-122).

Decisions about beginning or ending any treatment should be based on considerations of the patient's rights and welfare and, therefore, on the benefits and burdens of the treatment as judged by a patient or an authorized surrogate.

Sustenance Technologies and Medical Technologies

Debate also continues about whether there is a legitimate distinction between medical technologies, such as respirators and dialysis machines, and sustenance technologies, such as artificially administered nutrition and hydration. While we as a society still struggle with the question whether artificial nutrition and hydration should be obligatory or can be optional, court decisions, professional codes, and philosophical treatises agree that artificially administered nutrition and hydration may be foregone in some circumstances for every age group, as is true of any other life-sustaining technologies. The reasons, as summarized by Beauchamp and Childress, are (p. 125):

- No morally relevant difference exists between the various life-sustaining technologies.
- The right to refuse medical treatment for oneself or others is not contingent on the type of treatment.

This view remains controversial, and those holding the position that artificially administered nutrition and hydration can not justifiably be removed advance the following three arguments, again summarized by Beauchamp and Childress (p. 127):

- It is required because it is necessary for the patient's comfort and dignity.
- It is required because the provision of nutrition and hydration symbolizes the essence of care and compassion.
- Not providing it will lead to adverse consequences because society will not be able to limit decisions to legitimate cases.

Intended Effects and Merely Foreseen Effects

Finally, one additional attempt to specify the principle of nonmaleficence appears in what is called the principle or rule of double effect, which incorporates a pivotal distinction between clearly intended effects and merely foreseen effects. The principle or rule of double effect, as summarized by Beauchamp and Childress, has been invoked to justify claims that a single act, such as administering what may very well be a toxic dose of an analgesic necessary to control a patient's intractable pain, may have two foreseen effects: one that is good, relieving suffering, and one that is harmful, hastening death (p. 128).

Landmark Case: Karen Ann Quinlan

According to her parents, Karen Ann Quinlan was a pretty 21-year-old with an independent and adventurous spirit. A few nights after leaving home and moving to her own apartment in April 1975, Karen celebrated a friend's birthday at a local bar. After several alcoholic drinks, she complained of feeling faint, and friends took her home and helped her to bed. Shortly thereafter, they checked on her and discovered she was not breathing. Although emergency medical treatment restored her breathing, Karen never regained consciousness, and she was admitted to the intensive care unit of Newton Memorial Hospital in suburban New Jersey.

Why Karen lost consciousness is not known. Tests for barbiturates were positive, and she had been seriously dieting—perhaps even fasting—for several days before the night of drinking. Whatever the reasons, the cumulative effects likely suppressed her breathing, causing anoxia and resulting in irreversible brain damage. After many months, the family accepted the diagnosis of "persistent vegetative state" and decided to remove the respirator that was keeping Karen alive, believing that she would never want to live like she was living. Appeals to the lower courts, which generated immense publicity, and ultimately to the Attorney General of New Jersey were unsuccessful. Finally, in January 1976, the New Jersey Supreme Court ruled unanimously that Karen's father could serve as her legal guardian and that, at his request, the respirator could be disconnected and other support withdrawn.

The Quinlan case was a landmark legal decision because it held that it was legally permissible for a guardian to disconnect a patient's respirator and allow that patient to die. The court based their ruling on Karen Ann Quinlan's constitutional right to privacy (as exercised by her parents, using substituted judgment) that allowed for the removal of life support.[14]

Landmark Case: Nancy Cruzan

The first case ever heard by the United States Supreme Court on the withdrawal of treatment from formerly competent patients was *Cruzan v Director, Missouri Department of Health* in 1990. The case of Nancy Cruzan was essentially identical to that Karen Ann Quinlan, with one exception: Nancy Cruzan, also a young woman in a persistent vegetative state as the result of a 1983 car accident, required only tube feeding rather than a ventilator to survive. However, her parents also firmly believed that she would not wish to live under such circumstances, based in part on Nancy's own comments to her sister. For this reason, a trial judge authorized her parents, acting as their daughter's guardians, to have the artificially administered hydration and nutrition discontinued.

However, the Missouri Supreme Court reversed that decision, maintaining that Nancy's right to refuse treatment was personal and that no one, not even her parents, could exercise it on her behalf. On appeal, the U.S. Supreme Court held that a competent patient does have a constitutionally protected right to refuse life-saving hydration and nutrition, reflecting no distinction between medical and sustenance treatments.[15]

Summary of Beneficence and Nonmaleficence

What follows is an illustrative but selective list of the actions demanded by both the principles of beneficence and nonmaleficence[16]:

Beneficence

- Promote the well-being of others and oneself, using morally permissible means and not incurring disproportionate costs.
- Maintain one's competence; maintain and improve professional standards; maintain and improve working conditions.
- Make reasonable efforts to protect patients and the public from harm due to incompetent and unethical practice of other health-care professionals.

- Participate in efforts to promote the health needs of one's communities.
- Promote one's own mental, physical, emotional, and spiritual development.

Nonmaleficence

- Do not kill or physically harm others without justified cause.
- Do not impose unreasonable risk of harm. Negligence is conduct that falls below a standard of due care.
- Do not harm others by insult or ridicule.
- Do not break promises or agree to do something morally impermissible.
- Do not engage in sexual acts with patients.

Justice

"What we can do is to make life a little less terrible and a little less unjust in every generation. A good deal can be achieved this way."

Karl Popper, Utopia and Violence

Inequalities in access to health care and health insurance, combined with dramatic increases in the costs of such care and coverage, have fueled debates about what justice requires of and from us as a society. Justice is the ethics of fair and equitable distribution of burdens and benefits within a community. Classically defined as "giving each his or her due," theories of justice often debate about what is due and to whom it is due. In health care, the criterion of need is often the determining one for the distribution of services, yet even in the application of need, problems arise.

Distributive Justice

The term distributive justice, as defined by Beauchamp and Childress, refers to the fair, equitable, and appropriate distribution of all rights and responsibilities in society, including, for example, civil and political rights (p. 226). Problems of distributive justice arise when there is a scarcity of and competition for goods. For example, if there is enough fresh water to sustain urban and rural areas during drought, then restrictions on watering lawns or irrigating crops would not be necessary. Issues concerning the fairness of distribution generate questions about principles of justice. One principle of justice is formal, the others material.

Formal Principle of Justice

Common to all theories of justice is a minimal formal requirement traditionally attributed to Aristotle: "Equals must be treated equally, and unequals must be treated unequally." As Beauchamp and Childress describe, the principle is formal because it identifies no particular respects in which equals ought to be treated equally and provides no specific criteria for determining whether two or more individuals are, in fact, equal (p. 227).

An obvious problem with this formal principle is its lack of substance and specificity. That equals ought to be treated equally does not provoke debate in our society. But how do we define equality, and how do we identify which differences are the most relevant when we attempt to compare individuals and groups? As a democratic nation, we hold that all of our citizens should have equal political rights, equal access to public services, and equal treatment under the law. But how far should equality extend?

Material Principles of Justice
To distinguish between formal and material principles, Beauchamp and Childress specify the relevant characteristics for equal treatment as material because they identify the substantive properties for distribution such as need, which declares that the distribution of social resources based on that property is just (p. 228). To say that a person needs something is to say that, without it, the person will be harmed or affected negatively. However, as a society, we are neither required to nor capable of distributing all goods and services to satisfy all needs, such as cable television or cosmetic surgery. Presumably, then, our obligations are limited to more fundamental needs. For example, a person might suffer harm from malnutrition or nondisclosure of critical information.

Philosophers and bioethicists, including Beauchamp and Childress, have proposed the following as valid material principles of distributive justice (p. 228):

- To each person an equal share
- To each person according to need
- To each person according to effort
- To each person according to contribution
- To each person according to merit
- To each person according to free-market exchanges

Most contemporary societies invoke these material principles in framing public policies. For example, the opportunity for a basic education is shared equally by everyone; unemployment subsidies and welfare payments are distributed on the basis of need; jobs and promotions are awarded on the basis of merit; higher salaries are allowed on the basis of free-market wage scales and/or contributions to society.

Right to a Decent Minimum of Health Care
As Beauchamp and Childress point out, the questions about who will and who should receive what, if any, share of society's scarce resources generate controversy about a national health policy, about the unequal

distributions of advantages to the disadvantaged, and about the rationing of health care (p. 240). The primary economic barrier to health care access in the United States is the lack of adequate insurance. More than 40 million people lack health insurance of any kind; although the United States spends more resources on health care annually than any other country in the world, we are the only industrialized nation with less than half of our population eligible for public health insurance.

At the heart of the crisis is an excess of blame and a lack of responsibility. Both legislators and insurers act as though the uninsured and the underinsured are the responsibility of the other, and neither will shoulder the responsibility or take the lead to correct the current moral unfairness. As Beauchamp and Childress remind us, health care for the needy in former times was handled through institutions, such as charity hospitals. However, in our contemporary world of high technology and commensurately high costs, the virtue of charity and the moral ideal of equality have proved inadequate to the task of meeting many health care needs (p. 240).

Just access to health care and adequate financing of health care overshadow almost every other ethical and economic issue in the United States. Although every society must ration access through some mechanism or other, many societies can recognize a right to a decent minimum of health care within a framework for allocation that is both utilitarian and egalitarian.

Landmark Case: Tuskegee Syphilis Study
In late July 1972, Jean Heller of the Associated Press broke an extraordinary story: for 40 years, the United States Public Health Service (USPHS) conducted a study of the effects of untreated syphilis on poor, uneducated black men in Macon County, Alabama. Not since the Nuremberg trials of Nazi scientists and physicians had the American public been confronted with a medical scandal that captured so many headlines and provoked so much discussion. For many, it was a shocking revelation of the potential for scientific abuse in their own country, and Tuskegee immediately became one of the most condemned experiments of American medicine.

The study began in 1930 as a worthwhile project, funded by the Julius Rosenwald Foundation of Philadelphia and administered by the USPHS, to treat syphilis with the currently available therapy (arsenic-based) in areas in which venereal disease was extraordinarily prevalent. When funding became limited because of the Depression, only one site was chosen because it had an extremely high rate of syphilis, 40%. That site was Macon County, Alabama, whose largest town was Tuskegee. Financial support for diagnosis and treatment eventually disappeared, but by that time, many black men who had the disease had already been identified.

In 1932, USPHS decided that such identification presented a ready opportunity to study the natural history of the disease, and health-care professionals began a period of sporadic observation of 399 males. In order to determine how far the disease had progressed, painful spinal taps were conducted on men, who were induced to remain in the study with offers of hot lunches, free medical care, and burial insurance.

In 1943, penicillin was discovered, and when it became known that it was an effective treatment for syphilis, it became urgent for USPHS to justify continuation of the study and to ensure deception of the subjects involved in it. Consequently, the men never received penicillin, even in the 1960s and 1970s.

In 1966, Peter Buxton, a young researcher for the Centers for Disease Control, learned of the Tuskegee Syphilis Study and began a 6-year campaign to stop it. His protests were unsuccessful, but in the summer of 1972, he told the story to an Associated Press reporter on the East Coast, and the study came to a final, abrupt end. One year later, the United States Department of Health, Education and Welfare (HEW) issued a report in which it concluded: "The scientific merits of the Tuskegee Study are vastly overshadowed by the violation of basic ethical principles pertaining to human dignity and human life imposed on the experimental subjects."[17]

In essence, the Tuskegee Syphilis Study violated each of the four principles of health-care ethics described in this chapter. The two major violations of the principle of respect for autonomy turned on the issues of deliberate deception and informed consent. HEW concluded that informed consent was never obtained by the subjects and that submitting voluntarily to such a study was not informed consent. The major violation of the principles of beneficence and nonmaleficence turned on the issue of harm. The first topic of that issue was the harm caused by the spinal taps; the second, more crucial, topic was the nontreatment of syphilis; specifically, the withholding of penicillin. HEW concluded that withholding an effective treatment amplified the injustice to which this group of human beings had already been subjected.

Finally, the major violation of the principle of justice turned on the issues of racism and poverty. Was it simply a coincidence that all the subjects in the study were black males? To believe that the Tuskegee Syphilis Study was not racist as many have argued is to believe that some reason existed to study only blacks with untreated syphilis. Even though some physicians believed syphilis ran a different course in African Americans, why not include whites in both the infected and control groups? Apart from the issue of racism, the Tuskegee Study serves as a poignant reminder of the plight of the poor.

Summary of Justice
The following is an illustrative but selective list of the actions demanded by the principle of justice[18]:

• Promote treatment of all patients equally.
• Distribute benefits, resources, and burdens fairly.
• Advance policies and processes for fair access of health care to all members of the community.

References
1. Weiss J. Everyday Ethics. Dallas Morning News, 10 October 1998:1G.
2. Shanks T. Everyday ethics. Issues in Ethics, 1997;8:2.
3. Cohen R. The Politics of Ethics. The Nation, 8 April 2002:72-73.
4. Cohen R. Author talk. Retrieved October 10, 2004, from http://www.bookreporter.com
5. Beauchamp T, Childress J. Principles of Biomedical Ethics, 5th ed. Oxford: Oxford University Press, 2001:15.
6. See Jonsen A, Siegler M, Winslade W. Clinical Ethics: A Practical Approach to Ethical Decisions in Clinical Medicine, 3rd ed. New York: McGraw-Hill, 1992; Kornblau B. Ethics in Rehabilitation: A Clinical Perspective. Kentucky: Delmar Learning, 2000; Volbrecht R. Nursing Ethics: Communities in Dialogue. New Jersey: Prentice Hall, 2002.
7. Jonsen A, Siegler M, Winslade W. Clinical Ethics: A Practical Approach to Ethical Decisions in Clinical Medicine, 3rd ed. New York: McGraw-Hill, 1992:37.
8. White R. A demand to die. Hastings Center Report, 1975;5:119-120.
9. Kliever L. Preface. In Kliever L, ed. Dax's Case: Essays in Medical Ethics and Human Meaning. Dallas: Southern Methodist University Press, 1989:xv, xvii.
10. Englehardt T. Commentary: A demand to die. Hastings Center Report, 1975;5:121-122.
11. Englehardt T. Commentary: A demand to die. Hastings Center Report, 1975;5:122.

12. Volbrecht R. Nursing Ethics: Communities in Dialogue. New Jersey: Prentice Hall, 2002:55.
13. Volbrecht R. Nursing Ethics: Communities in Dialogue. New Jersey: Prentice Hall, 2002:50.
14. Pence G. Classic Cases in Medical Ethics. New York: McGraw-Hill, 1990:4-7.
15. Annas G. Sounding board: Nancy Cruzan and the right to die. New England Journal of Medicine, 1990;323: 671-672.
16. Volbrecht R. Nursing Ethics: Communities in Dialogue. New Jersey: Prentice Hall, 2002:55-56.
17. Pence G. Classic Cases in Medical Ethics. New York: McGraw-Hill, 1990:201-202.
18. Volbrecht R. Nursing Ethics: Communities in Dialogue. New Jersey: Prentice Hall, 2002:56

3

The Ethics of Everyday Practice: The Patient, The Virtuous PA, and the Physician

Michael Potts, PhD

Dilemma: Patient Self-Determination

You work as a physician assistant (PA) for an oncologist, Dr. Helen Jones, who gives her PAs a great deal of leeway. You have a closer relationship with some patients than does Dr. Jones. For this reason, Dr. Jones often allows you to be the one to give either good or bad news to the patients regarding results of surgeries, biopsies, and other tests. One of these patients is Juanita, a 24-year-old Mexican American woman, whose parents arrived in the United States when she was 6 years old and who are with her today, along with her two sisters. She was referred to Dr. Jones by her general practitioner after a pelvic examination revealed a mass in the area of the ovaries. You did the initial history and physical on Juanita, who is a pleasant woman with whom you developed an immediate rapport. You speak fluent Spanish. After an ultrasound and computed tomography scan reveal evidence of abnormal masses in the pelvic and abdominal region, Juanita is scheduled for an exploratory laparoscopy. After explaining the nature of the surgery, the possibilities of what could be revealed, and the organs and tissues that might need to be removed, you talk to Juanita's family. That is when the trouble begins. The family insists they should be told of her postsurgery prognosis first; if it is grave, they believe that Juanita should not be told. You try to explain the law and the concept of patient self-determination, but the family will have noth-

ing of that and still insists on knowing a negative prognosis first. Juanita has no problem with her family being informed of the results of her surgery, but she also has mixed feelings about whether you should inform her of the results. In one conversation she said, "You know, I'd want to know if I was going to die so I could make preparations for myself and my family." But in a later conversation, she said, "I really think my family should be the ones to tell me what's going on with my health. I know they would be reluctant to tell me bad news, but I would get it out of them eventually. Besides, I can read them pretty well if they leave something unsaid." You talk to Dr. Jones, who tells you, "I would inform the family and let them decide what to tell Juanita; you have to respect the family's culture." You disagree, believing strongly in patient determination, and when the surgery reveals that Juanita has stage IV ovarian cancer with multiple metastases with a very grave prognosis, Dr. Jones suggests you talk to the family first, then talk to Juanita without telling her the entire truth about her condition. You are irritated, thinking that Dr. Jones is living in the Dark Ages of medical ethics when patients were routinely not told of bad prognoses. Yet, you are uncomfortable going against your supervising physician. Should you or should you not tell Juanita the full truth about her condition?

QUESTIONS FOR DISCUSSION

1. What are the ethical issues and considerations in this case?

2. What are the legal considerations in this case?

3. How do you handle a disagreement with your supervising physician?

4. Should the patient's culture be a consideration?

5. Is there a "middle ground" for resolution?

This case is an example of one of many ethical dilemmas a PA may face during the course of practice. Most ethical issues a PA will face will *not* normally concern genetic engineering, in vitro fertilization, or euthanasia. Rather, they will concern "ordinary" matters such as respect for patients, truth telling, confidentiality, and informed consent. These are issues that involve "the ethics of the everyday" in medical practice. There is an ethical component to everything you do as a health-care provider. In some respects, these "everyday ethics" are the most important issues in medical ethics: they cut to the heart of the relationship between patient and medical practitioner. In order to explore how the PA should think about handling the situation with Juanita, this chapter will discuss the unique patient/PA relationship. It will then turn to a discussion of virtue and the PA. The third section will discuss the "ethics of the everyday" in terms of issues that PAs will likely face in the course of everyday practice, such as trust, truth telling, and confidentiality. The final section will discuss the chapter case study in more detail.

The Patient-PA Relationship

This relationship involves, first of all, a sick or injured person in need of help. The PA has the knowledge and ability to help this sick person. The patient's vulnerability is a key factor in the ethics of this unique relationship, as is the high level of trust required of the patient for the PA. An important feature of a PA's life, which will inevitably affect the patient-PA relationship, is the relationship between the PA and his or her physician-supervisor. For the PA, there is a three-sided relationship that involves every patient encounter and relationship: *patient-PA-physician.*

Sickness and Injury

Pellegrino and Thomasma[1] have argued that what is most central to medicine is the *relationship* between the patient and the health-care professional. Although they have in mind primarily the patient-physician relationship, their discussion can be applied to PAs and other health-care professionals. They begin with the patient, a person in need of help. While an illness or injury may be routine for those who work in health care, it is not so for the patient, because sickness disrupts routine. Sickness interferes with the course of a person's normal activities in life. The more serious the illness or injury, the more serious the disruption of routine. This is not a trivial matter. So much of human life is taken up with routine that any extensive disruption of that routine is a disruption of life itself. Major life plans and projects can be altered. A person may become too ill to hold a job. Plans to travel after retirement may have to be canceled. A promising football or basketball career may be ruined by a serious injury. Time that could be spent with a spouse, children, grandchildren, or close friends may be spent in hospitals; a sick person at home may remain too ill to interact with loved ones. Added to this is the pain, both physical and emotional, that often accompanies illness. It is not only difficult for the suffering person but for loved ones as well. The PA must recognize that sick people are suffering.

Perhaps the worst form of suffering a sick or injured person undergoes, as Pellegrino and Thomasma note, is the radical disruption in life meaning they experience. This is seen most clearly in life-threatening illness or injury. Questions such as "What does my life mean?", "Do I matter?", "Will death be the end of me?" arise along with the practical questions: "When I die, who will take care of my family?" "Should I revise my will?" and "What plans should I make for my funeral?" An uncertain prognosis may not make the situation any easier. Times of remission in a cancer, for example, may bring renewed energy to live life to its fullest as well as bring hope that the remission will last, but they may also carry with them fears that the cancer will return.

Even less serious illnesses carry with them their own existential anguish. A case of the flu reminds us that the body we often take for granted can hold us back and keep us from doing the things we are used to doing. Any illness reminds us that we are finite, limited creatures who will not live forever. The primal fear that something may be wrong that threatens a person's life keeps many people with symptoms from getting evaluated until it is too late. All health-care providers should be aware of the deep suffering, including fear, that may be going on beneath the surface of each patient. Such suffering and fear will be different for each patient, so the PA should be an empathetic listener to gain a sense of the patient's emotional state. Additionally, PAs should never lose sight of the fact that all these fears and concerns extend to those closest to the patient. Family and friends may be as deeply affected and involved as the patient. We hope that what drives these people is the well-being of the patient and that their actions are in the best interest of the patients.

Healing
Patients come to us for help. And it is a very special kind of help that the person is seeking. It is help to improve their lives; it is healing. Healing entails restoring the *person* to *wholeness,*[1] which involves both emotional and physical factors. Patients react differently to disease. Some patients may be happy with the penicillin to eliminate their strep throat and do not want further interaction with the health-care practitioner; they feel "whole" when they feel physically better and can do the things they did before their illness. Other patients may require emotional support to get through their illness. A patient may need encouragement to take needed medications. Needs are specific to the particular patient, and in order to heal patients, PAs must be able to learn the nuances of the patients they serve.

Knowledge and Power
Knowledge and power come into play in the relationship between patient and PA and, ultimately, the family. The PA generally has a great deal of training and medical knowledge that the patient does not have.

Although more and more patients are becoming better educated on medical matters, the PA still has formal training in medicine, as well as practical skills, that the patient lacks. This creates a disparity of knowledge between patient and PA, a necessary inequality arising from the very nature of the relationship. This inequality of knowledge also results in an inequality of power. The PA can not only diagnose the patient's illness but also prescribe powerful medications, order tests, draw blood, and in some cases administer invasive tests, such as cardiac catheterizations. This disparity of knowledge and power between patient and PA means that medicine, by its very nature, involves ethics.

One reason for this is the "vulnerability" of the patient,[1] a vulnerability enhanced both by the PA's greater knowledge and by the patient being weaker than normal due to illness or injury. Because the patient's illness interferes with normal everyday activities and, when severe, can interfere with major life plans, the patient may be and feel more dependent than usual. Dependence may be exacerbated by the PA as authority figure to the point that the patient feels powerless in the face of a health-care professional. Such disparity of power makes it easy for the PA to exploit the patient. The patient not only exposes his or her body to the PA but also reveals personal information that few others would know. From an ethical point of view, it is always wrong to take advantage of the patient's vulnerability. It is difficult for any kind of "consent" to be legitimate, given the power disparity of the relationship and the relative weakness of the patient. Regardless of this disparity, the patient must be given autonomy to decide.

Sensitivity to the patient's vulnerability also implies keeping patient information confidential. Some information, for example, information about a patient's prior use of illegal drugs or a patient's sexual practices, could harm the patient if released. A patient may also feel that he or she no longer can make his or her own health-care decisions. In the past, physicians used this fact as justification for taking a parentlike role with the patient, in which the physician informs the patient what to do and the patient follows the physician's orders. Unfortunately, this only made the power disparity between physician and patient wider. The contemporary emphasis on patient self-determination and informed consent is a way to partially bridge the power gap between the health-care practitioner and patient. This problem is complicated when there are family beliefs or personal beliefs that may be in conflict with the PA's basic concept of confidentiality.

Physician and Supervisor

The relationship between patient and PA is also one that involves the physician supervisor because the PA

and physician work together as a team. This three-way relationship and the notion that the PA is part of a health-care *team* is emphasized in the ethics manual for PAs developed by the American Academy of Physician Assistants: "Physician assistant practice flows out of a unique relationship that involves the PA, the physician, and the patient. The individual patient-PA relationship is based on mutual respect and an agreement to work together regarding medical care. In addition, PAs practice medicine with physician supervision; therefore, the care that a PA provides is an extension of the care of the supervising physician. The patient-PA relationship is also a patient-PA-physician relationship."[2]

The team approach to health care implies that both the physician and PA are working together for a common end, the good of the patient. The hierarchy of physician-PA should be understood in this broader context of cooperation. The PA must respect this hierarchy, because the PA's care is "an extension of the care of the supervising physician." The PA should recognize the limits of his or her scope of practice. If a PA is unsure about a diagnosis or course of treatment for a particular patient, the PA should consult the supervising physician. The patient should be aware of the physician's presence as part of the health-care team, even if the patient's primary care provider is the PA. In some cases, the supervising physician will meet with the patient periodically. Every successful PA-physician team must develop an appreciation and respect for what each does and contributes to patient care. An important component of this relationship is the ability to resolve problems and conflicts.

Virtue and the PA

Is technical skill the only thing that matters in being a good PA? Given the previous discussion, the clear answer is "No." But thinking this way is a temptation for PAs as well as for physicians, as both are trained in the predominately scientific "medical model" that often reduces real patients to disease processes and that emphasizes skill in using high technology. Despite the more frequent contact many PAs have with patients in clinical practice, they may fall prey to the trap of focusing only on this way of practicing even more easily than physicians. We may lose sight that ethics and our own morals play major roles in all that we do. Ethics are not always an emphasis in medical and PA education and training. In medical schools, where students have 4 years to work toward their degree, there has been an increasing emphasis on both medical ethics training and medical humanities courses to broaden the future physician's focus. At Bassett Healthcare in Cooperstown, New York, for instance, medical students are required to write either poems or stories about their experiences with medicine during their clinical training.[3] The training of a PA is far more condensed, with "approximately 26 months" being the average duration of a PA program.[4] With so much technical material to be covered in such short time, it is difficult to work ethics training into a PA program. Ethical issues might be discussed in the classroom in a medically oriented course, or students might take one ethics course in their program. The PA student may perceive ethics training as a minor part to what is really important. This is especially true given the PA student's heavy course load. Students rarely take kindly to writing a paper in an ethics class when an important pharmacology examination looms.

The truth is that ethics is at the very heart of medicine. Thus, it is vitally important for the PA student to study ethics. This involves relationships with patients and the ability to do good for these patients. It is important, then, for the PA to be an *ethical provider*. This does not imply that technical knowledge and skills are not important. As Pellegrino and Thomasma[1] note, a health-care practitioner who lacks the appropriate scientific knowledge and clinical skills is not only likely to harm patients (or at least not help them in an effective way) but is also engaging in a form of deception, claiming to be something he or she is not. An unknowledgeable and unskilled PA runs into the same ethical problems as any other "quack" in medicine.

PAs who have the requisite knowledge and skills still may not be good PAs. If a PA has a bad bedside manner and does not treat a patient with respect, for example, that patient will be unlikely to trust the PA. Such a patient will be less likely to tell the PA about symptoms he or she may be experiencing, and the PA will therefore not be able to provide effective care. A poor experience with a PA could also lead the patient to distrust the medical profession and not see a physician or PA when there is a real need to do so. A PA who is friendly and who takes the time to listen to patients (and who also has good technical skills) is likely to be more effective in diagnosing and treating illnesses and injuries. But it is not only good practical results that make it necessary for the PA to be an ethical person; it is also the requirement of the foundations of medicine itself. An ethical person is someone who has the virtues that facilitate human flourishing, which help to bring about human good. Much of what helps human beings to flourish, to be fulfilled, has to do with interpersonal relationships. A human society with individuals who have virtues such as integrity, respect, and compassion will flourish more readily than a society filled with persons who lack such virtues. If medicine is primarily a relationship between persons, then a virtuous PA will be able to do

more good for the patient than the vicious PA. For example, a PA is a better PA when he or she respects the patient as a person and treats him or her as such. If the fundamental end of medicine is healing a patient who is suffering, then the ability to truly care about the patient and develop empathy and trust will facilitate healing both of the patient's body and psyche. Being a good person, with virtues such as integrity, respect, and humility, is not something peripheral to being a good PA; it is a *sine qua non*, "without which, nothing."

Thus, virtues are necessary for good character, and good character is necessary for being a good PA. What is a virtue? A virtue is, first of all, a stable character trait developed by practice over time. But not all stable character traits are virtues: vices are also such traits. A virtue is a stable character trait, a "habitual disposition" that helps one "to act well,"[5] to act in ways that promotes human flourishing. For example, honesty is a virtue. An honest person does not have to think about whether to return a borrowed book; he or she will return it because he or she could not do otherwise. Honesty is part of that person's identity; it is a "second nature." One gains the virtue of honesty both by training and by practice. Early training in childhood in good moral values is important for the child's gaining the virtues. Also important is the parents or guardians setting a good example for a child to follow; part of developing virtue is following good role models. But ultimately, becoming virtuous involves more than being taught; it also involves practical activity, what Aristotle called "habituation."[6]

For example, suppose a child, Sue, has a lemonade stand. The child's parents teach her how to give correct change and emphasize that it is the right thing to do to be honest, for that implies respect for other people. Suppose the girl decides to cheat and not return sufficient change to some children. Their parents discover this and go to her parents, who punish her, explaining again why honesty is so important. Over time, Sue gets into the habit of giving correct change and understands why it is important to be honest. Eventually honesty becomes a permanent part of her character. Once that occurs, Sue does not consult rules or act from duty to be honest; she simply *is* honest. Suppose that Sue later becomes a PA. She is in a situation in which she makes a minor mistake that does not harm the patient, and this mistake could easily be hidden by falsifying the patient's chart. Because she has the virtue of honesty, the issue of whether to falsify the patient's chart does not arise for her; she automatically puts down the correct information.

Vices, like virtues, are developed, in part, by practice. To use the opposite of honesty, dishonesty, as an example, let's consider another PA, John. John has already developed the habit of being careless about charting; he takes few notes and often tries to write up his charts from memory at the end of a busy day. If he does not remember information about a specific patient, he will sometimes do some creative charting, such as writing the patient's family history from memory. For example, one day John remembered that Ed Jones had said something about heart disease in his family, but John did not remember the specifics, so he took a guess and wrote in the chart "No family history of CHD." It will not take long for this kind of "creativity" to become a habit for John; he is in the process of developing the vice of dishonesty, a vice that will likely be carried into areas of his PA practice other than charting.

Some virtues are necessary for anyone to be a good human being; others are more specific to the practice of medicine. For example, although it is a key virtue for medicine, it is also important for all persons to have the virtue of justice, of treating people fairly. But all of the virtues will enhance attainment of the fundamental end of medicine to help a person in need to heal. The following list of virtues is not meant to be exhaustive but is meant to cover the major virtues that affect the practice of medicine.

Integrity

"Integrity" includes honesty but is broader than honesty. It is the virtue that enables a person to be true to self when values are challenged, to hold one's own in the face of temptation to do wrong. A person of integrity is "predictable"; you can count on that person to act consistently with his or her moral values.[5] A PA with the virtue of integrity, for example, will resist the patient's repeated requests for antibiotics to treat a viral infection, even if this means the patient will become unpleasant or go to another PA or physician. Integrity implies a loyalty to the ultimate end of medicine to help the patient return to health, to wholeness. Prescribing antibiotics to a patient who does not need them is not helpful to the patient and may be harmful because of the greater risk of the patient contracting an antibiotic-resistant infection. Integrity also implies that if the PA is in disagreement with the supervising physician on an important issue in patient care, the PA will communicate his or her disagreement to the physician. Integrity to the profession also implies respect for the wisdom of the PA's supervising physician, so when the PA approaches the supervisor about a disagreement, it will not be in the presence of the patient, and the PA will discuss the disagreement in a respectful manner.

Integrity includes both being true to oneself and the profession and honesty. This implies, for example, being as accurate and truthful as possible in charting. Nevertheless, borderline situations may occur. Suppose you are a primary care PA and one of your long-time patients, David, 42 years old, comes to you with concern about an abnormally high blood pressure reading (146/92), preventing David from giving blood. David's blood pressure has always been in the normal range, but when you take it this time, it is 128/84, slightly up from previous readings. As you notice he is more nervous than usual, you believe that his elevated reading is because of his concern about the previous high reading. You talk to David and learn that, although he has always wanted to give blood, this was his first blood drive and he panicked, which could account for his abnormal blood pressure. You know that David's health insurance coverage has been sporadic because he has changed jobs several times in the last 5 years, and he will begin a new job in a month, with new insurance coverage at a small business in which each employee's coverage is individually underwritten. You are concerned that charting David's chief complaint as "abnormal blood pressure reading" will leave a paper trail that could affect David's insurance rates at his new job. David had also complained about feeling anxious and tired, and you consider listing those as his chief complaints. What should you do?

Our case study at the beginning of the chapter involves all of these issues and points. Dr. Jones disagrees with your desire to tell Juanita the truth about her grave condition before telling her family. Should you follow Dr. Jones' advice and tell the family first, even though this is contrary to your own moral position (as well as contrary to law and written policy on patient self-determination)? Or should you follow your conscience and tell Juanita first before informing the family? If you take the latter route, you would be in the difficult situation of doing something against your supervisor's suggestions. You would be duty-bound to tell Dr. Jones of your decision, and this could result in your receiving a reprimand or the loss of your job. What decision is most consistent with the virtue of integrity?

If one understands ethical decision making in terms of following absolute rules (in line with certain deontological theories, such as the moral theory of the 18th century philosopher Immanuel Kant), then what to do in David's case is easy: you chart the chief complaint as concern about the abnormally high blood pressure reading, without regard for how David's insurance company may react. In the case of Juanita, you would follow the rules on patient self-determination, inform her of the dire prognosis, and suffer the consequences. But if ethical decision making in line with integrity means putting the good of the patient above other ends, the right thing to do is not as easy to decide and may not be decidable in terms of formal rules. The focus of ethical decision making is on the concrete, particular situation rather than on principles or rules alone. One acts in accord with one's virtues, and there may not be one specifically right action that is the target of moral deliberation. Part of living in the real world is moral uncertainty, and medicine is no exception. This does not mean that moral decision making is arbitrary; the virtuous person will make better moral decisions than someone who is vicious. But there will be cases like David's in which the right thing to do is not clear; one could make a reasonable case that the PA of integrity will not chart the chief complaint as elevated blood pressure. But ultimately there are no algorithms from which one can derive a fixed solution to such situations.

Beside specific situations involving patients such as David's and Juanita's, there are other important issues relating to PA integrity. Part of being a PA of integrity is focusing on gaining both the medical knowledge and clinical skills needed to practice medicine in a way that best benefits one's patients. Being true to oneself as a PA involves making sure to gain the ability to help patients return to health. This is a professional obligation but is not divorced from morality. Many professional obligations are also moral obligations. A PA of integrity will be willing to examine himself or herself periodically to determine whether he or she still has good clinical skills.

Integrity is not limited to the patient-PA relationship; it should also characterize the relationship between the PA and the rest of the health-care team, including the PA's supervising physician. This means, among other things, that the PA must be truthful with his or her supervisor when the PA makes a medical error. It also includes truthfulness about other problems the PA may be having that could affect the PA's work, including sickness or severe personal problems. If a PA has integrity, then this will create trust between the PA and physician-supervisor and other members of the health-care team, thus facilitating the proper treatment of patients.

Respect

The PA should also possess the virtue of respect—having respect for all patients and colleagues as people of dignity and worth. Liszka[7] defines respect as "the tendency to regard another as having some worth, and, consequently, the desire to treat them with civility." Respect is important for ethics in general as well as for medical ethics. There are two levels at which one person may respect another. One, discussed by the German philosopher Immanuel Kant (1724-1804), is the position that we have a moral obligation to respect other people just because they are fellow human beings. An individual's worth as a human being is not based on wealth or contributions to the community but is inherent and fundamental.[7]

Various reasons have been presented for respecting our fellow human beings. In Judaism, Christianity, and Islam, such respect is considered due because human beings are made in the image of God and have the ability to make moral choices and respond to God. A secular reason for respecting other human beings was proposed by Kant: respect is due to human beings because they are rational beings. Kant also emphasized the free choices of rational beings with autonomy. It is this latter notion that has influenced contemporary notions of autonomy and self-determination and the idea that we should respect another person's autonomous choices.

A second level of respect is respecting individuals due to their status or position in a hierarchy.[7] This is a level of respect over and above the general respect we owe to human beings in general. For example, we respect the office of the President of the United States and, by extension, the person who holds that office. We respect an employer, both as a human being and as a supervisor. Both these forms of respect are important for medical ethics.

Respect is a particularly important moral virtue to hold in medicine for a number of reasons. First, showing respect for an individual reminds the PA that he or she is dealing with a human being, not a disease or an inanimate object. A patient is already in a vulnerable situation in relation to the PA; the last thing the patient needs is to feel devalued when a PA refers to the patient as a "disease" or is otherwise rude. Second, respecting a patient allows a physician to respect a patient's values and the patient's choices based on those values. A PA will almost never agree totally with a patient's value system. Yet the PA can still respect those values when the patient expresses them. Respect for patient autonomy flows from the respect that belongs to all human persons as rational beings capable of making their own decisions, including health-care decisions.

Respect for patients can be shown in a number of other ways; for example, in forms of address. Sometimes older patients consider it disrespectful if health-care providers address them by their first names. Doris Grumbach[8] tells of her anger at a receptionist in a physician's office who addressed her as Doris. She insisted on being addressed as Mrs. Grumbach. Grumbach believes that many health-care workers treat older patients like children, treatment that is incompatible with respect for them as persons.

Respect for the physician-supervisor and the position of authority he or she holds is also important. A good PA will address the supervising physician as that person prefers, especially in the presence of patients. Opposing the supervisor in the presence of others is disrespectful, except in very constrained circumstances (e.g., when the supervisor insists on committing gross malpractice even after the PA confronts the supervisor privately). Talking about the supervisor in a demeaning way behind the supervisor's back also reveals a lack of proper respect. The PA must realize that, although the physician and the PA are a team, the physician does have greater knowledge and training and should be respected as such.

In the dilemma with Juanita above, what is the best way to show respect to all parties involved? A strong argument can be made that the best way to respect Juanita is to tell her the truth about her condition so she can make her own health-care choices. One source for the doctrine of patient self-determination is the idea that the patient's choices should be respected, and in order for the patient to give informed consent for treatment or nontreatment, the patient must be given accurate information about the diagnosis, prognosis, and potential treatment. But this case is complicated by the patient's cultural background, in which the family is informed first of their family member's condition, and it is the family that makes health-care decisions. The family sincerely believes that it would be disrespectful to their culture for the PA to fail to tell them first about Juanita's condition. Finally, Dr. Jones may believe it disrespectful for a PA to fail to follow her advice. How can the PA show proper respect to all parties in this situation?

One possible way of handling this situation is for the PA to talk privately with Juanita again about her health-care values, then talk to her family, explaining the reasons that the PA believes it is best to inform Juanita of her condition first. The PA could also talk to Juanita and the family together. This would involve pointing out that it is Juanita who is ill and suffering and that it is only fair to let her know the truth about her condition before others, even her family members, know. The PA can then explain that the PA respects the high value placed on the family in their culture and knows that they will do their best to help Juanita in this difficult situation. If possible, the PA will meet with Juanita and the family as a group to ease any remaining hard feelings. In this way, respect is shown to both Juanita and her family. When the PA approaches Dr. Jones, the PA should still show respect despite their disagreement on Juanita's case: "I respect you highly as my physician supervisor, and I have learned a great deal from you in practice. I respect your wisdom and respect your opinion on what to do in the case of Juanita. I told Juanita about her condition before I told her family, not out of disrespect for their culture, but out of respect for Juanita's right to know. I met with the family and talked the situation out, and things have been resolved to everyone's satisfaction."

Respect is not incompatible with empathy for the patient, but it does also mean avoiding looking down on patients, regardless of their educational level or lot in life. The factory worker with a high school education should be treated with as much respect as the college professor or successful businessperson. In addition, respect means that the PA should treat patients as having intrinsic value even if their value systems differ from that of the PA. The suffering human being who comes for help needs that help regardless of beliefs or values. The PA does not have to agree with a person to respect that person's differing positions; the PA's job is to do what can be done to help restore that suffering human person to health, to heal the patient's illness.

Other PA Attributes

Respect includes respect for a patient's privacy, which can easily be violated in the impersonal setting of modern medicine. A visitor to a hospital may want time alone to deal with the loss of a loved one.[9] Patients need privacy as well. A woman who has just been told of metastasis to the liver from breast cancer should be offered some time to deal with that information in private. If a PA is at a sensitive part of a physical examination or test that exposes a patient uncomfortably, a professional, respectful attitude combined with a good bedside manner can alleviate the loss of dignity felt by the patient.

Respect should also be apparent in relations between members of the health-care team. There is a hierarchy among members of the health-care team, but if those who are at the higher end of that hierarchy are condescending and disrespectful to those in lower positions, it can destroy harmony between members. Comments such as "She's just an LPN," or "He's just a tech–don't ask him" do not show respect for other health-care workers or for the necessary positions they hold in the health-care team.

The PA should respect his or her physician supervisor, who in turn should respect the PA. In the case of a PA, respecting one's supervising physician involves, for example, addressing the physician as "Dr." in front of patients and respecting the rules the supervisor has set up for the practice. It also involves respect for the learning and experience of the supervisor. Respect for the supervisor does not mean that the PA will *like* his or her supervisor but that the PA respects the physician supervisor for his or her extensive training in medicine, authority, and responsibility for the practice and patient care.

Courage

Moral courage is the virtue that enables one to make difficult moral choices despite negative consequences. Courage was discussed in detail by Aristotle, who understood it in terms of bravery in the face of battle.[6] But courage can be understood more broadly; it can also apply to the ability to hold one's moral ground even if it leads to negative consequences. Such courage involves moral obligation, because it is necessary, in some situations, for a person to have courage to find the strength to do the right thing. It can be applied, then, to a wide variety of settings involving ethical choices, from the home to the office. In a home setting, it takes courage to stand up to a rebellious teenager who is violent or to turn in a family member who has committed a serious crime. In a work setting, it takes courage to become a whistleblower because this can cost someone a job or even a career.

Courage is required in many situations involving the PA-patient-family relationship (the courage to stand up to a difficult patient, for example). However, this section focuses on conflict between the PA and the supervising physician. Because of the authority the supervising physician has over the PA, it takes courage for the PA to question the moral or clinical actions of the supervisor. Fears regarding approaching a supervisor may range from fear of disapproval or censure to fear of getting fired. It is critical to choose battles carefully and not disagree over inconsequential acts.

But more substantive disagreements may require some boldness on the part of the PA. Suppose that you have just started a job working for an older primary care physician. A patient comes in complaining of symptoms that suggest acid reflux. You are aware of Drug A, which has recently been released. Human studies have shown that Drug A demonstrated good success in treating acid reflux disease, so you prescribe it for your patient, and at a follow-up visit your patient says the symptoms have been alleviated. Later, talking with your supervisor, the supervisor becomes upset with you, complaining that Drug A is overly expensive (even though you point out that your patient's symptoms have subsided and that the patient has good insurance coverage). The supervisor's patients have had good success with Drug B, and it is much less expensive than Drug A.

How should you handle that situation? You should be fair to your supervisor and listen to what the supervisor has to say. There may be a good case for preferring Drug B to Drug A. You might do research on the comparative benefits versus costs of the two drugs. If you are still convinced that Drug A is superior, and you are also reluctant to change a patient's prescription when what the patient is taking is working well, then you may have to muster the courage to challenge, in a polite way, your supervising physician. Your fundamental obligation in medicine is to work for the good of the patient, to restore some measure of health. If you believe your supervisor's behavior is not pursuing that end most effectively,

then courage is necessary for you to be able to challenge your supervisor.

There are more serious situations in which picking your battles may not be an option. If you notice clearly incompetent or obviously unethical behavior by your supervisor, then you are obligated to challenge your supervisor. For example, suppose several patients you know and trust complain to you that your supervisor is touching them inappropriately. Ignoring such accusations is not an option ethically, even if you are reasonably certain you would be out of a job if you bring the issue up with your supervisor. Courage to make such difficult choices must be a part of who you are as a person and a PA, or you will not find the strength to make the good and courageous choices when those choices could hurt your career.

Humility

Humility was not a part of ethics in the ancient world; Aristotle, for example, was not familiar with it. This virtue became a part of ethics primarily through the influence of the Christian tradition, which strongly emphasized humility. For a Christian writer such as Augustine, pride was the primal sin. But humility is an important virtue for ethics in a secular context as well. Humility has to do with recognizing one's limitations; it does not mean a lack of self-respect. A lack of humility can lead a person to go beyond ethical boundaries. A politician who lacks humility, for example, is tempted to go beyond his or her limits of power and abuse that power; the Watergate scandal is a case in point. Excessive pride is one vice that can lead persons in business to continue to take courses of action (such as ordering the writing of misleading financial statements to exaggerate the financial state of the company) that are clearly unethical. A father may have too much pride to apologize to his child he punished unjustly.

Applied to the PA, humility is the character trait through which the PA realizes that he or she is neither all-powerful nor all-knowing. An arrogant PA tends to deny his or her limitations, failing to recognize that there is always more to learn in medicine and that medicine is inherently uncertain. Such a PA may also fail to recognize that no matter how good he or she may be, all PAs make mistakes, some of which will harm patients. A humble PA will recognize that part of the education of the PA is learning from the patient, from what the patient tells the PA and from the patient's body.

A PA with the virtue of humility will not be condescending to a patient. The PA should not presume that the patient is unaware of options in his or her own health care; patients are much better read concerning medicine than previous generations. The PA should be open to the possibility that he or she could learn something useful about diagnosing or treating a particular patient from that patient.

A humble PA will also be willing to learn from other members of the health-care team. A PA who is too arrogant to think that he or she can not learn anything from his or her supervising physician has no business being a PA. To fail to understand that the physician has more extensive training and knowledge than a PA is to fail to understand the proper place of the PA in the health-care team. This does not mean a physician should not be open to learning from a PA. A humble PA will be willing to ask questions when he or she is unsure of how to diagnose or treat a patient. The PA should also be open to learning from other health-care professionals, such as nurses, who often have much to teach concerning basic patient care.

Empathy

Empathy is the virtue that helps us imaginatively to "put ourselves in the other person's shoes," that helps us to better understand another person's point of view. It is in part the ability to realize that we could, but for fortunate circumstances, be in a situation in which we are poor, disabled, sick, or injured. Empathy is one of the virtues that help drive compassion; if I am empathetic with someone who is in need of help, putting myself mentally in that person's situation, I can gain the compassion to drive me to help that individual. Because the PA is involved in treating those who are sick or injured, empathy is essential. A PA can recognize the danger of becoming too emotionally involved with patients but at the same time really care about patients and try to listen and understand what they are going through. Empathy includes compassion, literally, "feeling with" the patient. This is not strictly possible because no human being can literally feel another person's emotional states, but a PA can develop an ability to sense a patient's sadness or fear. The empathetic PA will recognize this and will listen carefully and communicate effectively with each individual patient so as to determine what is really happening in the patient's life. A PA must also be sensitive to the fear some patients experience when they have symptoms they feel are suggestive of a potentially serious illness. A patient with a chronic cough and shortness of breath may turn out to have bronchitis, but in that patient's mind are fears of the lung cancer that killed the patient's father. A patient with chronic stomach and intestinal problems may have acid reflux disease and irritable bowel syndrome, but the mind harbors fear of cancer. A woman, pregnant for the first time, may be thinking back to stories of her grandmother who died in childbirth. Listening to patients' stories gives the PA proper context to

understand their suffering. A PA who is not empathetic, who does not care to take time to listen to his or her patients, will miss out on these stories and will be unable to help patients heal fully. Because healing is the ultimate goal in medicine, a lack of empathy is incompatible with the good practice of medicine.

Empathy also helps the PA to interact effectively and develop trust with those from different backgrounds and cultures. Some cultures, for example, value modesty highly, and members of those cultures may be hesitant to undress for a medical examination. An empathetic PA will listen to a patient with such concerns and will gently explain the reasons for the patient to undress for the examination, doing as much as possible to preserve the patient's sense of modesty. Other cultures, as illustrated in the chapter case study, have different ideas about patient autonomy and truth telling. An empathetic PA will be willing to listen attentively to both the patient and the patient's family, imaginatively putting oneself into that person's culture and trying to see things from that patient's point of view. This does not imply that the PA will agree with the patient or agree with every aspect of the patient's culture. But if the PA sees the other patient's point of view as something to be taken seriously, then it will be easier to bridge the cultural gap that causes some of the ethical conflicts in medicine.

An area that could be overlooked is empathy between the PA and the health-care team, especially empathy with the PA's supervising physician. The PA who is empathetic with the supervisor will be able to work more effectively with the physician in patient care. If a PA sees that the supervisor is having a difficult day, the PA may be able to step up and see more patients that day. If a supervisor seems particularly harsh in criticizing the PAs, the empathetic PA will be better able to determine what might be going on with the supervisor behind the scenes. An empathetic PA will also be able to function more effectively as a health-care team member with nurses and technicians, treating them with respect and concern.

Benevolence

Benevolence is a stable character trait through which one not only wishes the good for others but also practically attempts to *do* good for others. It is a virtue at the very heart of medical practice. Because medicine has, as its fundamental end, the good of the patient, it is not possible for a PA or any other person claiming to be a medical practitioner to practice medicine without benevolence. A benevolent PA not only works for the good of the patient but also tries to avoid, at all costs, doing the patient harm (maleficence). Working with the patient by listening, giving advice on health care, prescribing appropriate medications and no more, and making appropriate referrals are ways the PA can work with the patient to facilitate the patient's restoration to health. In the case of patients who are terminally ill, the PA can give appropriate palliative care and reassure the patient that he or she will not be abandoned by the PA.

Benevolence puts the good of the patient above all other considerations; this can lead to some very difficult moral choices for the PA. For example, suppose a hypertensive patient's present medication is not working, and you wish to try Drug C. Drug C proves to be effective, and your patient does well. However, the patient's HMO refuses to pay for the drug, citing its expense, and will not change its mind despite you and your supervising physician's appeal. The patient cannot afford the medication, which costs $350 a month. You give the patient the samples of Drug C that are available, but they are only a 2-months' supply, and there is no guarantee that you will have more samples. In addition, other patients may need the samples, and your supervisor is concerned about your giving all the samples to one patient. You consider talking to your supervising physician about pushing the HMO some more, which takes valuable time, but which might benefit this patient. What should you do?

Acting in a benevolent manner for the good of the patient is difficult and is often more difficult in the age of managed care. A PA less concerned with the good of the patient in the above case might say, "That's tough; the HMO won't pay. Let's try something else now." But the benevolent PA may be able to come up with creative ways that can help this patient in this dilemma.

A benevolent PA will strive to keep his or her skills sharp; excellent clinical skills are for the good of the patient. This includes keeping up with the latest successful research in the medical field through both formal continuing education and through reading professional journals. Medical knowledge and excellent clinical skills are a fundamental part of practicing in a virtuous and ethical manner.

Finally, a benevolent PA will be concerned for the good of the health-care team with which he or she works. A smoothly functioning health-care team will work better for the benefit of the patient. A genuine concern for the good of one's supervising physician as well as for other members of the staff will do a great deal to make the office as a whole run more smoothly. This, in turn, will help lower the wait time for patients with appointments as well as improve the overall quality of their care.

Justice

Justice is related to fairness, to giving people what is due.[5] This implies that if we treat different people differently, it should be based on relevant grounds. Applied to the PA, justice is the virtue that enables a PA to treat patients fairly. It is most often discussed in medical ethics in the context of distributive justice or large-scale resource allocation issues. We focus here on the smaller-scale issues that involve everyday practice. Justice does not imply that every patient is treated in exactly the same way; after all, each patient is different and unique. But justice does mean treating patients who are in similar circumstances with the same standard of care. The PA must never discriminate against patients who are of a different sex or race, for example, because these factors are irrelevant to a person's worth and need for medical care. Suppose a female PA develops an intense dislike of men after a painful and bitter divorce. If she is treating a male patient, it would be unjust to allow her current dislike of males to affect the quality of care for that patient. The same would apply to a male PA who dislikes women. If the PA is able to treat a particular patient fairly and effectively, no matter what the PA may feel about the group to which that patient belongs, he or she is being a just PA. The PA should strive to overcome negative attitudes toward particular groups of people, but if that is not possible, he or she must set them aside while treating a patient.

Prudence

The virtue of prudence (the virtue the Greeks called *phronesis*) is a kind of "practical wisdom" that refers to a person's capacity to make the right moral choice in a given circumstance.[5] It is a skill that is developed, in part, by practice and goes beyond mere rule following. It is similar to a physician's or PA's clinical judgment, except that it is applied to ethics. Prudence is one of the most important virtues for anyone in the medical field to have. There is a clinical prudence that PAs develop over time, an intuitive ability to diagnose and treat individual patients that cannot entirely be subsumed under rules,[10] despite the proliferation of evidence-based medicine. Such evidence-based medicine, fueled by attempts to control heath-care costs and to provide efficient care, tends to ignore, as Erik Cassel[11] notes, the individual patient as person. Prudence, rather than focusing on principles and rules, is an ability to make the right medical decision with *this* patient with *this* particular condition and is a skill gained through many hours of clinical practice. Prudence in the moral sense works in a similar way; it is an ability to do the good thing in *this* moral situation with *this* particular person at *this* particular time. A prudent PA is also a PA of integrity, respect, courage, humility, empathy, and benevolence. Prudence allows a person to tie together all the other virtues to make a good moral decision. It is a form of practical reasoning akin to skilled intuition. For example, a prudent PA will know when and how to approach the physician-supervisor with a disagreement. It is prudence that accepts that the relationship between patient and PA is a form of friendship but does not allow that to go beyond the bounds of a professional relationship. Prudence does not mean that one is softening one's convictions or virtues; rather, it is a wise application of those convictions and virtues with careful attention to the uniqueness of a particular case.

Specific Issues in the "Ethics of Everyday"

The ethics of the everyday in a PA's practice will involve a number of relationships—with the physician supervisor, with nurses, with technicians, and office staff. But the most important relationships are those between each patient and the PA. As we discussed earlier, the patient, vulnerable and relatively weak, as compared with the PA, creates moral obligations for the PA to use his or her knowledge and power over the patient in a morally responsible manner. Virtues, stable traits of character gained, in part, by practice, are tools that help the PA to behave in an ethically proper way in practice. Returning to the case study, because you are Juanita's PA, you are already in a relationship with her, a relationship strengthened by your mutual rapport and your fluent knowledge of Spanish. In this situation, you have knowledge that she lacks—that she has cancer that will most likely cause her death. You also have power—both the power to tell her about her condition and the power to authorize specific treatment. This case is complicated by conflicting values: the values of the family, who believe that they should be informed of Juanita's condition and make health-care decisions for her; Juanita's values, of which she is uncertain; and your own values, which tell you that you should tell Juanita the truth first because you respect her right to self-determination. Your physician supervisor does not share your values. You have a deep concern for Juanita, partly rooted in empathy: you imagine what it would be like to be lying in bed after surgery, hoping for good news, only to hear what is, in effect, a death sentence. Because you are a benevolent PA, you want to do what is best for Juanita. You realize that Juanita trusts you, and you feel a sense of responsibility to do the right thing; you are a person of integrity. But you realize that if you follow what you believe to be right, this could result in a confrontation between you and Juanita's family and between you and your supervising physician. It will take courage for you to make a moral choice and stick to that choice. But you realize, being prudent, that there might be creative ways to do what is morally right while minimizing potential confrontations.

Virtues help the PA in everyday encounters with patients, encounters that involve a number of practical issues: establishing trust with the patient, protecting patient confidentiality, issues surrounding sex and relationships, dealing with difficult patients, truth telling, dealing with medical error, and informed consent.

Trust

Medicine is a practice involving a *relationship*, and this relationship is devoted to the particular goal of helping a patient return to health.[1] It is thus a cooperative activity between the health-care practitioner and patient; both patient and PA, ideally, work together for the patient's healing. Such cooperation involves establishing *trust* between patient and PA; without trust, the healing relationship cannot even get off the ground. Developing trust is a *moral* imperative of medicine; without it, the PA could easily hurt the patient, violating a fundamental axiom of medicine, "first, do no harm" (nonmaleficence). Without trust, the PA will not be able to help the patient effectively (e.g., the patient may refuse to take prescribed medication due to lack of trust in the PA).

One of the major positive results of establishing trust with a patient is obtaining a good medical history, a valuable tool in diagnosing a patient's condition. It is sometimes difficult, however, to get an accurate or complete history. There are a number of reasons for this, including unskilled use of questioning by the PA or the patient's being nervous. Another reason can be a patient's hesitancy to trust a PA. This is especially true of a first-time visit, when a more extensive history is required. Establishing trust can alleviate that patient's nervousness and allow the patient to feel comfortable and therefore to talk freely about his or her medical history. If there is uncomfortable or embarrassing information that a patient is tempted to withhold, trust can make the difference between a patient's disclosure or nondisclosure. For example, a man who is reluctant to tell his PA of sexual difficulties may find the strength to do so once he trusts his PA. A young woman who is being abused by her boyfriend is more likely to inform a PA she trusts of such abuse.

There are other situations in which trust can help the PA help the patient more effectively. A patient who is concerned about modesty during a sensitive part of a physical examination will be able to relax more with a trusted PA. A middle-aged man who has just taken a new job and is afraid of divulging his chest pains for fear of losing his job will be more likely to be forthcoming with a PA he trusts. A patient who trusts the PA is more likely to follow the PA's advice on health-care matters, take necessary medications, and follow through on referrals. Getting patients to trust the PA may be more difficult in pediatrics, due to children's fear of pain and medical settings. A child may resist when getting an injection or an IV; the PA should reassure and calm the child. But the PA should also be honest—if an injection is going to hurt, the PA should not lie to the child and say that it will not hurt.

How does a PA establish trust with a patient? There are practical ways that help, summarized in Box 3-1. Using making eye contact as an example, a patient, fairly or unfairly, may interpret a lack of eye contact as communicating a PA's lack of interest in the patient. A shy PA who has difficulty making eye contact should work on that skill to serve patients better. A benevolent PA's genuine concern for the patient's goodwill shines through the PA's demeanor and actions. Even small things like not making a patient wait for a long time past his or her appointment time can make the difference between a patient's trust and distrust. If the patient senses that the PA is on the patient's side, then most of the battle for the patient's trust has been won. Excellence in care is an important means of gaining a patient's trust. There is nothing more likely to destroy trust than a negligent error by the PA in the patient's medical care. A PA who fails to perform the proper neurological examination on a patient complaining of flulike symptoms with headache and stiff neck will likely not be trusted by that patient if it turns out that the patient has meningitis.

Empathy and good listening skills are also important in gaining a patient's trust. A PA who listens to a patient, not just to a list of symptoms, but to the patient as a person, is more likely to earn a patient's trust than a PA who talks over or disregards what a patient has to say. The PA should take the time and interest to ask the patient about a significant other, about children, about the patient's job, or about the patient's interests and hobbies. This is particularly true in the setting of primary care, in which there are often long-term relationships between particular patients and particular PAs. A personal rapport can often form the foundation of a trusting relationship.

In order for a patient to trust the PA, the PA must show him- or herself to be a person of integrity. The trust of a patient who believes the PA will tell the truth can be destroyed by one small lie. The author Stephen King[12] tells of a childhood doctor who told him that puncturing his eardrum would not hurt. King trusted the physician, but the puncture resulted in incredible pain. His trust in physicians was fatally damaged, even if the physician's motives were good. The physician had the option of telling the truth in a gentle way without overwhelming the child ("This will hurt, but it will help you feel better later"). This does not imply that it always morally imperative to tell the entire truth; it could be necessary to withhold information for the good of the patient. But generally, telling the patient the truth is the best option. Truth-telling in more complicated situations will be discussed in the next section.

If there is a specific problem with trust, such as a patient who is suspicious of medicine refusing to take medication, the PA should be tactful and sensitive yet truthful in informing the patient of the need to take the medication. Trying to understand the patient's point of view is helpful: "I understand that you've had some bad experiences with doctors and PAs in the past, Mr. Jones, but I can assure you that you need this medication. The reason is…."

Trust is not only essential to the patient-PA relationship; it is also essential to the PA-supervisor relationship. A physician needs to know she can count on the PAs who work for her. When she makes the decision to hire a PA, she is trusting the PA to have a minimal level of competence. She trusts the PA to ask her questions about what he does not understand and to ask for advice when he is not sure how to diagnose and/or treat a particular patient. She trusts him to inform her about mistakes he has made, especially those that harmed or could harm a patient. A trusting working relationship is absolutely essential for providing effective patient care.

Patient Confidentiality

Patient confidentiality has been a staple of medical ethics from the time of the Hippocratic school. The Hippocratic oath is very clear: "What I may see or hear in the course of the treatment or even outside of the treatment in regard to the life of men, which in no

| **Box 3-1** | **Establishing Trust with a Patient: Practical Suggestions** |

- Address the patient by name, using formal terms, e.g., Mr., Mrs., Miss, Ms., Dr.
- Maintain eye contact with the patient
- Use a pleasant tone of voice
- Smile
- Use humor
- Listen attentively to what the patient has to say
- Avoid showing frustration
- Respect the patient
- Be truthful with the patient
- Keep agreements with the patient; i.e., appointment times
- Provide competent health care

account one must spread abroad, I will keep to myself holding such things shameful to be spoken about."[13] As the AAPA ethics manual states, "If patients are confident that their privacy is protected, they are more likely to seek medical care and more likely to discuss their problems candidly."[2] And candid discussion is necessary for provision of good care. The patient is in the position of revealing some of the most intimate details about his or her body, and sometimes mind, to the PA, and that necessitates a trust that the PA will not reveal such information to others. Some information may result in discrimination against the patient if it becomes public knowledge[2]; other information may cause the patient embarrassment or social stigma. Even in cases in which there is little danger of social stigma from an illness, the patient may wish to tell family and friends only when he or she is ready to do so. The PA, of course, will discuss particular patients with the supervising physician and health-care team, but such discussion must take place in a private setting away from others' hearing. It is easy for the PA to be careless about confidential information; for instance, talking to staff about a patient within hearing range of other patients is a dangerous threat to confidentiality. PAs will often talk to other PAs or to other health-care professionals about patients. Sometimes they will discuss difficult or interesting cases, or a PA may want to relay a humorous story about a patient to relieve tension. The PA should remember that keeping a patient's information confidential is not only an ethical obligation but also a legal one; in fact, the legal strictures against disclosing patient information are much more stringent under the HIPAA regulations (Box 3-2). In talking about such matters, it is critical to omit any personally identifying information about a patient. If a PA teaches in a classroom or clinical setting, case studies should avoid presenting personally identifiable information. In small communities, it may be easier than the PA realizes to determine a patient's identity from information about the case. Proper care should also be taken with a patient's chart and other medical records; they should not be left in a place where unauthorized persons can view them (Box 3-3).

A number of situations raise issues of patient confidentiality in everyday practice. One complex set of issues revolves around sexually transmitted diseases. Suppose a long-time female patient is diagnosed with herpes. She tearfully confesses that she had a brief affair and thinks she caught the herpes from her lover. She begs you not to tell her husband, even though you both realize there is a chance that she has infected him. She says that her affair was due to a slip in emotional control, that she loves her husband, and she fears that telling him about her condition will damage

HIPAA: Health Insurance Portability and Accountability Act of 1996

- Patients have a right to access their own medical records; the medical practice may, if it so desires, charge the patient the cost of copying and sending the records
- Patients have a right to request that their medical records be corrected when they notice errors in the records
- The medical practice must provide to the patient a notice of privacy practices, informing patients of how the practice uses their personal information and the patients' rights to that information, including the patients' right to request further restrictions on the use of their personal information; however, the medical practice is not required to grant such a request
- Other than health-care providers sharing a patient's personal information in order to better treat the patient, in most cases a patient's personal information must not be released for non-health-care–related purposes
- There are limitations on using patient information for marketing; patients must give permission if their health-care information is being used for purposes other than treating the patients
- Even in the case of health-care–related purposes, the patient can request that personal health information not be shared with other medical staff, although the health-care provider is not required to grant that request
- Patients can request that the physician take steps to ensure that communication between the health-care provider and patient is confidential; e.g., allowing a physician only to phone a patient at home rather than at work
- Patients have the right to file a formal complaint if they believe their privacy has been violated
- For further information on HIPAA regulations, consult the U.S. Department of Health and Human Services Web site at http://www.hhs.gov/ocr/hipaa

or destroy their marriage. How should you deal with this situation?

This is a complicated situation; whatever the PA decides, it is likely that there will be some negative consequences. There are a number of plausible moral

Box 3-3	Keeping Medical Records Confidential

- Paper records should be kept in a secure location and locked when the office is closed
- Computer records should be accessible only to the physician, PA, and other authorized personnel
- Computerized medical records should be stored on a computer in a location separate from that of other information in the practice
- Computers should have the most updated security software
- Patient charts should not be left where unauthorized persons can see them; e.g., on the table behind the reception area where it is easy for patients to see them
- Staff who are authorized to obtain patient records should sign their name and record the date and times they had access to the records

options for the PA, but here is one possibility. Because your patient has been seeing you for quite some time and trusts you, you can talk frankly with her about the risks of her not telling her husband versus the risk of telling him. You could point out that if her husband is later diagnosed with herpes and discovers that she has not been honest, it could cause even more harm to the marriage. If the woman decides not to tell her husband, then you are legally bound to respect her wishes. From the standpoint of medical ethics, it will probably do more harm to the patient-PA relationship to tell her husband against her wishes—this can destroy trust and make the woman reluctant to be open with a health-care provider in the future.

The case of an HIV-positive patient is more complicated. If that patient has unprotected sex, the HIV virus can be passed on to the patient's partners. With the risk of HIV turning into AIDS, an often deadly disease, a patient's request not to tell his known sexual partners of his HIV-positive status is more problematic. This is a case in which legal and moral obligations may conflict. Suppose the legal requirement is that no one other than the patient can be told of his HIV status unless he gives permission for you to disclose such information. Suppose the patient refuses to give you such permission and tells you he is going to continue to have unprotected sex with his partners? Suppose you know the names of some of the patient's partners and could contact them if you wished. What should you do?

The PA could begin by talking to the patient concerning how his intended actions could infect his partners and appeal to his sense of concern for others. If he really cares about his sexual partners, would he want to infect them with HIV? If he insists on having unprotected sex, then it is difficult to know how to proceed ethically. You have fulfilled your obligation to diagnose and treat this individual patient—but do you have any moral responsibility to protect others that your patient could harm? Legally, you are bound to keep his HIV status confidential. It is difficult to determine what to do ethically, but one could argue that once you have fulfilled your medical obligations to the patient, you should maintain confidentiality, as confidentiality is essential to the trust needed for effectively caring for patients. However, it is not that simple; there are cases in which confidentiality can legally (and ethically) be breached; for example, if a patient were to confide in you that he committed a serious crime, such as murder or child abuse, then you would have an obligation to report that to law enforcement. The HIV case is a borderline situation, and a good moral case can be made either for disclosure or nondisclosure.

There are many other potential confidentiality issues in medical practice. Would you chart a first-time patient's cocaine use if the patient has been drug-free 10 years and if such drug use seems irrelevant to the current complaint? What if a 10-year old boy confides in you that he has been drinking alcohol but begs you not to tell his parents? What about the chapter case study—should you breach confidentiality and tell Juanita's family of her prognosis?

Confidentiality should be considered an essential part of good patient care rather than merely meeting a legal requirement. Care for confidentiality helps preserve that bond of trust between patient and PA, which is essential for the good of the patient's restoration to health.

Sexual and Other Relationship Issues

Sexual contact between patient and physician (and by extension, the patient and PA) has been strictly forbidden since Hippocratic times.[13] As the AAPA ethics manual correctly notes, "[s]uch relationships generally are unethical because of the PA's position of authority and the inherent imbalance of knowledge, expertise, and status. Issues such as dependence, trust, transference, and inequalities of power may lead to increased vulnerability on the part of current or former patients or key third parties."[2] In any of the helping professions, such as pastoral care, psychological counseling, or medicine, a client or patient may, due to emotional vulnerability, begin to have sexual feelings for the pastor, counselor, physician, or PA. These professionals are human as well, and it is often easy for them to allow their emotions to run out of control in such intimate contexts. But taking advantage of that for their own sexual gratification is just that: taking advantage of a vulnerable human being. It is thus both immoral and unprofessional. In medicine, the vulnerability of the patient is considerably increased: the physician or PA is allowed to view the most intimate parts of the patient's body as well as hear intimate secrets. Revealing oneself that way involves a tremendous amount of patient trust and gives tremendous power to the PA. The PA has the responsibility to use such power ethically. A medical relationship is not the proper context for a sexual relationship to develop. Any form of sexual advance or sexual comment by the PA is contrary to the good of the patient. As for a patient who makes sexual advances toward a PA, the PA should make clear that the relationship must remain professional, and the incident should be reported to the PA's physician supervisor.

The ethics manual also strongly discourages sexual relations between a PA and former patients as well as between "key third parties," such as a patient's "spouses or partners, parents, guardians, or surrogates," who "have influence over the patient."[2] If a PA wishes to date a former patient, it would be best to do so after considerable time has passed. Prudence is necessary in such situations. The PA should always consider first working for the good of the patient, which is essential to the integrity of the patient-PA relationship.

There are a number of specific situations the PA may face involving sexuality. Often a patient will transfer her feelings for a significant other to the PA because she regards the PA as a caring person who listens. This creates a dangerous situation, because the PA can be tempted to meet his own needs and sense of inadequacy at the patient's expense. For example, suppose that a young woman, Ann Jones, is a long-time patient of John Smith. Recently she has been coming in more often for minor complaints. At one appointment she says, "You know, John, you have been such a wonderful PA; you listen to me in a way no other man has listened before." Mr. Smith, who feels inadequate in his own life and suffers from low self-esteem, feels affirmed and enjoys the fact that Ms. Jones addresses him by his first name. He is already sexually attracted to her. He replies, "I'm glad we have such a good relationship, and I enjoy our appointments." He has already gone too far by referring to the "enjoyment" he feels—and Ms. Jones now believes she can go further—she places her hand on Mr. Smith's shoulder—and before long a patient is exploited, and a PA's career is ruined.

Mr. Smith should have taken steps early on to avoid a compromising situation. PAs are human beings and will have sexual feelings for some patients, but they must realize there is a fundamental difference between having feelings and acting on those feelings. Avoiding flirtatious conversation altogether—in the previous case, by changing the subject—would have helped Mr. Smith stay out of trouble. If he had replied to her first statement in a professional way ("Why don't we go back to your initial complaint of fatigue"), it would have sent the message to Ms. Jones that Mr. Smith wants to keep the relationship on a professional level.

Avoiding inappropriate touching is important. The PA sometimes has to touch sensitive areas of a patient's body, such as in a breast examination. How can he avoid problems? One practical way is to always have an additional person in the room when the PA examines someone of the opposite sex. If a man examines a woman, it is best to have a female nurse in the room. This not only protects the PA from false sexual harassment charges, it also makes it less likely that a PA who has difficulty controlling sexual feelings will behave inappropriately. If a PA feels sexually attracted to a patient during an intimate examination, it may be best for the PA to leave the room for a few moments; doing this without appearing awkward will take some skill, but it is better than a patient noticing the PA's attraction.

Even if a PA behaves in a professional manner, a patient will sometimes falsely accuse the PA of sexual harassment. If a patient makes a sexual advance to a PA and the PA responds in an ethically appropriate way, the incident should be noted in the patient's chart. It would be best if the PA also wrote a separate incident report and signed and dated it. If there were any witnesses, their accounts of what happened should also be included. Almost all problems involving sexuality in a PA's practice can be avoided if the PA behaves as a professional, recognizing the deep responsibility never to take advantage of a vulnerable patient.

Sexual issues are not the only relationship issues that arise between a patient and a PA. The relationship between patient and PA is a professional relationship, occurring in the context of the patient coming for help, but it can also be considered a form of friendship. An ethical PA will have concern, and sometimes affection, for patients. But close friendships with patients outside the medical relationship can be risky (in the same way that treating a close family member is risky) because the PA may be too emotionally involved to provide quality care. If the friend is treated differently or better than other patients, this can be construed as unjust as well as a conflict of interest.[2] In small, relatively isolated communities, such situations may be difficult to avoid; in such cases the PA should do his or her best to treat a patient who is a close friend in a fashion similar to that for other patients and not allow the emotional bond to harm the PA's "objectivity."

Dealing With "Difficult Patients"

No matter how benevolent or empathetic a PA tries to be, there will always be "difficult" patients. At one extreme are patients who are physically violent. No PA should feel obligated to treat a patient who makes the PA feel that he or she is in danger of being harmed. At a less intense level, some patients are obnoxious or complain constantly when they have no proper justification for complaint. A patient may be overly critical of everything the PA does or compare the PA unfavorably with physicians: "I'd rather see a real doctor, but I'd have to wait too long, so I guess I'm stuck with you." The patient may also unfavorably compare the PA with the patient's former health-care provider: "Where I used to live, Dr. Stone did a much better job than you." A patient may be personally rude in the course of an examination. Some patients may make snide remarks about the PA's race or gender; others may make lewd sexual comments.

Patients can be difficult in other ways. For example, they may not listen to the PA's advice, may keep smoking when they already have signs of bronchitis, or keep eating a high-fat diet despite grossly abnormal results from a lipid series. They may refuse to get prescriptions filled, be noncompliant in taking the prescriptions they have filled, or demand that a prescription for an antianxiety drug be renewed even though the patient is showing signs of becoming dependent on the drug. Patients may be uncooperative during an examination. Children can be difficult and uncooperative.

Difficult situations are all different, so handling them varies as well. The one overall principle stemming from the patient-provider relationship is for the PA to act for the good of the patient, to do what is best to heal the patient. Doing this sometimes implies that the PA must have a "thick skin" when dealing with difficult patients. If a patient becomes consistently belligerent to the point that the PA believes he or she is too much to handle, the PA can refer the patient to the supervising physician or to another PA or physician. Once a PA decides to treat a patient who is difficult or obnoxious, the PA must try to establish a healing relationship with that patient, because doing less is inconsistent with the fundamental goal of medicine to heal (Box 3-4).

Truth Telling

Whether to tell the patient the truth or deceive the patient is not just an issue that arises in extreme situ-

---

> ### Box 3-4 Tips for Dealing With Difficult Patients
>
> - Show concern for the patient, but also speak with confidence; be firm when necessary
> - Set boundaries with the patient on what constitutes unacceptable behavior and maintain those boundaries
> - Consider a psychological reason (e.g., clinical depression) as a cause of the patient's behavior
> - If you sense potential trouble, have someone else present with you and the patient
> - Have a specific plan beforehand to deal with a belligerent patient
> - If a patient becomes belligerent, speak in a calm but firm voice, informing that patient that such behavior in inappropriate
> - If you feel physically threatened, leave the room, and call law enforcement if necessary
> - Carefully chart every incident of a problem with a patient
> - Report all negative incidents to your supervising physician
> - If you feel uncomfortable treating a belligerent patient, ask someone else to take over care

---

ations, such as when a patient has a life-threatening illness. It is also an issue that affects the everyday practice of medicine, including the practice of a PA. Because developing trust is part of a healthy patient-PA relationship, and honesty is part of developing such trust, the general rule is that telling the truth is essential to the good of the patient. But it is not always possible or beneficent to tell the entire truth in every single situation. It is best to be as honest and open as possible, given the patient's level of knowledge and understanding.

The PA must also be careful to avoid being careless with the truth. For example, telling a patient with the flu, "You will be over this in a week," is something the PA cannot know for sure, and a statement like that can hurt the relationship if the patient is not better in a week. But if the PA says, "Most people's symptoms improve in a week, but if you're still having symptoms at that time, call me back," then the PA is taking care to be accurate and is modest about predicting the exact course of a patient's illness.

Truthfulness in charting is also important. In part, this is a matter of making sure the information in the chart is accurate. Taking detailed notes during a patient visit is important. When a PA in a busy practice sees a large number of scheduled and unscheduled patients, it may be difficult to remember details of the history and physical. There is a temptation to write something down for the sake of completeness even if the PA is not sure of the facts. Although the PA may do this without any intention of being untruthful, writing is still being careless with the truth. If a patient's chart reads "No family history of metastatic cancer" rather than "Father died of pancreatic cancer at 40; mother died of breast cancer at 35; sister currently being treated for breast cancer," this difference can make a great deal of difference in how the patient is managed.

Far more serious is willfully placing false information in a patient's chart. This can happen as a way to cover up medical error, whether the error be an action or an omission. The PA has a moral responsibility to accurately record what transpires between PA and patient, including any errors made. It is wrong for the PA to cover up his or her own error, and it is also wrong to cover up the error of someone on the staff, such as a nurse or technician. There is an aphorism in medicine that says, "If it wasn't written down, it wasn't done." But it does not follow that "If it was written down, it was done." Medication dosage errors, errors in information presented to the patient by the PA, errors in diagnosis—all should be recorded accurately in the chart. If a mistake is found in the chart itself, it should be corrected, but what was originally in the chart should be crossed out so that it is still readable. To cross out the mistake completely is a falsification of records, which is not only morally problematic but can get the PA into serious legal trouble.

Situations like the one in the case study, in which a patient's culture conflicts with truth telling, have gained the attention of some recent bioethicists. For example, Freedman[14] points out that there are cases, especially with cancer, in which a physician does not tell a patient the entire truth about his or her condition. Awkward situations can arise in the case of an incompetent patient who later becomes competent, with the family members already knowing the patient's terminal condition, and sometimes refusing to tell the relative or opposing the medical provider from so doing. With families from cultures that oppose telling the patient the truth about potentially terminal conditions, truth telling becomes an even more complicated issue. With the increasing pluralism in American society, there will be more and more chances for PAs to encounter patients from societies that do not share American individualism with its pride of autonomy over other moral values. Mexican, Filipino, Chinese, and Iranian cultures, for example, prefer that the patient's family hear bad news first, because bad news is thought to be disheartening to the patient. For such cultures, telling a patient with

cancer or some other serious illness of a poor prognosis would be "insensitive."[15] Thinking of the family as the primary health-care decision maker, even in the context of a competent patient, creates a conflict among the patient, the patient's family, the family's culture, and American law and bioethics. What should the PA do in case there is such a conflict?

One of the more promising approaches to this issue, although still couched in the language of autonomy, is Freedman's proposal of "offering truth" (Box 3-5).

An advantage of his approach is its focus on *conversation* between the patient and the health-care practitioner. Conversation implies relationship, and in a good conversation those involved respect one another and listen to each other. Empathy is important because it facilitates mutual understanding. Freedman's approach also recognizes that an individual's culture determines, to a significant extent, that person's values regarding health care and truth telling. It is more balanced than approaches that focus on telling the patient the whole truth about a terminal illness, even if the patient objects.

There remain, however, problems with Freedman's approach. Despite his concern for the cultural context of medicine, his position is overly individualistic, overemphasizing personal autonomy. There is little practical advice on how to deal with families who continue to insist that their loved ones should not know their prognosis. But Freedman's approach can be improved. His overly individualistic position should be softened to recognize that human beings are social beings whose health-care decisions involve their loved ones; the chapter case study is an example. Juanita is surrounded by her family, and their wishes

| Box 3-5 | Benjamin Freedman: "Offering Truth" |

- Focuses on the conversation between patient and health-care provider
- Recognizes that patients come from different backgrounds and cultures with different attitudes toward being told the truth
- Medical practitioners should "offer truth" to the patient—tell as much of the truth about the patient's condition that the patient is ready to hear
- If the patient is not ready to hear, the medical practitioner should back away for a while
- The medical practitioner persists in offering truth, but truth is never forced on the patient against the patient's will

regarding truth telling are part of what makes the case so morally difficult.

Freedman's proposal can also be strengthened at the practical level. Conversation with the patient over truth-telling should include not only talk about how much the patient wants to know but also conversation about the patient's family and their wishes. Taking Juanita's case study as an example, the PA (and most likely, in these cases, the supervising physician as well) should have conversations with her family, first, to try to understand their reasons rather than try to convince them of a particular point of view on truth telling. If Juanita wants to know her prognosis, she should be told, because respecting her wishes is part of a good patient-PA relationship. If she asks that the PA not tell the family that she has been informed of her condition, the situation becomes more difficult. Consulting the supervising physician in such cases is sometimes helpful, but in this case it is more difficult, given Dr. Jones' prior disagreement with the PA's values. If Juanita decides that she does not wish to be told of her condition and agrees with her family's position that they should be informed first, then withholding the truth from her may be the ethical way to proceed.

Dealing With Medical Error

Medical error gives rise to many ethical issues for the PA and deserves individual treatment in the chapter. The AAPA code of ethics makes it clear that the PA has a responsibility to "disclose to his or her supervising physician information about errors made in the course of caring for a patient."[2] But disclosure to the patient is only required "if such information is significant to the patient's interest and well-being."[2] This rule attempts to strike a proper balance between revealing all errors to the patient, which could be destructive of the patient-PA relationship, and not disclosing material errors that have harmed the patient. Not disclosing harmful errors can also damage the patient-PA relationship.

It is practically impossible to go through a career as a PA without making mistakes, either of commission or omission. There are probably minor improvements that the PA could make after every appointment with a patient. Some medical errors are ominous, with serious potential for harming the patient. They may involve misdiagnosis, such as a failure to diagnose a developing myocardial infarction in a woman who complains of fatigue or mistaking meningitis for influenza. They may involve omitting tests that are needed for a more accurate diagnosis or ordering a risky test for a patient who does not need it. They may involve medication errors. Mistakes may result from a failure to use prudence, failed judgment, or carelessness. Hilfiker[16] believes that the "worst kind" of

errors are "failure[s] of will…in which a doctor knows the right thing to do but doesn't do so because he is distracted, or pressured, or exhausted." A PA of integrity will strive to get beyond the pressures and weariness of a busy practice to make sure the right thing is done for a patient.

Should medical error always be reported to the patient? There is no doubt that the PA or supervising physician should inform the patient of errors that harm the patient. These could include prescribing the wrong medication, a medication dosage error, or negligent misdiagnosis. Medical practitioners, however, have found it difficult to openly discuss error, and Baylis[17] discusses three major reasons for such reluctance. First, some alleged errors are not real "errors," but chance events due to medical uncertainty. It may be difficult at times to distinguish "avoidable" medical errors from harms that are unavoidable. For example, a patient who comes in with symptoms suggesting a viral infection may develop complications causing major damage to organs such as the heart; this is something that cannot usually be anticipated by the PA. Another example is a case of surgery to repair an aortic aneurysm. First, if the aorta is thin or damaged due to atherosclerotic deposits, even a careful surgeon may not be able to avoid extensive bleeding or a postsurgical breach of the aorta. Second, there may also be concern that disclosure of medical error may damage the trust a patient has for the physician and/or PA. Third, there is the "fear of litigation."

Nevertheless, it will most likely destroy trust moreso if the PA and the physician do not reveal medical errors that cause harm to the patient. Disclosure is for the good of all, and it best preserves the fragile relationship between patient and medical practitioner. How should a PA disclose an error to a patient? First, the PA should be completely honest with the patient, avoiding euphemisms for error and avoiding speaking in the third person. Saying "I made a mistake and gave you too much heparin" is better than saying "A mistake was made." The former implies that the PA is taking responsibility for the error. Second, the PA should be apologetic; saying "I'm sorry" is essential. The PA should tell the patient exactly what harm resulted from the error; for example, "The medication error caused the bleed in your stomach."

The PA cannot control the patient's reaction; even with an honest apology, the patient may react in a hostile manner. The patient may no longer wish to be treated by the PA. The most serious consequence is litigation by the patient. Yet it is better to inform than for the patient to later discover that the PA has made an error that caused harm. The PA must not violate the trust required between PA and patient necessary for good medicine.

But what if an error does not harm the patient or has little chance of harming the patient? Suppose that a medication dosage error occurs that is so minor the patient is not harmed? The PA has the responsibility of noting the error on the patient's chart, but it is not clear that the patient should be told in this case. The AAPA ethics manual is correct on this point. Informing the patient of every minor error can undermine the patient's confidence in both the PA and the health-care system. When telling a patient about an error is more likely to do more harm than good, the PA has no ethical obligation to do so.

There may also be situations "in the middle," in which the patient is only slightly harmed, or there is a small potential for harm due to medical error. Ordering too much of an anticoagulant that carries only a slightly increased risk of bleeding is one example. The PA must weigh the potential harm of informing the patient of the error against the potential of a patient complication and the patient later discovering the error. A good maxim in such cases is "When in doubt, inform the patient."

If a patient is badly harmed, the PA will require emotional support to be able to go on and treat future patients effectively. This is particularly important if a patient dies as the result of a PA's error. It is here that a good, trusting relationship with the supervising physician can be invaluable for the PA's survival. The PA will need the courage necessary to keep on practicing medicine in such situations.

The PA has a responsibility to report all medical errors to the supervising physician. The relationship between PA and physician-supervisor is one in which the PA acts under the authority of a physician yet has some autonomy. Such autonomy implies trust in the PA by the physician. If the PA refrains from reporting medical errors, and the physician discovers this, it violates that trust. It could also create legal difficulties for the physician. If a patient is harmed by an error, litigation is possible, even if the PA is honest with the patient. Because the PA is an extension of the physician, the physician supervisor will certainly be named as a party to any litigation in the case of a PA's medical error. The physician needs to know about a PA's error, at the very least, in order to be prepared in case litigation occurs.

Informed Consent

The issue of informed consent is largely parallel to the issue of truth telling, as informed consent can be construed as a form of advance truth telling. Like truth telling, informed consent was emphasized in medical ethics quite late, making its first appearance in U.S. law in 1957.[18] By the end of the 1970s it was well established, at least in law. Dealing with informed consent is an everyday part of the PA's life. The AAPA code of ethics strongly emphasizes the importance of informed consent. It defines informed consent as "provid[ing] adequate information that is comprehendible to a competent patient or patient surrogate."[2] The information provided the patient should include "[a]t a minimum...the nature of the medical condition, the objectives of the proposed treatment, treatment options, possible outcomes, and the risks involved."[2] The manual has a healthy and holistic view of the concept of "shared decision making" between patient and PA, noting that it "involves assisting patients in making decisions that account for medical, situational, and personal factors."[2]

The PA works with informed consent every day; the attempt to explain a diagnosis to a patient or to give a patient information about a prescribed drug are examples. As is the case with truth telling, the primary justification offered in the bioethics literature for requiring informed consent is patients' autonomy to make decisions affecting their own bodies.[18,19] Whereas this was an important corrective to the paternalistic "doctor knows best" view in the past, the strongest justification for informed consent is found in the patient-medical practitioner relationship.[1] The physician or PA has much more medical knowledge than the patient as well as power over the patient. This creates a fundamental inequality between the patient and the medical practitioner. The gap in both knowledge and power can be narrowed by informed consent by giving the patient some knowledge of the disease or injury as well as of treatments and their attendant risks and benefits. The patient is then empowered to make a reasonably informed decision concerning health care. Although the health-care practitioner-patient relationship is never one of equals, informed consent, rightly understood, preserves as much of the patient's dignity and free choice as is possible when the patient's normal life, perhaps even sense of identity, is threatened by illness.

Too often, however, informed consent has been considered a hurdle to be overcome, a rule to be followed to keep the physician or PA out of legal trouble and safe in the event of a lawsuit, rather than something essential to the relationship between patient and provider and central to the ethical practice of medicine. To cover every possible treatment option, no matter how little support there is for its efficacy, and every possible problem that could arise from each option, is an astronomical task impossible to perform in practice. The physician or PA must present as much information as he or she feels is needed to cover oneself from potential lawsuits (again placing the focus on one's own legal protection rather than on what is good for the patient). As an alternative, Brody[19] suggests a modification of Katz's "conversational model."[20] A conversation has a certain "open-endedness" missing in a legalistic approach, and the patient is free to ask questions; the physician or PA is free to answer the patient's questions, though the answers will not be as structured as they would in a more formal setting. A conversation cannot be governed by a "list of rules."[19] Brody's difficulty with a pure conversational model is that he does not believe it has the legal backbone to be a sound legal standard of informed consent. He prefers what he calls "the transparency standard," in which, during the course of a conversation with a patient, the physician makes his or her reasoning about treatments "transparent" to the patient. The physician is, in effect, "thinking out loud." This also allows room for questions by the patient and for the physician to answer them.

While still focusing on legal protection for the physician, Brody's transparency model fits the nature of the relationship between patient and medical practitioners better than the other models. First, like Katz's conversational model, it emphasizes what is central to medicine: the relation between patient and health-care practitioner. It also recognizes that conversations in the context of real human relationships cannot be subsumed under formal rules; there is an openness in conversations that parallels the openness in other human relationships, such as friendships. Brody's model focuses on the patient and the illness as the medical practitioner attempts to make his or her reasoning transparent concerning the patient's diagnosis, prognosis, and, in particular, treatment options. This does not imply that the physician or PA is merely presenting a mechanical list of treatment options; the physician or PA is stating the reasoning for what the best treatment options are for this particular patient. This would include whatever reasoning is based on good scientific grounds, such as results of clinical trials. It would also include the unique factors affecting a particular patient, which can only be gained by a trusting relationship between patient and practitioner. Once the practitioner can say, "Here's my reasoning on what I think is best for you given what I know of your situation; now do you have any questions?" then the conversation is off to a good start. The patient has time during the conversation to interject comments and ask questions.

Despite the advantages of Brody's view, its greater emphasis on a legal standard of informed consent, while practically necessary in order for the physician or PA to avoid liability, carries with it the danger of shifting the practitioner's focus too much toward the legal end of informed consent. Despite Brody's claim that the medical practitioner's making his or her reasoning "transparent" should avoid this problem, the practitioner may still wonder later, "Did I mention this possibility to the patient? Am I covered on every point? Was I right not to mention every treatment option to the patient, no matter how unsupported it may be?" Perhaps such fears are unavoidable in a litigious society in which fears of legal liability and malpractice suits paralyze physicians and can affect PAs as well.

Although fears concerning informed consent may be unavoidable even in the best of models, Brody does bring out one key point, which may mitigate such fears and also work for the good of the patient: "Informed consent is a meaningful ethical concept only to the extent that it can be realized and promoted within the ongoing practice of good medicine."[19] As good medicine can be practiced only in the context of a trusting relationship, informed consent, rather than being thought of as a legalistic requirement, should be considered an essential part of such a relationship.

For example, suppose a long-time patient, Ann, a 40-year-old woman, visits her PA, Mary, with a chief complaint of palpitations. In the course of the history, Ann mentions that she has been under considerable emotional stress due to a sudden and unexpected decision by her husband to leave her. Mary also knows from previous conversations with Ann that she has three children and has a full-time job. EKG results are normal, and Mary doubts that a referral to a cardiologist would be helpful in Ann's case. Mary also considers options such as recommending that Ann get counseling to deal with her situation or placing her on antianxiety medication. Mary wants to cover the relevant options, but in a way that is fitting for Ann's situation. After evaluating the EKG and consulting her supervising physician, Mary tells Ann, "Your EKG is perfectly normal, and while I could refer you to a cardiologist for further tests, I don't think that will be necessary. However, if it would put your mind at ease about your heart for me to refer you, I will; it's up to you. I know from our previous conversations how much you love your husband and understand that the stress from his leaving you must be overwhelming. I suggest that you consider professional counseling to help you through this crisis as well as talking to other family members who I know have supported you in the past. Another option that could relieve some of the physical symptoms of anxiety, such as palpitations, would be an antianxiety drug. I will be happy to suggest an option with minimal side-effects that has helped a number of people. Let me know what you believe is best for you. If you have any questions, feel free to ask."

Normally this conversation would be interrupted by Ann's comments or questions. But Mary takes account of the medical facts concerning Ann, as well as her life situation, and is engaging in a conversation with her, in the course of which informed consent can take place. In such a conversation, the patient and PA deliberate together concerning the best course of treatment.[21] Mutuality, respect for the patient's values and choices, and a trusting relationship are present.

Another problem that can arise, even in the above model of informed consent, is that an experienced PA may not depend wholly on formal rules to diagnose or prescribe for a patient.[10] In addition, no matter how good the patient-PA relationship is, no individual can exhaustively know another's deepest feelings; the PA cannot know the patient's "innermost feelings about...life, health, disability and pain." Nor can the patient know the PA's "innermost feelings about the preferred therapy based on a lifetime of experiences with similar patients."[10] It may be good for the PA, after giving the treatment options and the pros and cons, to say openly, "My feeling is....." or "My sense is...."

There are other practical issues that arise concerning informed consent. Some individuals cannot give informed consent, such as children or those who are mentally unable to do so due to severe injury or neurological deficits. In the case of children, the PA should still try to explain procedures to them as clearly as possible if they are old enough to understand, even if they are not the ones giving legal consent. Normally, parents or guardians give consent for the treatment of minors. Recently, the notion of informed assent has come into vogue.[22] This means that the medical practitioner explains the child's diagnosis, prognosis, and treatment options to the best of the child's ability to understand. The child then gives or refuses assent for that treatment. In most cases, refusal to assent to treatment is not binding (medical research is an important exception). But informed assent gives the child as much share in decision making as the child can handle.

In the case of neurologically impaired patients, health-care decisions are made by a guardian. The guardian can be a parent, a loved one with legal guardianship, or the state. The patient may, if there is sufficient cognitive capacity, be able to give informed assent to a treatment. Some patients who are competent but later become neurologically impaired may have living wills, which express their wishes concerning life-sustaining treatment. Other patients may have someone designated as having medical power of attorney, in which case the proxy makes health-care decisions when the patient becomes incompetent.

With adult patients who are competent, the PA should be able to adjust to a patient's educational level. Some patients in contemporary practice are very well read concerning medicine, especially those with chronic illnesses. The PA should be respectful of such knowledge, never condescend to a patient, and be willing to correct inaccuracies in a kind way. Other patients know very little about medicine, and the PA may have to work hard to simplify language in order for the patient to have some understanding of what is going on. The PA should realize that the knowledge gap between patient and PA will be greater for some patients than for others. The PA should also recognize that some patients prefer a more paternalistic health-care provider. Such patients may say, "Just tell me what's wrong with me, and give me something that will help. I don't want to hear all this other information." In adjusting to these patients, the PA may be in the position of offering truth, while still giving the patient as much information as possible to make an informed choice. In the case of medications, the PA can suggest that the patient read the material on safety provided by the pharmacist if the patient is not willing to listen to the PA. In any patient-PA situation, informed consent should take place in an atmosphere of concern for the patient, integrity, trust, and mutual respect.

CASE STUDY DISCUSSION

We have discussed a number of attributes that contribute to the ethics of PA practice and relationships. Let us return to Juanita's case (which started our discussions) to reconsider it as a whole in light of the prior discussion. Sometimes it is easy to miss the obvious and most fundamental consideration that Juanita is ill and has come to you for help. If possible, you will work with her to restore her to bodily health. If this is not possible, you will do what you can for her good, such as offering palliative care to help Juanita deal with the physical pain of cancer, and as much emotional support as you can professionally muster to help her through the emotional struggles of dying. You are a PA who has the virtue of benevolence; you are genuinely concerned for Juanita. You are also empathetic and have a sense of her present struggles with the uncertainty of not knowing her prognosis. You also recognize her family's love for her and their desire that she not be told bad news if her cancer turns out to be terminal. You respect both Juanita and her family and realize that they are concerned for her good, as you are. You are concerned about the family and care for their feelings, but you realize your ultimate duty is to Juanita, for it is *she* who has come to you for help.

You know that Juanita has mixed feelings about being told her prognosis after her surgery by someone other than a family member. You also realize that after you brief the family on the surgery and prognosis, they will insist that you not tell Juanita. A complicating factor is the important relationship you share with Dr. Jones, which has been cooperative and productive. You have worked well with her in the short time you have known her and are concerned about damaging that relationship.

That being said, some general advice may guide the PA in this case. You should certainly try to talk with Dr. Jones again privately before the surgery takes place to express your concerns and your view that you or she should tell Juanita of her prognosis, whether that prognosis is good or bad. Both you and Dr. Jones can be "transparent" concerning your reasoning and intuition on the good thing to do for Juanita. Dr. Jones may change her mind, in which case there is no longer a conflict between your desires and hers. But she may hold her ground and insist that if you talk with Juanita that you not tell her if the prognosis is terminal. Another, and probably more likely option, given that Dr. Jones knows the intensity of your feelings, is that Dr. Jones would insist on talking to Juanita if there is a bad prognosis. This creates its own set of problems: how would Juanita and her family react if they are used to you providing information instead of Dr. Jones? Should you tell Juanita anyway, risking your relationship with Dr. Jones and perhaps your career as a PA, especially given Juanita's earlier ambivalence? What would this do to the trust you and Dr. Jones have had for each other? Would another option be talking with Juanita informally so that she can let you know whether she is ready for bad news?

If Dr. Jones still wants you to talk with Juanita and her family, you will be in the position of telling them how her surgery went and how her future looks, since this reflects Juanita's desire that her family know her condition. Then you can broach the subject of whether to tell Juanita again, basing your case not on abstract principles such as autonomy but on what you know about Juanita as a person. You should be open to listening to her reasoning and concerns, even if they seem irrational to you or are opposed to your own positions on medical morality. You should keep in mind that you continue to have a relationship with the patient's family.

In dealing with Juanita, assuming her prognosis is grave, probably the best range of actions in this situation is to offer to tell her the truth about her condition. Perhaps you could say: "Juanita, you made it through the surgery just fine. Would you like to know what we found?" If Juanita says, "No, not now; maybe later, please," then the door remains open for talking with her later. If she says, "I don't know what you should do," then it may still be best to say, "That's OK; I'll talk to you later about this when you've decided what is best." But if Juanita replies, "Yes, I want to know, good or bad. I know what my family thinks, but I really want to know the truth," then the best option is probably to tell her the truth. Juanita is the person in need; she is the one who is dying, and she is the one who should have the ultimate priority of decision making on what she wishes to know about her condition. If Dr. Jones disagrees, this may be one of the situations in which you will have to act for the good of the patient against your supervisor's desires. It is a difficult call, on which even virtuous PAs may disagree. Whatever is done should be for the good of the healing relationship between PA and patient and should help Juanita in her time of greatest need.

References

1. Pellegrino ED, Thomasma DC. A Philosophical Basis of Medical Practice. New York and Oxford: Oxford University Press, 1981.
2. American Academy of Physician Assistants. Guidelines for ethical conduct for the physician assistant profession. Adopted May 2000. Retrieved June 8, 2004, from http://www.aapa.org
3. Svahn DS, Kozak AJ, eds. Let Me Listen to Your Heart: Writings by Medical Students. Cooperstown, NY: Bassett Healthcare, 2002.
4. American Academy of Physician Assistants. Information about PAs and the PA profession. Alexandria, VA: American Academy of Physician Assistants, 2004. Retrieved June 8, 2004, from http://www.aapa.org/geninfo1.html
5. Pellegrino ED, Thomasma DC. The Virtues in Medical Practice. New York and Oxford: Oxford University Press, 1993.
6. Aristotle. Nicomachean ethics, Ross, WD, trans. In McKeon, R, ed. The Basic Works of Aristotle. New York: Random House, 1941.

7. Liszka JJ. Moral Competence: An Integrated Approach to the Study of Ethics, 2nd ed. Upper Saddle River, NJ: Prentice-Hall, 2002.

8. Grumbach D. Excerpt from Coming into the end zone. Reprinted in Reynolds R, Stone, J, eds. On Doctoring: Stories, Poems, Essays, 3rd ed. New York: Simon & Schuster, 2001;158-65.

9. Drane JF. Becoming a Good Doctor: The Place of Virtue and Character in Medical Ethics, 2nd ed. Kansas City: Sheed & Ward, 1995.

10. Dreyfus HL, Dreyfus SE. Mind Over Machine: The Power of Human Intuition and Expertise in the Era of the Computer. New York: The Free Press, 1986.

11. Cassel E. The Nature of Suffering and the Goals of Medicine, 2nd ed. New York: Oxford University Press, 2004.

12. King S. On Writing: A Memoir of the Craft. New York: Scribner, 2000.

13. The Hippocratic Oath. In Temkin O, Temkin CL, eds. Ancient Medicine: Selected Papers of Ludwig Edelstein. Baltimore: Johns Hopkins University Press, 1967. Reprinted in Steinbock B, Arras JD, London AJ, eds. Ethical Issues in Modern Medicine, 6th ed. New York: McGraw-Hill, 2003; 55.

14. Freedman B. Offering Truth: One Ethical Approach to the Uninformed Cancer Patient. In Steinbock B, Arras JD, London AJ. Ethical Issues in Modern Medicine, 6th ed. New York: McGraw Hill, 2003; 76-82.

15. Galanti G. An introduction to cultural differences. Western Journal of Medicine, 2000;172:335-336.

16. Hilfiker D. Mistakes. In Reynolds R, Stone J, eds. On Doctoring: Stories, Poems, Essays, 3rd ed. New York: Simon & Schuster, 2001; 325-336.

17. Baylis F. Errors in medicine: Nurturing truthfulness. Journal of Clinical Ethics, 1997; 8:336-340. Reprinted in Steinbock B, Arras JD, London AJ. Ethical Issues in Modern Medicine, 6th ed. New York: McGraw Hill, 2003; 107-111.

18. Katz J. Informed consent–must it remain a fairy tale? Journal of Contemporary Health Law and Policy, vol 10. Reprinted in Steinbock B, Arras JD, London AJ. Ethical Issues in Modern Medicine, 6th ed. New York: McGraw Hill, 2003; 92-100.

19. Brody H. Transparency: informed consent in primary care. Hastings Center Report, 1989;19:5-9.

20. Katz J. The Silent World of Doctor and Patient. New York: Free Press, 1984.

21. Emanuel EJ, Emanuel LL. Four models of the physician-patient relationship. JAMA, 1992;267:2221-2226.

22. Committee on Bioethics, American Academy of Pediatrics. Informed consent, parental permission, and assent in pediatric practice. Pediatrics, 1995;95:314-317.

GLOSSARY

autonomy "self-determination"; applied to medical ethics, refers to the patient's right to make choices concerning his or her health care without interference from others.

benevolence a virtue through which one desires the good for other people and actively tries to bring about that good through action; applied to medical ethics, it is an active concern for the patient's well-being that leads to action designed to help that patient.

courage a virtue that can be understood broadly to refer to having the strength to make difficult moral choices despite negative consequences.

deontological refers to moral theories that hold that some actions (or rules) are right or wrong in themselves regardless of consequences.

empathy the virtue that allows a person to better understand another person's point of view.

habituation the process by which one gains a virtue; it primarily involves practicing virtuous activity until it becomes a permanent part of one's character.

HIPAA Health Insurance Portability and Accountability Act of 1996; a law, designed to protect the patient's privacy rights, that strictly regulates how a patient's health-care information can be shared with others.

humility the virtue that allows one to recognize one's own limitations, to recognize that no one is all-powerful or all-knowing.

informed assent usually applied to children, this refers to the ability of children to give approval to treatments once these treatments have been explained. As parents or guardians grant formal consent for treatment, a child's refusal of assent is rarely binding except in the case of a child's decision to participate or refrain from participating in medical experimentation.

informed consent the patient's grant of approval to a treatment based on sufficient information about that treatment provided by the health-care practitioner.

integrity the virtue that enables a person to consistently behave in accordance with his or her moral values.

justice as a virtue, justice is the character trait that enables a person to be fair to others.

prudence the virtue that refers to the "practical reason" needed for a person to make the right moral choice in a given circumstance.

respect the virtue that enables a person to treat other human beings as persons having intrinsic worth, who deserve to be treated with propriety.

virtue a stable character trait, developed by habituation, that enables one to act in a way that promotes human flourishing.

Clinical Ethical Case Discussions

F.J. Gianola, PA-C

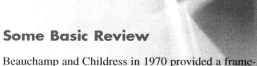

This special section presents five case studies that involve ethical dilemmas. These cases are preceded by introductory material, some of which is presented in more detail in other chapters. A good approach for you or your class is to hold group or class discussions about the cases, the ethical and professional issues involved, and possible solutions or resolutions. There may be some redundancy in the cases and overlap of issues. Remember, no patient will come to you with a single diagnosis, and no ethical/professional problem will involve just one issue.

All clinical and ethical problems must be placed and evaluated within a patient's narrative and life context. By doing so, one may find that, even in similar cases, the treatments and answers to ethical conundrums may vary. But the data should always be collected in the same way and in a manner that is reproducible.

How can busy physician assistants (PAs) and PA students gather their thoughts and address ethical issues within their practices and study? One approach is to gather data in the same way one would do a physical examination or collect information from a patient history. We tend do a physical examinations the same way every time. We ask every patient the history of present illness in the same manner to collect all the data we need to make an appropriate assessment and provide the proper treatment. When assessing an ethical dilemma, the same principles can be applied.

Some Basic Review

Beauchamp and Childress in 1970 provided a framework that clinicians can use to recognize ethical principles. In *Principles of Biomedical Ethics,* they defined the basic principles as:

- Autonomy: respecting the decision-making capacities of autonomous individuals
- Nonmaleficence: avoiding the creation of intentional, needless harm or injury to the patient, either through acts of commission or omission
- Beneficence: being of benefit to the patient, taking positive steps to prevent harm to and remove harm from the patient
- Justice: allocating benefits, risks, and costs fairly

To apply these principles to a specific case is easier said than done. Jonsen, Siegler, and Winslade (a philosopher, a physician, and a lawyer), in their text *Clinical Ethics: A Practical Approach to Ethical Decisions in Clinical Medicine,* created a clinical approach to addressing ethical issues that is practical, user-friendly, and accessible to all clinicians. Their (casuistic) case-based paradigm consists of four topics that are fundamental and essential in every clinical encounter where an ethical issue may be identified. See Box 1-1.

- Medical indications (beneficence and nonmaleficence): What is the clinical presentation, including prognosis, diagnosis, and treatment?

Box S-1   A Clinical Approach to Ethical Issues

Medical Indications

The Principles of Beneficence and Nonmaleficence

1. What is the patient's medical problem? history? diagnosis? prognosis?

2. Is the problem acute? chronic? critical? emergent? reversible?

3. What are the goals of treatment?

4. What are the probabilities of success?

5. What are the plans in case of therapeutic failure?

6. In sum, how can this patient be benefited by medical and nursing care, and how can harm be avoided?

Patient Preferences

The Principle of Respect for Autonomy

1. Is the patient mentally capable and legally competent? Is there evidence of incapacity?

2. If competent, what is the patient stating about preferences for treatment?

3. Has the patient been informed of benefits and risks, understood this information, and given consent?

4. If incapacitated, who is the appropriate surrogate? Is the surrogate using appropriate standards for decision making?

5. Has the patient expressed prior preferences, e.g., Advance Directives?

6. Is the patient unwilling or unable to cooperate with medical treatment? If so, why?

7. In sum, is the patient's right to choose being respected to the extent possible in ethics and law?

Quality of Life

The Principles of Beneficence and Nonmaleficence and Respect for Autonomy

1. What are the prospects, with or without treatment, for a return to normal life?

2. What physical, mental, and social deficits is the patient likely to experience if treatment succeeds?

3. Are there biases that might prejudice the provider's evaluation of the patient's quality of life?

4. Is the patient's present or future condition such that his or her continued life might be judged undesirable?

5. Is there any plan and rationale to forgo treatment?

6. Are there plans for comfort and palliative care?

Contextual Features

The Principles of Loyalty and Fairness

1. Are there family issues that might influence treatment decisions?

2. Are there provider (physicians and nurses) issues that might influence treatment decisions?

3. Are there financial and economic factors?

4. Are there religious or cultural factors?

5. Are there limits on confidentiality?

6. Are there problems of allocation of resources?

7. How does the law affect treatment decisions?

8. Is clinical research or teaching involved?

9. Is there any conflict of interest on the part of the providers or the institution?

Jonsen AR, Siegler M, Winslade WJ. Clinical Ethics: A Practical Approach to Ethical Decisions in Clinical Medicine. 5th ed. New York, NY: McGraw-Hill; 2002.

- Patient preferences (autonomy): What are the patient's goals? What would the patient like done in this situation? With all clinical encounters, the patient's values are integral to ethical decision making.
- Quality of life (nonmaleficence, beneficence, and autonomy): What signs and symptoms will affect the patient's quality of life? The objective of all clinical encounters is to improve, or at least address, quality of life for the patient.
- Contextual features (justice): What is the context for this clinical encounter? We must consider the patient's family, insurance coverage, hospital policy, legal constraints, and additional matters outside our and the patient's control.

If we are aware of the data needed to assess ethical issues, it becomes much easier to include all the information required for a proper assessment.

In the ethical cases presented in this text, we will try to demonstrate how the data allow us to begin our case analysis. At the base of our efforts is "What is the ethical question?" Many times this is not clear. The initial step is to try to identify the ethical question or professional issues in a sentence or two. This will help clarify the dilemma or disagreement. The next step is to try to ascertain if this problem is similar to other cases we have encountered. What are the similarities or differences? Are there comparable cases in the community, and is there community or professional agreement? The answers to these questions may help us, but our decision will depend on the facts of our specific case. Be willing to explore these issues beyond this text. Go to other resources; look for different viewpoints. Discuss them, debate them, and revisit them when you have more experience as a student or PA.

These ethical cases are real. The identities and places been have changed to protect the patients.

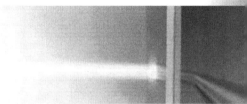

CASE 1

Compelled Birth Control in a Minor

Case Presentation

Ms. L is a Native American woman who presented in clinic with her 12-year-old daughter D, who was complaining of abdominal pain. A limited interview with both mother and daughter was conducted. During that time the ground rules of confidentiality were discussed and agreed to by daughter and mother, the rule being anything the daughter told the provider was between the provider and daughter unless suicide or homicide was at issue. The mother was then asked to step out of the examination room, and a complete history was obtained, and a physical examination was performed.

D reported no past illness other than colds and flu. She had no past surgeries and was not taking any medications. Her immunizations were up to date. Her review of systems was negative. Her age of menarche was 10 years old, with 28 days between menses. Flow is moderate and not painful, although she has some premenstrual cramping. Her last menses was 10 days ago.

She complained of some vaginal discharge and confided she has been sexually active for the past year with two male partners. Her sexual activity has been by mutual consent. She has had unprotected intercourse on numerous occasions. She had just returned home after running away and living with her boyfriend for about 2 weeks.

Upon physical examination, D is a well-developed, well-nourished 12-year-old Native American adolescent. She is a normal female, a Tanner stage B4, P4 with an unremarkable physical examination, with the exception of her pelvic examination: an abnormal discharge was noted. No pelvic or abdominal pain was noted upon examination. Gonorrhea and chlamydia cultures were obtained.

After the history and physical examination, D was counseled about her sexual activity and the risk of sexually transmitted disease. She wants to share this information with her mother and would like to do it in the office with our presence for support.

Ms. L returned to the office and, after hearing of D's sexual activity, requested that D be placed on birth control immediately. Ms. L specifically requested Depo-Provera. D protested that she does not want to be on birth control. Ms. L stated, "I am your mother and your legal guardian, and you *will* have the Depo-Provera." After calming Ms. L and D, other birth control methods were discussed (oral contraceptives, diaphragms, spermicides, condoms, and absti-nence). D refused the oral contraceptives, diaphragm, and abstinence. She stated she might consider condoms.

Ms. L became even more upset and stated, "As long as you live at home and as long as I am responsible for your welfare, I have the right and responsibility to decide the method of your birth control and what tests you will have." Ms. L again insisted on the Depo-Provera injection for her daughter.

QUESTIONS FOR DISCUSSION

1. What are the ethical, legal, and professional issues in this case?
2. Can a minor be compelled by a parent to take a birth control medication?
3. Who can speak on behalf of 12-year-old D?
4. Can D refuse treatment?
5. Can Ms. L's demand for treatment override D's refusal?
6. What are the laws governing treatment of minors in your state?
7. What would you do in this case?
8. Does being Native American change your thoughts on the issues?
9. From a medical standpoint, what else should you do in D's assessment and management?

Medical Indications (Beneficence, Nonmaleficence)

D is a healthy, sexually active Native American adolescent. She may have a sexually transmitted disease. After confirmation from her laboratory tests whether there is a sexually transmitted disease, treatment with the proper agent would follow. There are many concerns about sexually active young adolescents. At 12 years old, many are concrete thinkers but are generally unable to think abstractly or to hypothesize. At the same time, these adolescents are trying to decrease family dependency. Often encompassing all of this is the "myth of immunity" in which the teen believes "it won't happen to me." Elkind's[1] concept of the "personal fable" expresses teen feelings of immortality and invulnerability.

Sexual activity and risk taking have not been uncommon experiences for adolescents in the United States during the 20th and the beginning of the 21st centuries. Numerous papers have been published about "teen pregnancy" and its effects on the adolescent and society. However there have been very few studies of Native American adolescent pregnancy. One study funded by the Indian Health Service (IHS) provided a grant to the Adolescent Health Program at the University of Minnesota.[2] Fifty tribes throughout the United States participated, and about 14,000 Native American adolescents were surveyed between 1988 and 1990. The survey queried feelings about a number of subjects, including sexual health and risk-taking behavior. The Native American adolescents generally answered the same as other adolescent groups more often than giving different responses.

In this survey, 56.8% of the adolescent girls and 65% of the adolescent boys had sexual intercourse by the 12th grade. Adolescents who were sexually active had their first intercourse at 14.2 years for the girls and 13.6 for the boys. It should be further noted that 20% of Native American births are by adolescents. This has been a fairly constant figure from 1980 to 1996.[3]

The PA described the benefits and risks of contraceptive technology. This is well described in the literature. The methods include abstinence, male condoms, other barrier methods, oral contraceptives, contraceptive implants, and contraceptive injections.

Depo-Provera (medroxyprogesterone) is the only injectable hormonal contraceptive available in the United States. Side effects include irregular menstrual bleeding. Within 12 months, more than 50% of women report amenorrhea and, with longer use, 75% report amenorrhea. Other side effects include weight gain, bloating, mood changes, depression, and headaches.

One concern in use by adolescents is that fewer than 50% of young women return for a second injection, and fewer than 33% return for a third injection. This may be due to the variability of sex partners and frequency. Side effects of weight gain and mood changes may also be a cause for decreased use. Adolescents in the United States tend to use contraceptives inconsistently. This may well be due to conflicting messages they receive about sexuality from the media.[4] Behavioral factors that increase risks for sexually transmitted diseases (STDs) include multiple partners, partners who themselves have multiple partners, and erratic use of condoms. The use of alcohol and other drugs leads to poor use of contraceptives and a decrease in inhibitions and may increase the number of partners.

Studies show that pregnant American adolescents younger than 17 years have a higher occurrence of medical problems than do adult women.[5] This includes complications with pregnancy and birth and medical problems for the infant. The complications include prematurity, low birth weight, and infant mortality three times higher than for adult women. Maternal medical problems include poor maternal weight gain, pregnancy-induced hypertension, and anemia.[5]

Frasier et al,[6] in a 1995 study of white women younger than 18 years with adequate prenatal care compared with mothers 20 to 24 years, showed a risk (relative risk, 1.9) of premature infants or an infant weighing less than 2500 g at birth (relative risk, 1.7).

Patient Preference (Autonomy)

D was adamant about not wanting birth control. Her mother was just as adamant about D being given a Depo-Provera injection at this visit. D does not want an injection because it would hurt, and the medication has such a long-term effect. She does not want birth control pills because she is afraid she will forget to take them and that all her friends will find out she is taking them. She thinks a diaphragm is strange and that it is unlikely she would use it in front of a boy or ever. An IUD was discussed. She was very sure she did not want anything in her uterus and was very afraid of the procedure. The female condom was new to her, and she thought it looked a bit large and awkward, and she would never buy and use one. D declared abstinence would never happen.

"Informed *consent or dissent*" is a key question in this case. Informed consent is the permission of a patient or patient's representative for treatment. In the treatment of an adolescent, this consent is confounded by the developing competency of the adolescent. Traditionally, children below the age of majority have been presumed unable to make treatment deci-

sions, and parents have had the power to consent for their treatment. Over the past 30 years, an increasing understanding of the cognitive skills of children and adolescents has developed, with the result that parents, health-care providers, and the courts acknowledge that many adolescents have the capacity to take part in some decisions about their health care.[7,8]

When assessing cognitive development and capacity for informed consent or dissent of adolescents, the ability to reason and understand and the voluntariness of the treatment need to be evaluated.[9] The American Academy of Pediatrics (AAP), in its 1995 Statement on Informed Consent, Parental Permission, and Assent in Pediatric Practice, provides the following guidelines:

1. Helping the patient achieve a developmentally appropriate awareness of the nature of his or her condition.
2. Telling the patient what he or she can expect with tests and treatments.
3. Making a clinical assessment of the patient's understanding of the situation and the factors influencing how he or she is responding (including whether there is inappropriate pressure to accept testing or therapy).
4. Soliciting an expression of the patient's willingness to accept the proposed care.[10]

The AAP goes further to address issues of assent (dissent): "The clinical situation in which a persistent refusal to assent (dissent) may be ethically binding."[10] Although some consider this a vague statement, it gives a sense of priorities.

This seems most obvious in the context of research (particularly that which has no potential to directly benefit the patient). A patient's reluctance or refusal to assent should carry considerable weight when the proposed intervention is not essential to his or her welfare and/or can be deferred without substantial risk. Medical and nursing staff should respect the wishes of young patients who withhold or temporarily refuse assent in order to gain a better understanding of their situation or to come to terms with fears or other concerns regarding proposed care. "Coercion in diagnosis or treatment is a last resort."[10]

Two other legal concepts must be evaluated in the issue of informed consent of a minor. First, an "emancipated minor" is any minor who is self-supporting, not living at home, married, pregnant or a parent, in the military, or declared by the court to be emancipated. These minors are to be treated as adults on the question of informed consent. Second, a "mature minor" is an unemancipated minor who has decision-making capacity and to whom state law has granted decision-making power for treatment of specific medical conditions, such as sexually transmitted disease, pregnancy, mental health services, and drug or alcohol treatment. There appears to be no legal risk to the provider in honoring a mature adolescent's informed consent if the patient is older than 14 years old, the patient demonstrates maturity and decision-making capacity, intervention is neither a major one nor for the benefit of another, and these points are documented in the medical record.[11]

D is only 12 years old and is not an emancipated minor, and it is not clear whether she is a mature minor in this case. However, the AAP has articulated a clear position on issues of assent (dissent): "The clinical situation in which a persistent refusal to assent (dissent) may be ethically binding." The question is: can D understand the impact that nontreatment (no contraceptives) will have? Does this 12-year-old have the capacity to view her future as a mother?

Is the "substituted judgment" doctrine applicable in this case? Can the mother's demand for contraceptives for her daughter be affirmed? Lord Eldon created the substituted judgment doctrine in 1816 to permit substitute judgment for an incompetent person. Since then, it has found its way into American law. "In theory, the doctrine of substituted judgment looks to the individual to determine what she would do in a particular situation if she were competent. This doctrine works well in the situation where a person, once competent, is rendered incompetent to consent to a medical procedure."[12]

In this case, D is developing competency, including morals, beliefs, and her sense of self. At her age, without injury she cannot have obtained competency and lost it. She is in the process of gaining competency. Substituted judgment cannot be used in this case.[13]

Is the "best interest standard" applicable in this case? This standard is considered the choice a "reasonable person" would make if she were able. In the context of this standard, can D's mother demand treatment for D? The mother has determined that treatment is in D's best interest, after considering all the risks and benefits of contraceptive therapy. If D has the cognitive skills to understand and articulate her dissent from care, our Western culture recognizes that D's rights and interests must be acknowledged.[14] To uphold D's dissent or refusal of treatment depends on her ability to comprehend and appreciate her situation. It is not clear yet if the best interest standard can be applied in this case.

Quality of Life (Nonmaleficence, Beneficence, Autonomy)

Conflict between parent and adolescent is not uncommon as the adolescent develops into a young adult. As the adolescent grows, there are tremendous physical and psychological changes from ages 11 to 21 years. Becker describes four major developmental tasks:

1. Gaining independence from parents
2. Accepting body image
3. Establishing a peer group
4. Developing an identity (including a sexual, moral, religious, and vocational identity)[15]

Becker further divides psychological development of female adolescents into three categories: early adolescence, 11 to 13; middle adolescence, 14 to 17; and late adolescence, 18 to 21 years. This case focuses on the early adolescent.

Becker describes early adolescence as characterized by:

1. Decreased dependence on family
2. Body image concerns resulting in preoccupation with comparing oneself to others to answer the question "Am I normal?"
3. Increased interest in peer group (which usually involves same-sex friendships)
4. Early identity development with the first thoughts regarding future plans.[15]

These groupings may seem rigid; however, it is important to remember that some children will pass through these categories chronologically earlier or later, depending on the individual child and her or his experiences and biology.

D is 12 years old. As an early adolescent, she is seeking decreasing dependence on her family. This, in itself, can create conflict within the family. D has increased concern about body image and concern if she is "normal." She has more interest in her peer group and is affected by peer pressures. She has also started sexual experimentation and has engaged in frequent unprotected sexual intercourse with at least two males in the past year.

D has been engaging in "high-risk" behavior that can have considerable negative health outcomes. Having early sexual intercourse is frequently associated with other high-risk behaviors, such as alcohol, drug, and tobacco use. By having unprotected sexual intercourse, D is engaging in high-risk behavior that may result in a sexually transmitted disease, and she has a greater risk of becoming pregnant.

Stevens-Simon notes that adolescents who become mothers prior to age 16 have higher-risk pregnancies and their children are also at higher risk. Young adolescent mothers have higher incidence of anemia, pregnancy-induced hypertension, lower genital tract infections, cephalopelvic disproportion, puerperal complications, obesity, and hypertension. These adolescents tend to be underachievers or school failures and experience social isolation, stress, depression, and repeat pregnancy. The child of a young adolescent is more likely to be premature, have more accidental trauma, be underimmunized, and face increased risk of sudden infant death syndrome.[4]

D denies she is engaging in other high-risk behaviors. She does not smoke, drink, or use drugs. She does not engage in these activities because she does not think they will make her feel any better and she has seen how drinking and drugs have not had a good effect on some of her friends. She enjoys sex because it makes her feel good, and she finds it "wonderful." She likes being touched, close to someone, and cared for by a boy.

D's quality of life may, however, be negatively affected if she continues with her high-risk activities and if she does not avail herself of some form of birth control and protection. STDs, high-risk pregnancies, and effects on a very young mother's health have been discussed previously.

The socioeconomic impact on D if she becomes a parent at such a young age could be overwhelming for her. If she becomes pregnant, will the boy help support her and the child? How will the young man be able to provide for D and the baby? Most younger women who become pregnant and care for their children have a lower educational level and do not return to school.

Contextual Features (Justice)

Ms. L and her daughter are Native Americans and members of a small urban tribe. They live in a high-crime, low-income area of the city. Ms. L is a single mother of three children, a 17-year-old son, 12-year-old D, and another daughter who is 3. Ms. L is employed in a minimum-wage job. Their health care is provided by a tribal clinic that is operated and owned by the tribe. Tribal law is noted to have a no emancipated minors statute without exception. Unmarried pregnant adolescents become wards of the tribal court.

Just prior to coming to the clinic, D had run away from home, and Ms. L found her living with her boyfriend. Ms. L had asked D not to see the boyfriend, but D did not pay attention to the request. Ms. L was pregnant at the age of 16 and is very concerned that D not have the same difficult life Ms. L has had. Ms. L explained this to D, and D's response was that she does not mind if she gets pregnant. Many of her friends' sisters have had babies by the time they were 16.

Case Recommendations

This case presents an issue of parental concern and responsibility: the parental view that the adolescent

needs to receive a specific birth control method and the legitimate assertion of a young adolescent to refuse. The adolescent struggle for independence and the parent's concern for a responsible adolescence are an ever-present reality. However, at the beginning of the 21st century, the pressures from an ever-changing civilization and the speed of those changes have added tremendous stresses to parents and adolescents.

In this case, D is a 12-year-old sexually active adolescent engaging in frequent unprotected sex. Her mother has demanded at this clinic visit that her daughter be given Depo-Provera injections. D vigorously refuses. The ethical issues (and to some extent, legal issues) present are whether the mother of a 12-year-old can require that she receive a birth control method that the daughter has refused, and is the provider required to administer this therapy?

Because this is not a life-threatening situation, initiation of treatment can be delayed. This will give the mother, D, and the health-care provider time to further discuss the issue of contraceptives. It will also give the health-care provider time to further evaluate D's understanding of the situation.

Applying the AAP guidelines on informed consent would give D the ability to reach an appropriate developmental understanding of the nature of her condition. It would allow the provider to assess if D understands all the options of birth control, including side effects and risks. D needs to further understand the concerns about STDs and pregnancy in young adolescents. The provider can judge D's understanding of her situation, evaluate her refusal of this particular birth control method, and offer other methods she could choose. A meeting with the mother to discuss the development of cognitive skills in adolescents may help in providing the daughter a decision-making opportunity.

D has come to the provider as a patient and should receive support from the provider. The provider-patient relationship obligates the provider to be D's advocate. If the separate meetings do not resolve this situation, the provider must act as D's advocate and support the adolescent's preference and evolving autonomy[5] and her refusal of treatment.

Discussion of Mature Minor Doctrine

The focus of this discussion is to review the issue of the "mature minor" doctrine and how it affects adolescents, families, and PAs. Over the past half century, the mature minor doctrine has evolved as part of common law (law that is based on judicial cases when no statute or code exists). In recent years, many state and federal laws have codified some variations on the mature minor concept. The ethical rationale for this concept is rooted in the principle of *autonomy*, analyzed as *patient preference*, and applied as *informed consent*.

Autonomy is the principle that competent persons should be permitted self-determination.[16] An autonomous decision is one that is intentional, that is understood by the person making the decision, and that is not controlled by others who might influence and determine the action. Patient understanding does not mean complete understanding of the biomedical science. A patient usually cannot be expected to understand the full range of the biomedical spectrum of a disease. However, the patient should have a substantial comprehension of the medical choices at hand. That is your responsibility as a PA.

The PA's respect for autonomy obligates him or her to make known to the patient all the information about the issue, to make sure the patient understands the choice and its implications, and to provide a reasonable number of options to encourage effective decision making. The special fiduciary relationship developed between patient and provider obligates the provider not only to disclose information but also to provide an opportunity for dialogue; a give-and-take conversation with the patient. Autonomy also requires the provider to respect both the affirmation of treatment as well as the informed refusal of unwanted treatment.

Informed consent is the application of autonomy in the health-care setting. Reich suggests that "informed consent is a concept whose force should come not primarily from its legal necessity but rather from enhancement of good medical care."[17] Informed consent has two aspects: the process that entails *autonomous authorization for* medical intervention and the paperwork that is represented by *the social rules of consent* in institutions that must obtain written legal consent prior to a medical procedure. The two components of informed consent are analytic, including a determination that a judgment is based on competence, disclosure, understanding, voluntariness, and consent as well as a legal contract that attests to such a determination.

Competence in its core meaning is the ability to perform a task. In ethical analysis, the presumption of competence has evolved to mean a decision-making ability to agree to a specific treatment. Competence is specific to decision making rather than a global concept.[18] The competence of a person to authorize or refuse an intervention should be determined by whether that person is autonomous. Further, competence is the ability to understand the therapy, deliberate regarding the major risks and benefits, and make a decision after such deliberation.

The mature minor doctrine allows adolescents who are mature to give consent for medical care if they are able to understand the treatment and conse-

quences of medical intervention. This doctrine is an exception to the general parental consent rule. Parental consent originated from the concept of "children as property." During the Industrial Revolution, child labor and protection laws were enacted requiring parents to support, educate, and act in the child's best interest. A general rule emerged that minors were legally incompetent to make medical decisions on their own without the consent of parents.[19]

The mature minor doctrine has been addressed by the courts in decisions limiting parents' unconditional best interest rights. The Supreme Court of the United States in 1976 stated: "Constitutional rights do not mature and come into being magically; it comes about only when one attains state-defined age of majority. Minors as well as adults are protected by the Constitution and possess constitutional rights."[20]

Specific state statutes include the following criteria when defining a mature minor:

- The patient is older than 14 years.
- The patient demonstrates maturity and decision-making capacity.
- The intervention is neither major nor for the benefit of another.

The AAP, in its 1995 Statement on Informed Consent, Parental Permission, and Assent in Pediatric Practice, created a guide that provides direction for pediatricians when treating their minor patients.[10] The statement encourages decision making by older children and adolescents and recognizes that assent and refusal of assent in treatment empowers children to the extent of their capacity.

There are some concerns in the ethics community (Hardwig,[21] Nelson,[22] Foreman,[23] and Ross[24]) about the mature minor doctrine, the lack of families incorporated into the ethics paradigm, and the policy statement by AAP. These criticisms raise the issue that the concepts of best interest and autonomy are being misapplied.

Oberman[25] is concerned that the laws governing minors have evolved with societal perceptions of adolescent health-care needs and do not incorporate a comprehensive theory of adolescent capacity. There is no easily identifiable and consistent definition of maturity. Maturity is a concept influenced by many factors and consequently is difficult to measure. Oberman presents three subsets of health situations for consideration: maturity in healthy adolescents, maturity in chronically and/or critically ill adolescents, and adolescents and medical research. In presenting the three subsets, the principles of substitute judgment and autonomy are addressed. The conclusion of this analysis appears to be that without standardized criteria to evaluate maturity in an adolescent, the only way in which to apply the principles of substitute judgment and autonomy is on a case-by-case basis.

In Ross'[24] criticism of the AAP statement on informed consent,[10] the ethical principle of autonomy is argued. Ross asserts the need for *family interest* and autonomy to be present in a patient's health care decision-making. The initial criticism is that American ethical analysis places *patient autonomy* as the prime ethical principle and, in so doing, it excludes parents from participation in decisions regarding the health care of their children. The nucleus of the Ross position is that all decisions should be made within the family unit, and within that unit parents are preparing their children for adult long-term autonomous decision making. Intrusions by health-care providers and/or the state on the decision should be opposed, with the only exception being in cases of abuse or neglect. To support this position, Ross notes that no criteria exist to measure maturity or decision-making capacity. Further, for consent to be "informed," competence, disclosure, understanding, and voluntariness need to be present. Competency is context-specific, and there is no test that measures competency uniformly. Such a test is unlikely to be developed.

Ross contends that children have traditionally been considered incompetent. Respect for autonomy in health-care decision making is based both on competence and age. Three reasons to limit a child's autonomy are provided. First, children need protection while developing autonomy, and the age of emancipation is a proper age of minimal accomplishment of that task. Second, a child's lifetime world experience is limited by age. Parental assistance in acquiring world knowledge and setting life plans is an essential element in moving to autonomy. Third, when the family is "intimate," parents should have extensive options in goal setting that may "compete" and "conflict" with a single member's choices, even if those choices are apparently made with "competence." Parental decisions in the family unit for the betterment of the family should triumph over those of an individual nonemancipated member.

The essence of the Ross argument in a parent-child disagreement in health-care decisions is that third-party involvement in the decision-making process *undermines the family*. A health-care provider is concerned only for the child's transient medical needs whereas the parents provide for all the other needs and are responsible for raising a responsible child who will become an autonomous decision maker.

Hardwig[21] presents the theory that benevolence and patient autonomy are rooted in fidelity. Benevolence and patient autonomy must be rejected or drastically changed to support family values and incorporate the family unit into the ethical analysis of treatment decisions. The focus of the health-care provider must move from single-patient orientation to family orientation. Hardwig argues the interests of the family and patient are morally equal.

Nelson[22] essentially agrees with Hardwig and argues that present-day biomedical ethical analysis obscures the family. The family unit should have a major moral weight. Nelson presents the questions of why families matter, the vulnerability of family values, medical decision making as if relationships matter, and reviews the incompetence and intimacy concerns. The center of Nelson's line of reasoning maintains that decision making in health care makes a difference to the family unit and that ethical analysis must include families in the paradigm.

Foreman[23] takes the involvement of family into the analysis one step further in the British health system and provides a theoretical "family rule" and "framework" to acquire ethical consent from children. The family rule states that "informed consent in children and their families should be regarded as shared between children and their families, the balance determined by implicit, developmentally based negotiations between child and parent."[23] The family rule "diffuses" the child's right to consent by deliberations between the parent and child. Foreman argues that this diffusion allows respect for the child's autonomy within the parameters of "the rule."

Alderson[26] comments that Foreman's "family rule" will interlope on already complex and diffuse laws and weaken the competent minor status, especially in cases of parent-adolescent conflict. The criticism continues that "family rule" complicates matters by "increasing adult power over children" and decreasing dialogue with children. The outcome of this could be forced treatment of children who dissent "it seems up to the age of 18 years."[12]

The essence of Foreman's[27] reply to Alderson is that the "family rule" would provide a structure of professional practice that would address her concerns. Ultimately, "[T]he law can then step in, as in other circumstances, when this practice has been negligently observed."

Hardwig, Nelson, Foreman, and Ross present an alternative or addition to the present structure of bioethical analysis, which includes the family unit as an intricate party in the decision-making process and suggests that family be incorporated into the paradigm.

Conclusion

The issues of the "mature minor" doctrine and how it affects adolescents, their families, and PAs is very complex and often similar to watching a movie of the adolescent's life, but needing to take a snapshot of a specific heath-care incident that depends on the child's maturity and decision-making capacity at that moment. In respecting the autonomy of the adolescent, numerous factors need to be assessed in the ever-changing internal environment of the adolescent and the external environment of the family and society. If respect for adolescent autonomy is the goal, the health-care provider and the family need to work collaboratively to fulfill that goal. In evaluating competency, decision-making capacity, and maturity in a health-care setting, it is incumbent upon the PA to make available to the adolescent all the information needed in a dialogue that enables the adolescent to make the decision in an informed and consensual manner. This includes the ability to weigh information and consider the future impact of the decision.

Families cannot be ignored in the process. However, incorporating the family into the ethical paradigm, especially when a parent-adolescent conflict exists, is problematic. The intimate family unit has more than one member, and all members do not have an equal voice. By adding the family to the paradigm, would the family unit be analyzed as a single voice in the analytic process? This is unclear. Traditionally, in American bioethical analysis, autonomy and patient preference have rested on the one-to-one dialogue between the patient and provider. To require the addition of a third party, the family unit, into the final decision making would demand a major change in the paradigm.

The "mature minor" doctrine applied in family practice with a parent-adolescent conflict is not an unusual situation. The provider must ensure that the adolescent understands the treatment (or nontreatment) and consequences of medical intervention.

The provider should evaluate this on a case-by-case basis. The inclusion of the family should be made to the extent possible. This is a natural part of a family practice. The conundrum presented in a family practice, however, is how to respect the wishes of all the members of the family. The AAP policy statement[6] provides a guide. When parent-child conflicts exist, the provider must respect the adolescent's autonomy. In family practice, the ongoing relationship of the provider, family, and individual family members is usually stable. The dialogue with the family will continue. If the parent-adolescent health-care conflict is not life-threatening, a delay in the decision may well assist in the dialogue and strengthen the understanding of both the adolescent and parent. This approach will maintain respect for the autonomy of the adolescent. Embracing and incorporating a family rule in this process would undermine an already tense relationship among the provider, the adolescent, and the family.

In the case analysis of D and her mother, sparse literature exists on refusal of contraceptive care for a minor when the parent demands a specific treatment be given. If the provider acquiesced to the request of the mother and administered this treatment while the adolescent adamantly refused, the further issues of battery and abuse could be raised in this case. Alderson[27] made an eloquent statement about refusal of treatment by adolescents: "It is frequently remarked 'children cannot refuse treatment.' Of course they can refuse, no law can stop them. The question is whether the doctor should override their refusal, legally or morally." This is a tremendous issue for all health-care providers and for patients and their families.

CASE 2

Somatizing Patient

Case Presentation

Ms. A is a 40-year-old woman who has been a patient in a managed care organization (MCO), more specifically a nonprofit health maintenance organization (HMO). She has a long history of unexplained, persisting medical complaints consisting of abdominal pain, pelvic pain, nausea, vomiting, dehydration, fatigue, lightheadedness, and depression. Her abdominal and pelvic pain

started 2 years ago. She has had multiple abdominal surgeries, which include a laparotomy, appendectomy, and cholecystectomy.

She has been seeing her psychiatrist weekly for the past 7 years. The psychiatrist is not a provider member of the HMO; however, the HMO approved this care. She reports a long series of hidden memory recoveries in therapy. These memories include both emotional and physical abuse by family members, teachers, professionals, and tradesmen. She reports having developed a very dependent feeling for the therapist.

Ms. A has described some of these hidden memories to her primary care provider. Some examples are: "The bus driver was so mean today. I remember him molesting me when I was a child." and "I saw a man selling vegetable peelers on TV. I remember him molesting me." At her most recent physical examination Ms. A's data were: blood pressure 130/88, pulse 90 and regular, respirations 16, temperature 98°F, weight 220 pounds, and height 61 inches. She is oriented to time, place, and person. When she first appeared for her examination, she was on the table sobbing, partially doubled over and gripping the sides. When the examination started, she stopped crying and started discussing her newest stuffed animal. Her examination results were normal, except for the abdominal portion. Her protuberant abdomen has well-healed midline and left lower quadrant surgical scars. No masses or organomegaly were noted. There was tenderness in the left lower quadrant on superficial palpation. On deep palpation with the patient distracted, there was no pain. No rebound tenderness was present. Psoas and obturator signs were negative. There was no costovertebral angle tenderness. The pelvic examination was benign, with no masses or tenderness. The stool guaiac result was negative.

Ms. A has had extensive diagnostic testing for her past abdominal and pelvic pain. The tests included multiple abdominal and pelvic ultrasounds and CT and MRI scans, all of whose results were negative.

Ms. A's daily activities include walking in malls, shopping, preparing her own meals, and doing some light housework (dishes, dusting, and laundry). She lives with her elderly mother, whose relationship she treasures, and she is single.

Her problem list includes depression, somatoform disorder, false memory syndrome, and obesity. Because of a gait disturbance caused by foot pain secondary to obesity, she was put on 100% disability by the non-HMO psychiatrist 6 years ago.

Her medications include Compazine 5 mg qid, Imodium 2 mg qid, Prozac 20 mg qd, Imipramine 75 mg HS, Tylenol 325 mg, three prn for pain.

Ms. A frequently refuses to cooperate with the primary care team in the investigation of pathology or to establish new therapeutic goals, such as rejoining the workforce. Ms. A cites the advice of her therapist as the rationale for refusal. She averages four to six medical care visits per month. She has refused all efforts by the primary care team to refer her for re-evaluation to the HMO mental health services.

The question asked by the primary care providers is would it be ethical to interrupt the outside psychiatric care, reevaluate, and potentially refuse further reimbursement outside the HMO?

Medical Indications (Beneficence, Nonmaleficence)

Ms. A's diagnoses of depression, somatization, and false memory syndrome carry significant morbidity and potential iatrogenic ramifications. Somatization is the occurrence of unintentional, unexplainable physical symptoms because of emotional distress or stressful life situations. The physical symptoms have no physiological explanation. Somatization is not a discrete disease but rather a group of symptoms that are not reflected in objective evaluations. Manifestations of somatization can range from minimal (overstated complaints of common stress-related symptoms of headache, low back pain, or lightheadedness) to severe, causing debilitating and overwhelming pain and disability.[1,2] In almost all cases, the symptoms appear in healthy-looking individuals. The diagnosis of somatoform disorder must include the presence of three or more vague or exaggerated symptoms, often in multiple body systems. Their occurrence must be chronic.[1] Ms. A's chronic symptoms described in the case presentation included abdominal pain, pelvic pain, nausea, vomiting, dehydration, fatigue, and lightheadedness. This fulfills the criteria for somatization.

The pathophysiology of somatization is not clear, and there are no apparent studies that identify the etiology of such pathophysiology. There are four mechanisms of symptom formation that are frequently identified.[1,3] The four mechanisms appear to apply in Ms. A's case:

1. The "amplification of bodily sensations" refers to common minor body irritations that the patient magnifies so much that they become unpleasant, intense, and disturbing.

2. The "identified patient" occurs when a family structure under stress identifies a single member as a patient in order to stabilize the family structure. The family member assumes the role of a chronically ill patient.

3. The "need to be sick" causes somatizing patients to prefer the sick role during stress because it can relieve unattainable interpersonal expectations. In many societies the "sick role" produces caring and support. The need to be sick is not malingering (knowingly faking symptoms). The patient is not aware of the process that causes the symptoms and cannot will them away; the patient sincerely suffers. Barsky expresses the dilemma of the somatic patient and provider: "There is no pill that can cure, and no surgery that can excise, the need to be sick."[3]

4. "Disassociation" is the mind's ability to have sensation in the absence of actual sensory stimulation. This can include feelings of depersonalization (feeling one is not oneself) or out-of-body experiences. The somatizing patient tends to experience disassociation more often than other psychiatric conditions.

It is not uncommon for providers to find the "reverse funnel-down effect" in somatizing patients. In the normal process of diagnosis, the provider funnels to fewer and fewer diagnostic possibilities as the inquiry proceeds. In the somatic patient, the further the investigation goes, the greater the number of possible disorders that are found.[4]

The first obligation of Ms. A's providers in managing her somatization is to understand and truly appreciate that the patient is suffering from an illness. Although the symptoms may appear overstated, the suffering is at all times real. The treatment plan should consist of regularly scheduled clinic visits. Patient adherence to the schedule is important. In the beginning, visits may need to be more frequent. The provider should explain to the patient that consistent, regularly scheduled visits are necessary to address the present symptoms and any new ones. This will provide the patient with boundaries while allowing interaction with the provider and the "laying on of hands," which in itself is therapeutic.[5] The BATHE technique[6] is a helpful way to structure the visit.[5]

Treating the somatizing patient such as Ms. A is a challenge for most primary care providers in this time of short visits and production quotas. However, a solid relationship with a single provider, often in consultation with a mental health provider, is the basis for successful management of somatizing patients. Prognosis for a cure is poor. Longitudinal follow-up studies have confirmed that 80% to 90% of patients initially diagnosed with somatization disorder maintain a consistent clinical picture.[7,8] Coping with the symptoms through a supportive provider-patient relationship decreases morbidity and potential iatrogenic complications.

Patient Preference (Autonomy)

Ms. A strongly believes her sessions with the psychiatrist are helpful. She has told her primary care provider that she has recovered a number of "hidden memories" during her session with the psychiatrist and has worked with him on how best to address those memories.

Ms. A finds the care of the primary care team members more than acceptable, believes she can confide in them, and trusts their medical care. She disagrees with the primary care provider's suggestion about her mental health care. Her concern is that she will not receive the same amount of care by the HMO mental health service equal to that of her present psychiatrist. She is very concerned about establishing a trusting rapport with a new therapist. It has taken 7 years to create a trusting therapeutic relationship with her present therapist.

She refuses to go to the mental health service within the HMO for a second opinion and possible therapy within the HMO. She has been referred a number of times by various providers without success. Ms. A believes that her psychiatrist understands her and she sees no reason to leave his care.

Quality of Life (Nonmaleficence, Beneficence, Autonomy)

Ms. A has been a member of the HMO for over a decade. The primary care team at the HMO has provided her continuity of care. A non-HMO psychiatrist has provided her mental heath care for 7 years.

She has been diagnosed with somatoform disorder and depression. Her depression is being treated with medication and talk therapy. The primary care team is addressing her somatization, but with minimal success. As a result of foot pain caused by her obesity, her psychiatrist has placed her on 100% disability. Her foot pain is constant, and she is unable to walk more than 50 feet. She must stop to allow her pain to decrease to a tolerable level before walking again. The pain started about 6 years ago. After a significant work-up including x-ray and MRI, no pathology was identified. Her job had included significant walking and time on her feet.

Ms. A's quality of life is severely affected by her physical and psychological afflictions. If effective therapy is not identified, Ms. A has the potential of iatrogenic complications. She is also at a higher risk of morbidity from undiagnosed true pathological conditions. This would further cause deterioration in her quality of life.

Contextual Features (Justice)

Ms. A averages four to six patient care visits per month. In the course of addressing her primary care complaints (which usually involve some variant of emotional crisis or abdominal or pelvic pain), the providers were frustrated by her refusal to cooperate with follow-up investigation of suspected pathology. The staff and providers dread her visits. The visits frequently go beyond the allotted appointment time. This tends to bog down the schedule and cause appointment delays for other patients. Ms. A frequently bursts into tears at the visits when describing a personal unfairness suffered during the week or another hidden memory revealed during therapy.

There is also serious tension between the psychiatrist and the primary care team. The therapist's advice has constantly countered the primary care team's advice. The primary care team provided two examples.

First, the primary care team would set a goal for Ms. A, such as returning to the workforce. It appeared to the primary care team that if Ms. A was able to walk the malls and shop for 3 to 4 hours per day, this activity was consistent with the ability to work at least part-time and gradually increase to longer hours. In telephone conversations and written communications with the primary care team and in sessions with the patient, the therapist would dismiss the idea. The therapist insisted that such a goal would place unrealistic and counterproductive expectations on Ms. A.

Second, the therapist advised Ms. A that whenever she was nauseated, she was probably dehydrated and should go the HMO urgent care center for rehydration. This resulted in repeated visits to the urgent care center. Upon arrival, Ms. A would be evaluated for dehydration, which was never present. When the negative results of the evaluation were presented to the patient, she created such a scene demanding intravenous fluids that it became easier to give her intravenous fluids than to continue unsuccessful dialogue. This resulted in petulant phone calls from the urgent care center to the primary care team. A patient care conference with the urgent care team, the primary care team, and the psychiatrist was arranged. The psychiatrist refused to attend. The consensus at the conference was that the driving force behind Ms. A's visits to the urgent care center was the psychiatrist's advice. Dialogue between the teams and the psychiatrist to limit the urgent care visits was unsuccessful.

QUESTIONS FOR DISCUSSION

1. What are the medical and ethical issues in Ms. A's care?
2. Does the primary care team have a "right" to require Ms. A to see HMO psychiatrists?
3. Is it ethical to put limits on her care outside of routine visits?
4. How would you handle a patient ethically who does not follow your recommendations?
5. Is there something that can be done about the outside therapist's unwillingness to meet with the primary care team? (This is more a professional and legal question but a valid one.)

Case Recommendations

Continuity of care for patients with somatization is essential for proper management of this condition. The tension between the HMO and the psychiatrist is not beneficial for Ms. A. The main ethical issue to be addressed is, as stated earlier, would it be ethical to interrupt the outside psychiatric care, reevaluate, and potentially refuse further reimbursement outside the HMO?

There are two ethical principles in this case; First is the principle of autonomy,[9] and the second is justice.[10] The issue of autonomy requires that Ms. A be given a choice about her care. The principle of justice, fairness, what is deserved, and entitlement requires a look at the issue from within the nonprofit HMO providing care for the patient. A nonprofit HMO, unlike for-profit managed care systems, accommodates the need of human biology, with a perspective toward the full life span. Success is best defined by healthy outcomes and improved quality of life.[11]

Three distributive justice theories should be considered when investigating the nonprofit HMO's distribution of health resources. They include the utilitarian theory, the libertarian theory, and the egalitarian theory.

In applying the theories to the nonprofit HMO and its members, the following applies. The utilitarian theory considers that the welfare of the members takes precedence over the welfare of the individual.

The egalitarian theory holds that all members are created equal and deserve to share resources equally or that resources should be given to the members who have the greatest need. The libertarian theory provides access to benefits available based on members' ability to pay.

Providing full-spectrum care within the nonprofit HMO system reflects two of the six material principles of justice, "to each person an equal share" and "to each person according to need." Care is provided to all members of the HMO system within the budget of the system. Care outside the system is discouraged and must be approved by the organization. Justice to each member of the HMO requires that all members have equal access within the system but not necessarily outside the HMO organization.

Taking the principles of autonomy and justice and applying them to Ms. A's case, the following points should be considered.:

1. One primary care provider is selected as Ms. A's only primary care provider.
2. A mental health provider within the HMO is to be assigned to Ms. A.
3. The primary care provider, the mental health provider, and the non-HMO psychiatrist meet at the request of the ethics committee in order to:
   • Explore with Ms. A her choice to work within the HMO system for her care
   • Address all the issues involved in continuing to see the non-HMO psychiatrist and the possibility that this would be at her own expense.

This recommendation also ensures that Ms. A has mental health care coverage as needed. By providing Ms. A with a single primary care provider, in consultation with an HMO mental health provider, she will have a better chance of continuity and consistency in the management of her somatoform disorder and other health-care needs.

Discussion Point

Does this approach seem reasonable to you? What do you believe are other options?

Case Discussion

MCOs are providing a substantial portion of health-care delivery in the United States at the beginning of the 21st century. A question that continues to agitate providers is how can the patient-physician relationship continue to be an ethical undertaking in a managed care system?

MCOs attempt to modify the behavior of physicians and consumers in the delivery and consumption of health care. MCOs by their nature undertake the task of health cost containment within their organization. This can change the traditional patient-physician relationship to the physician-payer-patient relationship. This is the essence of the ethical question.

The patient-physician relationship can be strengthened or weakened by any of the reimbursement schemes within an MCO setting. Under the traditional fee-for-service system, the physician was not limiting care. But one major focal point within MCOs is to reduce patient health-care costs.

The ethical principle of fidelity and the accepted tenet of veracity are the bedrock of the patient-physician relationship.[12] Fidelity is often used within the context of the principles of justice, autonomy, and utility. Fidelity in an ethical framework is classically associated with voluntary promises, commitments, and oaths. Being true to one's word is the core premise of fidelity. The standard of fidelity rests on the values of loyalty, trust, and promise-keeping. In the physician-patient relationship, truthfulness and confidence are combined with fidelity to form the basis of the relationship.

Contained within the patient-physician relationship is a contract that the patient makes with the physician to secure the rights to truth in connection with diagnosis, prognosis, procedures, and treatment. The physician's contract with the patient requires the right to truthfulness from the patient.

Veracity within the relationship relates to *any* truthful and honest management of information that may affect a patient's comprehension or decision making. It is not limited to informed consent.[7]

Fiduciary and loyalty responsibilities consist of two parts. First, the physician assistant (PA) removes self-interest in any conflict with the patient's interests. Second, the patient's interest takes priority over the interests of any others. This applies not only to the physician's personal interest but also to the interests of other patients.[13,14] The patient's interest is primary because the power relationship between the physician and the patient is inherently unequal. The patient lacks access to and knowledge of diagnosis and therapy.

The physician's fiduciary responsibility and veracity are put to the test in MCOs where dual loyalties present themselves. With limited resources, the physician must balance the loyalty required by individual patients with the needs of other patients within the practice. On the other hand, the physician's personal financial needs depend on the financial incentives of the MCO. Many times these incentives include bonuses for keeping costs down. This increased pressure to ration care puts the physician in an ethical predicament.

Physicians who are placed in the situation to make these "bedside" rationing decisions are at a significant disadvantage. They usually do not have all the information needed to make such decisions. The decisions can be inconsistent from physician to physician, and physicians have no special expertise in how to ration health care. As each physician is compelled to make these rationing decisions, patients soon understand the situation and become distrustful of the provider. The patient's trust in the physician is damaged. Traditionally, physicians in a fee-for-service system have not been placed in this situation.

Conversely, the traditional notion of the physician being unaware of the benefits or risks of the costs of therapy may no longer be valid. Escalating healthcare costs and a cost-containment frame of mind make it necessary for physicians to be aware of these factors and to disclose them to individual patients in their shared decision making. In today's environment, it is the physician, not the manager, who should make the rationing decision, even at the bedside. The physician at the bedside should make the overriding ethical rationing decisions while considering his or her fiduciary and loyalty responsibilities.[13]

The traditional patient-physician relationship has been gravely altered by managed care as it exists today. There will be many more patients joining MCOs as Medicare and Medicaid persuade higher enrollment of their beneficiaries. This will affect more and more patients and providers. The patient-physician relationship for the past hundred years has been a one-to-one fiduciary relationship where veracity was paramount.

If one were to look at that relationship in geometric terms, it has been a linear, two-dimensional relationship. In today's climate, the relationship is now three-dimensional, a patient-payer-physician triad. In a linear two-dimensional relationship, all the geometric space is covered by the physician's fiduciary relationship. In the new three-dimensional configuration, not only are there three parties but also the area the relationship covers is cubed. The increased depth of space is much larger than the fiduciary relationship can cover. This is especially true in a for-profit managed care system. In that system, the patient-physician relationship has been turned into a commodity. The space within the cube, if not enclosed by ethical responsibility, is a void waiting to be filled, ethically or not.

There have been numerous papers written about managed care in the 1990s. There have not been many that have addressed how to fill that void in an ethical manner. However, a few papers have looked at ethical models to address this issue. Smith[15] describes 10 goals MCOs should adopt:

1. Place patient interests above all.
2. Promote personal and longitudinal relationships between patients and physicians.
3. Value the collaborative relationship between primary care and subspecialists.
4. Be committed to caring for the needs of a stable group of patients over time.

5. Communicate with patients in terms they can understand.
6. Focus on disease prevention.
7. Consider high-quality care to be both effective and affordable.
8. Measure outcomes to monitor and improve quality of care.
9. Base financial incentives on patient outcomes instead of on quality of care.
10. Value and support education and research.

These goals could fill the void and provide an ethical patient-physician relationship.

Christensen[16] presents an ethical model that would provide quality care. The institution should be nonprofit to remove shareholder and profit maximization. Physicians should be salaried to reduce the issue of bedside rationing. Group- or staff-model HMOs fulfill these criteria. Share the risk of capitation across a large group of physicians. Physicians should manage clinical practice. Physicians need to be involved with utilization review and quality management. Physicians should be closely involved in the creation and implementation of practice guidelines. Patients or members of the MCO should be involved in the operations of the organization at multiple levels.

This model would also reduce the ethical pressure on the patient-payer-physician triad in an MCO to ration at the bedside by implementing guidelines that assist in rationed care.

Emanuel and Dubler[17] provide an "ideal" ethical conception of the patient-physician relationship in an MCO by six Cs: choice, competence, communication, compassion, continuity, and (no) conflict of interest.

Choice is essential in an ethical patient-physician relationship. The choices include choice of practice, primary care physician, specialist, and treatment alternatives if there is more than one treatment with equivalent outcomes for a condition. Competence includes four elements: a good fund of current knowledge, technical skills, clinical judgment, and known limitations with a willingness to consult. Communications consist of the physician listening and understanding the patient and communicating that understanding. The patient is able to tell the physician what information he or she does and does not want or need to know. The physician has the ability to tell patients in an comprehensible way the nature of the disease, diagnosis, and treatment as well as how the treatment supports or undermines the patient's core values. Compassion consists of an empathetic physician who understands the patient's troubles. Continuity offers a relationship that continues over time, and the physician recognizes the changes that evolve in the patient's values and feelings. (No) conflict of interest means that the physician's primary concern is for the patient's well-being, even though the physician may have obligations that conflict. These obligations could include caring for another patient, interests of a third party, or the physician's own interests, especially financial considerations.

Smith, Christensen, and Emanuel present similar and complementary models for implementation of an ethical way to deliver health care that preserves the principle of fidelity and the precept of veracity, which are the foundation of the patient-physician relationship. The commonality among all three is that they are patient-centered and eliminate or minimize conflicts of interest. If these were the concepts used to fill the void, a reasonable "ideal" within the MCO environment may possibly be achieved.

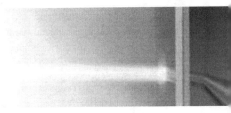

CASE 3

Addiction and Autonomy

Case Presentation

Ms. Z is a 50-year-old single woman who is a patient at a community health center clinic. The clinic staff has cared for her for the past 5 years. Before that time, she had her health care provided by the county hospital. Ms. Z has had an alcohol addiction (abuse) problem since the age of 18. Her present multiple medical problems can be attributed to her 32-year history of alcohol abuse. She is currently skeptical about long-term (1-year) inpatient treatment of her alcoholism.

Since she has been a patient at the community health center clinic, she has been admitted to the hospital 23 times, has visited the emergency room at least 14 times, has had 5 ICU admissions, has been at the alcohol rehabilitation center for 30-day treatment 3 times, and has attended extended-care facilities for medical rehabilitation 3 times. She has had visiting nurse services almost continuously for the past 3 years.

Her latest admission was for a gastrointestinal bleed. Her problem list at discharge included the following: seizure activity secondary to decreased calcium and magnesium, aspiration pneumonia, hypertension, Kisselman's syndrome, acute and chronic alcohol abuse, chronic pancreatitis with malabsorption, multiple fractures due to falls: femoral fracture in 1997, humeral fracture in 1999, pubis fracture in 2000, and head trauma due to falls; glaucoma; cholelithiasis, postmenopause, tobacco use 25 pack years, history of esophageal cancer, status post esophagectomy and gastric pull through 1997, history of pneumonia resulting in adult respiratory distress syndrome (ARDS), chronic renal insufficiency, and anemia.

Her current medications include Lansoprazole 30 mg qd, Atenolol 100 mg qd, folic acid 1 mg qd, multivitamin 1 qd, amlodipine besylate 5 mg qd, Prempro 0.625/2.5 mg, Pancreatin 1 qd, magnesium oxide 420 mg tid, Timoptic eye drops both eyes qd.

Ms. Z's activities of daily living have been diminished due to her pubis fracture. She has an unstable gait. She also has hygiene challenges and needs reminders by a visiting nurse service about self-care issues.

The clinic staff is concerned about Ms. Z's competence. On her admission to the county hospital in 2003, she had a complete psychiatric evaluation. The psychiatrist believes she understands that her alcohol dependence has grave medical complications and risks. The psychiatrist believes she is competent and can refuse a 1-year inpatient alcohol treatment.

The physician assistant at the community health center clinic is frustrated in her effort to provide the best care for Ms. Z, and she asks the question: "Can we ethically admit her to a 1-year inpatient alcohol treatment center against her will when we think it is in her best interest? We have a good idea from our experience that she will die of alcohol-related complications if they are not treated. Is someone who is dependent/addicted to alcohol able to make such a decision?"

Medical Indications (Beneficence, Nonmaleficence)

Ms. Z has had an alcohol dependence problem for 32 years. Her present medical condition and complications can be attributed to her alcohol use.

Alcohol dependence is defined in the *Diagnostic and Statistical Manual of Mental Disorders,* Fourth Edition (DSM-IV). The definition states that physiological dependence on alcohol is indicated by evidence of tolerance or symptoms of withdrawal: "Dependence is described as a maladaptive pattern of substance use leading to clinically significant impairment or distress."[1] Three or more of the following seven factors occurring in a 12-month period are indicative:

- Tolerance needing increased amount of substance to maintain desired effect or diminished effect using the same amount of substance
- Withdrawal
- Increased amount of substance taken over a longer period than intended
- Persistent desire or unsuccessful efforts to cut down on use
- Significant time is devoted to obtaining substance
- Reduction of or giving up occupational, social, or recreational activities because of use
- The substance use is continued despite knowledge of having persistent psychological or physical damage caused or exacerbated by substance

Diamond and Jay[2] describe alcoholism as characterized by addiction to ethanol. They describe alcoholism in the medical setting as a chronic disease in which the patient craves and consumes ethanol uncontrollably and has signs and symptoms of withdrawal when drinking ceases.

QUESTIONS FOR DISCUSSION

1. Does Ms. Z meet these criteria? Describe the points in her history that support your answer.

2. Is Ms. Z competent to make her own decisions (autonomy)?

3. Does inpatient treatment offer any advantages over outpatient treatment? (Look for data that support you answer.)

4. Considering her current health status, will inpatient treatment prolong her life?

Continued Discussion

Ms. Z fulfills the diagnostic criteria for alcohol dependence/addiction. Treatment for her chronic alcoholism could decrease some of her present disease state. She could decrease her falls, electrolyte imbalances, seizures, aspiration pneumonia, and many of her other problems.

Inpatient and residential treatment for at least 1 year has been recommended. Hanna[3] suggests that inpatient treatment has no distinct advantage over outpatient treatment, except in special cases. Such cases include people who are medically compromised by complications of alcohol abuse and those with disintegrated social networks. Walsh and others[4] conducted one of the few recent randomized clinical trials of alcohol treatment and explain the successful inpatient treatment of specific populations.

Weiss[5] presents the rationale for inpatient treatment of substance-dependent patients. Medically managed intensive inpatient services can provide top-quality medical supervision for multiple medical problems in combination with alcohol detoxification. Mee-Lee et al[6] identified six areas to assess for admission for inpatient treatment: (1) acute intoxication and/or withdrawal potential, (2) biomedical conditions and complications, (3) emotional and behavioral complications, (4) treatment acceptance or resistance, (5) relapse potential, and (6) recovery environment. One final consideration when assessing inpatient treatment is whether the patient poses a threat of harm to self or others and what is the likelihood of achieving treatment success in a less restricted environment.

Medically managed intensive inpatient services usually consist of stabilization of medical conditions including detoxification, nutritional deficiencies, and organ damage secondary to ethanol intake. Intensive psychotherapy treatment with individual and group therapy, and often peer confrontation, are included. In addition, combined pharmacotherapy for anxiety and depression is prescribed. Bunn and colleagues[7] found that patients who completed an extended formal inpatient alcoholism treatment had lower mortality rates 3 years after discharge than patients who had shorter inpatient stays. This coincides with Simpson's[8] findings that inpatient or outpatient treatment of fewer than 90 days resulted in more frequent relapse than those of more than 90 days.

Ms. Z has grave chronic medical illnesses. She has multiple hospital admissions and emergency room visits, intensive care unit admissions, 1-month alcohol rehabilitation admissions, and admissions to extended-care facilities for medical rehabilitation in the past 5 years, and she continues to drink alcohol. Without discontinuation of her alcohol intake, she will most likely die from the resulting organ damage.

Her best chance to control her alcohol dependence is admission to medically managed intensive inpatient services, followed by supervised residential placement. To date, she has refused long-term inpatient therapy.

Patient Preference (Autonomy)

Ms. Z has been seen in clinic on at least a monthly basis requesting treatment of her health problems. She has been admitted to the emergency department and hospital numerous times in the past 5 years seeking treatment of the presenting medical condition. On her recent admission to the hospital the issue of resuscitation was discussed, and she requested all means of care be given to her in regard to mechanical therapeutics to keep her alive.

In addition, an evaluation by a psychiatrist found her oriented to time, place, and person. The psychiatrist further believes Ms. Z understands that her long history of alcohol dependence has led to grave medical complications and that she faces risks from continued use. She is able to describe the consequences of *not* receiving long-term inpatient treatment, including death from potential complications of her alcohol dependence, such as pneumonia and acute respiratory distress syndrome. The psychiatrist believes she is competent and can refuse a 1-year inpatient alcohol treatment. There has been no change in that opinion to date.

Ms. Z has had at least three admissions to month-long alcohol treatment centers for her alcoholism, and each time she relapsed after discharge. It was recommended to her after the last hospital admission and clinic visit that she be admitted to an inpatient and residential treatment center for at least 90 days and up to 1 year. Her response was "no." Her rationale was that a 1-month treatment had not worked, so how could a longer admission and treatment help?

Ms. Z, at some level, wants good health as demonstrated by coming to the clinic. However, she also demonstrates poor health, as shown by her behavior of alcohol abuse. On the surface it may appear rational; Ms. Z argues she can have alcohol only if she refuses inpatient treatment; so she refuses inpatient treatment. In a broader sense, she wants good health *and* bad health. This is in keeping with addictive judgment. Hazelton, Sterns, and Chisholm[9] discuss in great detail decision-making capacity and

ethical considerations in their paper "Decision-Making Capacity and Alcohol Abuse: Clinical and Ethical Considerations in Personal Care Choices." This paper indicates that people who abuse alcohol frequently deny abuse or the consequent health problems. It is unclear if this is solely related to the patient's personal defense mechanism or the toxic effect of alcohol on the nervous system.

"Competency" and "capacity" are frequently used interchangeably, and this can cause confusion. They are not the same. Competency is a legal process presented and determined in a court of law evaluating the individual's ability "having significant ability…possessing the requisite natural or legal qualifications" to engage in a given endeavor.[9,10]

Capacity may be a part of that process. A healthcare provider, usually a psychiatrist, assesses an individual's ability to form a rational decision. Capacity is the ability to take in information, understand, assess, and form a rational decision from that information.

Capacities should be evaluated for specific tasks or responsibilities. One of these tasks is executive cognitive function: the ability to organize and plan, foresight, self-regulation, and self-awareness. In chronic alcohol abusers, this executive cognitive function is often significantly impaired.[11] The evaluation of executive brain function as part of an assessment is of value.[12] Language and visual-spatial function in the alcohol abuser are spared in the majority of cases. When the mental status test is performed, an assessment may be overestimated. Nadler, Richardson, and Malloy[12] have shown that executive cognitive function deficits have a predictive value in personal care competency. This executive cognitive function may well effect readiness to change drinking behavior.[13] Thus, poor executive functioning will usually have poor personal care competency. This may be the issue in Ms. Z's case.

She has been encouraged by her sister, primary care provider, psychiatrist, social work caseworker, and nursing staff to be admitted for the extended alcohol treatment, and she continues to refuse to do so.

Quality of Life (Beneficence, Nonmaleficence, Autonomy)

Ms. Z's quality of life is impaired by her alcohol abuse. Quality of life is an observation of another. Nevertheless, the observation has a subjective analysis by the provider who has knowledge of the physical costs of continued alcohol abuse in this case, which must be addressed to the family and patient in as detailed a manner as possible. Ms. Z finds her quality of life acceptable if she is able to continue to drink just some alcohol.

If Ms. Z's alcohol dependence is not treated, she will continue to deteriorate. The consequences to her quality of life may include the following sequelae of alcohol damage to her body and mind. If she continues to have acute intoxication episodes, she will have more blackouts, a condition when she will appear to be alert and functioning but does not have an active memory of or ability to recall events for some period. Motor impairment will result in falls and head injuries, with possible subdural hematoma. Losing consciousness will increase the potential of aspiration pneumonia. Her chronic alcohol use can result in Wernicke-Korsakoff syndrome, a condition with cerebellar degeneration, peripheral neuropathy, cerebral atrophy, and dementia. Her liver disease will cause further deterioration, with alcoholic hepatitis, portal hypertension, cirrhosis, and hepatic encephalopathy. Hepatic injury can also decrease clotting factors and, with esophageal varices and bleeding, can cause her death. The increased incidents of withdrawal bring with them the expectation of the full syndrome of delirium tremens (DT), which has a 10%-15% mortality rate.

The rate of esophageal cancer is increased by 75% in chronic alcoholism. Ms. Z has had one episode of an esophageal tumor. There also appears to be a link with chronic alcoholism and increased incidents of breast, colon, and liver cancer. Psychiatric complications are significant from chronic alcohol ingestion, which include chronic depression with increased incidents of suicide. In Ms. Z's present alcohol-dependent state, her quality of life appears to be worsening and without successful treatment will continue to deteriorate.

Medically managed intensive inpatient services will include detoxification. Detoxification can be very uncomfortable if the patient is not cared for and well managed. Of patients being detoxified, about 5% suffer from DT.

There are frequently minor withdrawal symptoms, which can include insomnia, tremulousness, mild anxiety, gastrointestinal upset, headache, diaphoresis, palpitations, or anorexia. Symptoms are usually present within 6 hours of the cessation of drinking and may develop while patients still have a significant alcohol level in their blood. Findings resolve within 24 to 48 hours.

Withdrawal-associated seizures in long-term alcohol abusers are not uncommon and are generalized tonic-clonic convulsions that usually occur within 48 hours after the last drink and may occur after only 2 hours of abstinence.

Alcoholic hallucinosis develops within 12 to 24 hours of abstinence and resolves within 24 to 48 hours. Hallucinations are usually visual, although auditory and tactile phenomena may also occur.

In the short term, Ms. Z's quality of life will be negatively affected by withdrawal. In the long term, she could face intensive psychotherapy treatment with individual and group therapy and often peer confrontations. Her end organ alcohol damage will not resolve. Again, Ms. Z considers her present quality of life reasonable if she has her alcohol.

Contextual Features (Justice, Loyalty, and Fairness)

The contextual features of this case can be divided into three categories:

1. The effect on Ms. Z's family
2. The tension with the clinic and staff
3. The pressure of finite resources in her community

Ms. Z is single, her parents have died, and her sister, Ms. Y, is her only living relative in the community. Her sister has found Ms. Z in various degrees of disarray. The most recent incident occurred when Ms. Y, unable to contact Ms. Z by phone, went to her sister's home and found her unconscious, incoherent, and smelling of alcohol in a fecal- and blood-smeared apartment. Ms. Y called the paramedics, who transported Ms. Z to the county hospital. After cleaning the apartment, Ms. Y is at her "wit's end" and not sure how much longer she can be of assistance if her sister does not comply with treatment.

Clinical staff members, including her PA, nurses, and other support staff, are concerned about Ms. Z but find her frustrating. Ms. Z misses appointments because of her drinking and is noncompliant in taking her prescribed medications. The staff is also concerned about the inordinate amount of emotional, fiscal, and clinical resources Ms. Z is consuming. They believe that if she would comply with inpatient treatment, her prognosis would improve.

There is pressure on the finite resources in her community at large, in this case Washington State. The community is so concerned that the response of local elected officials to the dilemmas caused by patients like Ms. Z in similar circumstances is an attempt to expand the involuntary commitment law.[14]

This legislation addresses the fact that the present chemical dependency involuntary treatment law only allows a 72-hour hold for evaluation and petition for involuntary commitment. A person must meet two criteria for incapacitation: the inability to make rational decisions about his or her need for medical treatment and a likelihood of committing serious harm to self or others. A person must meet both criteria for involuntary treatment, and very few people who need it have qualified for treatment under this law.

The bill includes persons who are incapacitated, which is defined as those who are gravely disabled or at substantial risk of serious harm. "Gravely disabled" is defined as "a person in danger of serious physical harm resulting in failure to provide for his or her essential human needs of health or safety" or "[one who] manifests severe deterioration in routine functioning evidenced by a repeated and escalating loss of cognition or volitional control over his or her actions and is not receiving care essential for his or her health and safety." "Serious harm" is defined as an individual inflicting harm upon others or himself, such as suicide or other physical harm, or harm to the property of others. "Alcoholic" is defined as one who suffers from the disease of alcoholism.

Ms. Z has had such a strong impact on the medical staff that one member has been designated to present Ms. Z's case (with complete anonymity and privacy maintained) as part of the open hearing on the legislation.

Case Recommendations

The concerns of the clinic staff, PA, and especially Ms. Z's sister should be taken very seriously. Their questions are: "Can we ethically admit her to a 1-year inpatient alcohol treatment center against her will but which we feel is in her best interest? We have a good idea from our experience that she will die of alcohol-related complications if she is not treated. Is Ms. Z, who is dependent on/addicted to alcohol, able to make such a decision?"

Ms. Z's stated preference is not to be admitted to an inpatient treatment facility to treat her alcohol abuse. The principle of autonomy[15] in our North American culture provides the individual the right to decide his or her medical fate even if it means death is a result of that decision. However, in making an autonomous choice, the chooser must act intentionally, with understanding, without controlling influences. In this case, does Ms. Z have a comprehension or understanding of her condition and fate?

The recommendations include the following: Ms. Z has not had a formal psychiatric evaluation since 1999; her health condition has continued to decline; she has been in the hospital since 1999 with head trauma, fractures, electrolyte imbalances, and alcohol liver disease.

- She should have a competency evaluation by a designated chemical dependency specialist. A part of this evaluation should include determining her capacity for her personal care choices and evaluating her executive cognitive function.
- During evaluation, she should continue to have home health care for treatment and continued evaluation.

- Members of the clinic team should meet with Ms. Z, her sister Ms. Y, and the home health-care team member to discuss Ms. Z's prognosis. In the discussion, the do-not-resuscitate orders, living will, power of attorney, and other end-of-life issues should be presented to her.

Throughout the meeting, the providers should be noncoercive, caring, and objective.

At present there is a penumbra of law in Washington State, and it remains to be seen how cases similar to Ms. Z's will be decided. Consequently, at this moment under present law, if Ms. Z is competent, comprehends her circumstances, and does not present serious harm to herself or others, she has the ethical and legal right to choose not to be treated in an inpatient facility.

Much will depend on Ms. Z's irrational desires for alcohol. A competent person can possess irrational desires driven by addiction, as in this case of craving for alcohol and a desire for health and life. Here are some question s to consider and discuss:

- Does addiction affect Ms. Z's competency for choice, with self-deception, denial, personal identity, and self-control?
- Does addiction affect her ability to take in information and be able to understand, assess, and form a rational decision from that information?

Discussion of Autonomy and Alcoholism

What follows is a further discussion of the biomedical principle of autonomy and the diagnosis of alcoholism. Today in the United States, a debate continues about the use and abuse of alcohol, its impact on society and on the alcoholic. This debate in the modern era started with the enactment and repeal of the 18th Amendment to the Constitution (the prohibition of alcohol) and continues through the present. The intention of this discussion is to address one of the ethical dilemmas of that debate: alcohol addiction and autonomy. The discussion of alcoholism must start with a basic question: is chronic alcohol abuse a disease or a self-controlled behavior?

The Behavior Theory

Schaler[16] describes abuse of alcohol in the following manner. The disease of alcoholism was first described by Benjamin Rush in 1774 as having four criteria for diagnosis. He identified the causative agent as alcohol, described the condition as loss of control and declared it as a disease, and described the cure as abstinence. Those who see alcohol abuse as a behavioral state believe there is no scientific evidence to support the claim that alcoholism is a disease. The modern alcoholism movement was initiated by Jellnick in 1952 in his description of alcoholism as phases experienced by an alcoholic, with the initial description "one drink sets into motion a series of physiological events that deprive them of control over drinking."[17]

Schaler contends that a disease has a scientific pathological classification of disease nosology. Pathologists describe the pathology of specific conditions and record it in texts. Alcohol abuse results in physiological damage to tissue, but this is from the effects of ethanol, not from the disease "alcoholism." It is further suggested that standard medical practice diagnoses a physiological disease by signs (objective data) and symptoms (subjective data). Symptoms alone cannot define a disease. There must be some objective data to provide physical evidence of pathology. The disease of alcoholism is diagnosed by symptoms only. Those who classify alcoholism as a behavior believe alcoholism is not a mental illness.[18] Addiction is not a disease. It is an intentional and willful act. One chooses an activity. The Temperance Movement was the political outgrowth of the view that alcohol abuse results from loss of control rather than disease. "Nothing inherent in the word 'addiction' assumes disease."[16] Behaviors cannot be diseases. Diseases have specific signs that people exhibit involuntarily. Behavioral actions are something people do voluntarily, based on human ethical values. Alcoholism could be considered a metaphorical disease rather than a literal one. The behavioral group maintains that something is not a disease if it can be reversed by an act of will. Because drinking is a behavior that can be controlled by the individual who can stop the behavior, alcoholism is not a disease.

Disease Theory

Reznick[19] describes the medical disease model. He explains that Jillnek defined the concept of the disease in 1952. "The disease conception of alcohol addiction does not apply to excessive drinking, but solely to the loss of control which occurs in only a small group of alcoholics that does not occur in a large group of excessive drinkers. [This] would point toward a predisposing X factor in addictive alcoholics."[18]

Alcohol dependence is defined in the *Diagnostic and Statistical Manual of Mental Disorders,* Fourth Edition (DSM-IV).[20] The definition states that physiological dependence on alcohol is indicated by evidence of tolerance or symptoms of withdrawal. "Dependence is described as a maladaptive pattern of substance use leading to clinically significant impairment or distress."[20] Three or more of the following seven factors occurring in a 12-month period are indicative:

- Tolerance needing increased amount of substance to maintain desired effect or diminished effect using the same amount of substance
- Withdrawal
- Increased amount of substance taken over a longer period than intended
- Persistent desire or unsuccessful efforts to reduce use
- Significant time devoted to obtaining substance
- Reduction of or giving up occupational, social, or recreational activities because of use
- Substance use continued despite knowledge of having persistent psychological or physical damage caused or exacerbated by substance

In 1996 the AMA stated that alcoholism[16] is an illness characterized by preoccupation with alcohol and loss of control over its consumption such as to lead usually to intoxication if drinking begins, by chronicity, by progression, and by tendency toward relapse. Alcoholism is typically associated with physical disability and impairment and emotional, occupational, and/or social adjustments as a direct consequence of persistent and excessive use.

The medical/disease mode considers alcohol dependence as a disease that is a physical addiction, with psychological dependence and compulsive behavior.

Some examples of recent studies of brain change revealed by PET scan[21] show neurotransmission, usually found in abundance in frontal lobes, is significantly decreased in a person with 20 years of alcohol abuse. This neurotransmission system is involved in the modulation of logical decision making, impulse control, and management function. The medical model/disease group contends alcohol intake is a choice, but as dopamine depletion continues over a period, there is a change from that of choice to being biologically driven.[16]

The two theories create significant tension when considering treatment for chronic alcohol patients. They create further friction in the discourse of the principles of autonomy, beneficence, and justice. This friction exists in evaluating the case of a 50-year-old single African American woman with a 32-year history of alcohol abuse and her ability to make an autonomous decision. There is more information that should be considered.

Women and Alcohol Abuse

Until recently, gender-specific research was woefully deficient for women. It now appears that 2%-5% of women in the United States abuse alcohol,[22,23] with white non-Hispanic women most likely to drink alcohol. African American and Latino women exercise the highest rates of abstention. However, those African American women who do drink tend to drink heavily and have more alcohol-related problems. Of women who drink heavily, 37% have comorbid mental health illness, most commonly major depression and major anxiety disorder, and specific organ damage including cirrhosis and alcoholic hepatitis. Poor progression in liver disease is accelerated in women, who die earlier than men with their liver disease from alcohol abuse. There also appears to be a gender difference in metabolism of alcohol.

Women are more likely to be poor and without insurance. Men outnumber women with alcohol problems by a ratio of 2:1. However, the treatment ratio of males to females is 4:1.

Minorities and Alcohol Dependence

Black and Hispanic youth and adults[24-26] disproportionately experience negative effects of alcohol, including physical, mental, and social consequences, although use is lower than among white Americans. The physical damage includes cirrhosis of the liver, esophageal cancer, hypertension, obstructive pulmonary disease, and severe malnutrition. In recent studies, there appears to be a social economic status correlation with substance abuse.[27] Relative to whites, black Americans have lower incomes, are more likely to be underemployed, have less wealth, receive less pay for equal years of education, and are much more likely to live in poverty. The risk factors when combined with alcohol,[28] including individual factors, interpersonal factors, and the contextual factors, increase socially negative consequences. Contextual factors include availability of alcohol in poor neighborhoods, more advertising, more package liquor stores, and more availability than in other neighborhoods.[28]

Autonomy, Justice, Beneficence Behavior Theory

The tension in the discourse of the principles of autonomy, beneficence, and justice in the treatment of the alcohol-abusing patient is decreased if it is looked at from the perspective that alcohol abuse is a behavior by an individual that is conducted by choice. The outcome as presented by Shelton[29] in his discussion of individual or collective nonmedical liberty theory appears to be congruent with Schaler[16] and the behavior theory. In both cases, the patient has the right to refuse. Society has no responsibility to care for the individual who refuses to stop drinking and accept the consequences. In this case, Ms. Z will most likely die form her alcohol abuse.

Autonomy, Justice, Beneficence in the Medical/Disease Theory

The same tension in the discourse of the principles of autonomy, beneficence, and justice in the treatment of the alcoholic patient in the medical/disease model is much more difficult to resolve. Autonomous[30] persons must be able to express their personal values and make their own decisions. Beneficence[31] requires assessing capacity, and if the patient is incapable, society must protect the patient from harm to him- or herself or to others.

The beneficence/autonomy[30] struggle can be resolved by assessing capacity. Capacity is an abstract concept representing a normative process. A person must understand the information to make a decision and understand the consequences of the decision. The present use of capacity is the process of the ability to make the decision, not the decision made. There are only two outcomes in the present model—capable or incapable—but in reality capacity is on a continuum. A boundary is crossed at a point to make one incapable, and although it may fluctuate, in an alcoholic capacity is usually on a decline.

Justice/Alcohol Addiction

Justice requires that everyone in society be treated fairly,[31] and the Material Principle of Justice specifies the relevant characteristics for distribution of substantive properties. Limited resources in health care should be allocated justly. Nearly 8% of the U.S. population is alcohol-abusive, alcohol-dependent, or both. The cost to society from their health problems, lost productivity, crime, accidental death, and fire is estimated to be $165 billion. Treating alcohol problems and their medical consequences costs $20 billion. Direct costs for medical care are $15 billion.[32] If these costs result in harm to others in society, then we should look at how to reduce the cost and how to reduce the subsequent harm to society and its members. Ethically, the principle of justice may well require treatment of alcoholic patients to reduce the end cost to society.

Conclusion

Jonsen observes in his paper, *Why Has Bioethics Become So Boring*, "American individualism was the product of having to make a world from scratch but that it was an individualism that could not have succeeded without cooperation."[33] The issue of autonomy of the alcohol-abusing patient should be considered in that light.

In American society, there appears to be disproportionate dependence on autonomy rather than an attempt to apply the principles of justice and benevolence as a balance to individual rights. Responsibility to and for the community needs to be integrated into ethical analysis. The challenge is how to define unacceptable risk for the alcoholic patient. Health-care providers cannot compel their treatment decisions on the capable patient unless society decides that the greater good of protecting individuals and society outweighs the autonomy of the patient in this specific situation.

Ms. Z has been using alcohol for 32 years. If the behavior theory is applied to her situation, the providers would not treat her further, and she would most likely succumb to her alcohol consumption. If the medical/disease theory is applied, her present condition must be evaluated to assess her competency and capacity. Does she understand her medical situation? Does her addiction and deteriorating condition prevent her from making an informed decision? If by her condition, Ms. Z is seen as a gravely disabled person, the application of the autonomy principle creates an unacceptable risk to her and society.

Discussion Point

In light of Ms. Z's contextual factors regarding minority women and alcohol abuse, would the application of the principles of justice and beneficence compel treatment?

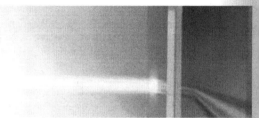

CASE 4

Informed Consent, Culture, Sex, and Language

Case Presentation

A 16-year-old Guatemalan Mayan Indian female (Ms. B) came to the community clinic today for her first visit, complaining of vaginal bleeding for the past 4 days. She speaks neither English nor Spanish. Her husband, also a Guatemalan Mayan Indian (Mr. B), is serving as the interpreter, using Spanish to speak to the Spanish-speaking, bilingual PA student. The student, in turn, interpreted for the attending physician. Mr. B stated that Ms. B had a birth control injection about 3 months ago and that she is now bleeding. The couple is living and working in the United States illegally and has no medical insurance. Her initial examination was provided by the PA student and presented to the attending physician.

Ms. B denies abdominal and pelvic pain, fever, malaise, nausea, vomiting, or diarrhea. She has used three to four tampons a day for the past 4 days for the vaginal bleeding. She has no history of pregnancies, abortions, or venereal disease. She has had only one sexual partner, Mr. B.

During the physical examination, Ms. B sits quietly, eyes downcast. She is a well-developed, well-nourished young woman in no apparent distress. Her development is that of a normal female, a Tanner stage B5, P5. The physical examination is unremarkable. The results of the laboratory tests, including complete blood count, chemistries, and liver function tests, were normal. The urinalysis was normal, and pregnancy test was negative. The assessment is that her vaginal bleeding was most likely caused by depletion of Depo-Provera.

The options for her care were then discussed with Ms. and Mr. B. She was informed that the bleeding was most likely caused by withdrawal of hormone therapy. She was also informed of other birth control methods, but she gave no response. The attending physician then asked the couple if they wanted to get pregnant. Without hesitation and without translating for Ms. B, Mr. B said yes. The attending physician then explained to Mr. B that a short time was needed to regularize her menstrual cycle, then the couple could proceed with their family plans.

The attending physician is a white male in his mid-40s, and the PA student is a Hispanic male in his late 30s. Ms. B never made eye contact or spoke directly with either provider. The student was very concerned about what appeared to be the lack of a truly informed consent of care by Ms. B. He was also concerned about what appeared to be a lack of cultural understanding by either provider about the two very young Guatemalan Mayan Indian patients.

The ethical question is: How can a patient truly be informed if the provider cannot speak the patient's language or understand the patient's culture?

Medical Indications (Beneficence, Nonmaleficence)

Ms. B is a healthy 16-year-old woman who has a high potential of becoming pregnant. She has no health problems. However, her age and low-income status may well be negative factors in a potential pregnancy.

The goals of medicine in this case are to inform and reassure Ms. B about her vaginal bleeding, inform her of birth control methods available, and help her understand the risks of pregnancy at a young age. The goal of medicine in this case may also be to support her in becoming pregnant.

American adolescents younger than 17 years have a higher occurrence of medical problems involving pregnancy, birth, and infancy than do adult women. These complications include low birth weight and infant mortality rate three times higher than for adult women. Maternal medical problems include poor maternal weight gain, prematurity, pregnancy-induced hypertension, and anemia.[1]

Frasier et al,[2] in a 1995 study of white women younger than 18 years with adequate prenatal care compared with mothers 20-24 years, showed a risk (relative risk 1.9) of premature infants or an infant weighing less than 2500 grams at birth (relative risk 1.7). The risk factor could be much higher for Ms. B if she does not have adequate prenatal care and adequate nutrition.

Ms. B is not only an adolescent but also an undocumented immigrant. This factor can create significant health risks for mother and infant. Undocumented immigrants are reluctant to see and are cautious of health-care providers because of concerns of being reported and deported.[3] Children of undocumented immigrants who are born in the United States are U.S. citizens. In spite of this, the pregnant woman is ineligible for prenatal care. This creates a higher risk pregnancy.[4]

Other types of birth control are available to Ms. B. However, it is unclear because of the language barrier whether she could avail herself of them and would want to use them.

Patient Preference (Autonomy)

Ms. B's preference to become pregnant is unclear. Mr. B reports that his wife want to become pregnant. The major question is: is she fully informed?

Informed consent consists of the ability of the patient to fully comprehend and understand the medical situation and agree to the medical plan and treatment. Informed consent is rooted in the principle of autonomy.[5] Childress and Beauchamp further identify five elements that should be engaged if one is to give informed consent. These components include competence, disclosure, understanding, voluntariness, and consent. These elements are combined as follows: "One gives an informed consent to an intervention if (and perhaps only if) one is competent to act, receives a thorough disclosure, comprehends the disclosure, acts voluntarily, and consents to the intervention."[5]

These elements are further categorized into three sections.

1. Threshold elements (preconditions)
   • Competence to understand and decide
   • Voluntariness in deciding
2. Information elements
   • Disclosure of material information
   • Recommendation of a plan
   • Understanding disclosure and recommendations
3. Consent elements
   • Decision in favor of or against plan
   • Authorization of the chosen plan

All the elements and categories are based on understanding and choice. To make an informed refusal, one must acknowledge comprehension of the choices available. Ms. B had very little direct interaction with the providers, either verbally or with active body language. All her interaction was through Mr. B. This is not to say that Mr. B believed his intentions were in Ms. B's best interest. However, it appears that she is competent to understand, in spite of a language barrier, but it is not clear if this is a voluntary decision on her part. In reality, Ms. B's preference is not known.

A significant issue in this case is the problem (or potential problem) when a family member or friend acts as an interpreter for the patient. Communication is often contaminated by the imposition of the related interpreter's values. It is not known if Ms. B wants to avoid pregnancy—she is on Depo-Provera, while her husband wants her to become pregnant. In almost all cases it will be recommended that a nonrelated interpreter be identified for follow-up visits. In this case, it may be difficult to find an interpreter who speaks her native language.

Quality of Life (Nonmaleficence, Beneficence, Autonomy)

A 16-year-old woman in a new country who speaks neither English nor Spanish and is an undocumented immigrant faces significant quality-of-life issues. In this case, nothing is known from the patient about her present quality of life. She is healthy and is without any medical problems. Nevertheless, she faces hardships of poverty in the United States and potential deportation. It is unclear how financially dependent Ms. B is on her husband. It is also unclear how pregnancy may complicate her life. As much as possible, she should be kept from harm.

Contextual Features (Justice)

From the little information the couple has shared with the health-care providers, it appears that Ms. B spent a majority of her life in Guatemala. As a Mayan Indian growing up in Guatemala, she was in the middle of a civil war whose violence was focused on the Mayan Indian population.

From 1960 to 1996, a 36-year internal war existed, during which 140,000 civilians were killed. A majority of those were Mayan Indian: 250,000 children were orphaned, 45,000 disappeared, a million people were displaced, and 440 Mayan villages were destroyed. Presently 89% of the Guatemalan population lives in poverty.[6]

In Guatemala, a Mayan's mean life expectancy is 45 to 50 years; 35% of children die before the age of 5, and the infant mortality rate may be as high as 100-150 per 1000 births.[7]

Many Mayans from Guatemala have fled to Chiapas, Mexico.[8] One major aspect of the civil war was the silencing of the population, especially the children. Lykes[9] describes the tragedy of the civil war with this insight, "The state silences the population through terror, exploiting fear in a particular way."

Many Mayans left Guatemala and are still afraid to share their personal tragedies with anyone.

Contraceptive use in Guatemala is varied. As of 1985, the major form of contraception is sterilization, with female sterilization at about 10% and male sterilization at 35%. Together, this accounts for 45% of the birth control used in Guatemala. Approximately one fourth of the females in relationships use contraception methods. Only 5% of the Mayans use birth control.[10,11]

Mayan women view pregnancy as a normal life process and not an illness. A study by Princeton University, RAND, and Instituto de Nutrición de Centro América y Panamá found 85% of common pregnancy care for Mayan women was by traditional midwives, and birthing rarely occurred at a medical facility.[12] The three fundamental premises of childbearing for these traditional women were:

1. A sense of the sacredness of childbearing
2. The need for reliance on God to ensure positive outcomes
3. The bittersweet paradox of childbirth

Sacredness and the essential nature of childbearing are core values for these women. Privacy and being cared for by other women were also apparent. Another strong belief is that childbearing women and the unborn child are in a physically and spiritually weakened state and are susceptible to illness and evil forces.

Husbands are not present for the births. Masculinity and virility in this culture are believed to be determined by the number of children a man can father. Many husbands refuse to allow their wives to use birth control even if their health is at stake.[13]

Other contextual issues include Ms. B's status as an illegal immigrant, which affects her qualifications for Medicaid and financial and social resources available to her as an indigent woman. Congress in 1996 enacted the Personal Responsibility and Work Opportunity Reconciliation Act. This act denied federally subsidized health coverage to illegal aliens, which includes Medicare. However, in the act, states could obtain a federal waiver that would allow the state to provide state-funded health coverage to a narrow spectrum of illegal immigrants "Permanently Residing Under the Color of Law" (PRUCOL). This is the condition in which the person is in the United States illegally and the Immigration and Naturalization Service knowingly permits him or her to remain. In 2000 the U.S. federal courts ruled infants of illegal +immigrant parents until 1 year of age are eligible for Medicaid.[13]

There are presently more than 8.7 million illegal immigrants in the United States: 84% live in eight states: Massachusetts, Arizona, New Jersey, Illinois, Florida, Texas, New Mexico, and California. A majority live at or below the poverty line. They are eligible only for free emergency care and often visit the emergency room for nonurgent care.[13]

These contextual cultural features have a significant impact on Ms. B and how she can and will relate to the issues in this case. Even though they may not be aware of them, the providers, too, are affected by these issues.

QUESTIONS FOR DISCUSSION

1. Identify and discuss the ethical issues involved with this case.

2. Identify and discuss the legal aspects of this case.

3. What options are open to addressing the ethical issues?

4. What do you do as a student if the preceptor says "Just let it go. She will be fine."?

5. What would you do for Ms. B and for her husband?

Case Recommendations

This discussion will address the issue presented by the PA student: "How can a patient be truly informed if the provider cannot speak the language of the patient or understand the patient's culture?" The cultural diversity within the United States has enriched and defined our society for over 200 years. The dominant Western European culture has influenced the direction and basis of U.S. institutions. The influence of other cultural groups is creating a change in the expectations and responsibilities of the citizens and health-care professionals. A prime example of this change is seen in the population groups in California. The most recent census finds there is no dominant ethnic population, and by 2025 the Hispanic population will be between 41.5% and 49.3%[14] of the population of the state. California has been an indicator of future trends for many years and is again pointing the way to the future. This may well be a considerable dilemma for a monolingual and culturally unaware provider.

As discussed earlier, there are five elements needed for informed consent or refusal. These are competence, disclosure, understanding, voluntariness, and consent. The goal is for Ms. B to trust the provider and share her preference of care. To enable this, the provider should work with Ms. B to understand her social and cultural history.

- The first recommendation is to identify a female primary care provider, nurse, or social worker to work with Ms. B and to consider her cultural background.
- The second recommendation is for the provider to obtain ethnographic data by performing an ethnographic interview as described at the Ethno-Med Web site.[15]

- The third recommendation is to provide an interpreter through the community or the telephone translation service, which provides over 140 different languages.[16] The reason for this recommendation is that untrained interpreters often make errors that can seriously impair the physician-patient relationship. Relatives of the patient many times filter the translation to the provider and to the patient based on the relatives' own biases.[15]

There are several state and federal laws, including Title VI of the Civil Rights Act of 1964, that require linguistic services in the medical setting. The Office of Civil Rights unswervingly has taken the position that the Hill-Burton Act covers linguistic services. Medicaid requires beneficiaries be informed orally and in writing in a language they understand. Federal Categorical Grant Programs, which include Community Health Centers and Migrant Health Centers that receive federal funding, agree to provide "services in a language and cultural context most appropriate to their patients."[15] Although the laws and regulations exist, many times they are not enforced or are ignored. To provide Ms. B the ability to make an informed decision in her health care, these services are essential.

Discussion of Informed Consent, Culture, Sex, and Language

The focus of this discussion is a look at the principle of autonomy in relationship to cross-cultural ethical conflicts in the case of Ms. B.

In the fifth edition of *Principles of Biomedical Ethics*, Beauchamp and Childress respond to some criticism of the order of the presentation of the four principles of bioethics and the fact that they had stressed autonomy over the other principles. They responded, "Although we begin our discussion of the principles of biomedical ethics with respect for autonomy, our order does not imply that this principle has priority over all other principles."[5] Nonetheless, it appears that the principle of autonomy in applied bioethics in the United States reflects a rugged individualism.

Autonomy can be defined as "self-rule, free from controlling influence of others and from inadequate understanding that prevents meaningful choice."[5] American informed consent typically requires that full information be presented to the individual, including relevant benefits, adverse effects, and risks of treatment or research. The individual must be legally competent and understand the information presented. The choice of treatment must be voluntary and free of undue influence or coercion.[5]

A culture is defined as a shared system of values and learned patterns of behavior, including the customary beliefs, social forms, and material traits of a racial, religious, or social group. When there are differences between the prevailing culture and a minority cultural group, noticeable ethical and interpersonal tensions can develop.[17] The previous definition of autonomy can create profound issues for some of the cultures that make up the multicultural society of the United States. The components of this rigid interpretative approach to the principle of autonomy can create significant obstacles for some cultures. Full truthful disclosure can be in conflict with the wellness and stamina of a culture's members. For example, in Carrese's study of Navajo reservation life and Western bioethics found in Navajo culture, it is understood that thought and language have the power to shape reality and control events.[18] Carrese further clarifies this by quoting anthropologist Gary Witherspoon's observation, "In the Navajo view of the world, language is not a mirror of reality, reality is a mirror of language."[18] In Navajo culture, language forms reality. Full truthful disclosure for Navajo patients can be potentially harmful.

Similarly in Thai culture, Buddhism believes the mind and thoughts have a direct effect on the body. The first verse of the *Dhammapada* includes "we are a result of our thoughts." Meditation provides mind-body relaxation techniques, which enable one to obtain a healthy mental state, which has significant effect on health.[19]

Coward and Ratanakul describe the dilemma of the vigorous North American autonomy as "I-self," separating from others in one's family and society. The "I-self" is competitive, separating one from other humans and from the environment. "I-self" tends to promote one's self-interest. The "I-self" viewpoint, if taken to its end, can put human beings at odds with the sustainability of nature.[19]

The opposite is the "we-self," which many Eastern cultures, such as Hindu, Buddhist, and Chinese societies, view as the extension of self to society. The "we-self" sense of personhood provides expansion to the family, nature, and the cosmos. This perspective tends to de-emphasize the individual and emphasize the responsibility to the whole.[19]

Cultural beliefs affect how people perceive bodily functions, make medical decisions, and expect health providers to behave, to classify disease, to make prognoses, and to make medical decisions.[20]

Jecker, Carrese, and Pearlman present an approach to tackling these cross-cultural quandaries.[17] It consists of three steps.

1. Identify goals
   - Collect data about the patient's values and cultural orientation
   - Collect data in an ethnographic manner, being astute to particular details
   - Be self-reflective of the purpose of the encounter, thus clarifying the provider's goals and the patient's goals.
2. Identify mutually agreeable strategies
   - Identify alternative mutually agreeable strategies
   - Identify a consultant familiar with the patient's culture, language, and customs
3. Meet ethical constraints
   - Means chosen to achieve goals must be compatible with the provider's values
   - Means chosen to achieve goals must be compatible with the patient's values and the values of the patient's culture.[17]

This is one way for providers to understand what autonomy means within the patient's culture and if the concept of autonomy as known in our dominant culture exists in that culture at all. It also provides for an understanding of the decision-making process within the patient's culture.

Not everyone agrees with a multicultural approach to ethical dilemmas. Catherwood argues "that it may well be that only culture is morally justified in its traditions and the other is just morally wrong no matter what its opinion or cultural context."[21] His argument continues that multicultural pluralism cannot defend the proposition that two cultural ethics are right. One must be wrong. He continues that moral claims have a burden and substance that demand and require that they be enforced on others. Resolving ethical cases requires one principle to be dominant and to be the moral thing to do. Whatever that true thing to do is, it then becomes universally applicable. A common moral and cultural basis is needed.

The argument continues that in a lenient multicultural pluralism there is no room for individualism. The "demand" for single guiding principles and the need for a coherent universal constancy in their application are incompatible with tolerance. "Intolerance of some cultural traditions is morally required…forging of a moral mono-culture is preferable." Catherwood suggests the way to address the multicultural differences is through "allowing those skilled in the Western analytical philosophical tradition free rein in tackling opinions and traditions of other cultures."[21]

The struggle between a monoculturalist and multiculturalist, pluralist, ethical theory has existed for many years. The dominant culture in a society needs to attempt to understand and appreciate minority cultures and to apply their cultural ethic whenever possible within the context of applied clinical bioethics in the patient-provider relationship.

Clinical bioethical values can be applied from the viewpoint of the provider or the patient. In the case of cultures where autonomy is from the viewpoint of "we-self" and the provider culture is "I-self," the tension is apparent. The patient's perception of reality is paramount: it is the patient who lives with the final decision.

Beauchamp and Childress add to the discussion of autonomy by clarifying their position, "Respect for autonomy is not a mere *ideal* in health care; it is a professional *obligation*. Autonomous choice is a *right*, not a duty of patients."[5]

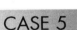

CASE 5

Pain and Suffering in Cancer Clinical Trials

Case Presentation

Ms. C is a 27-year-old woman with acute promyelocytic leukemia (APL). She participated in a research protocol, receiving an unrelated matched peripheral blood stem cell transplant. A consult 75 days post transplantation was requested from the pain team because of poor control of back pain. Ms. B had a history of spondylolisthesis after an injury as a teenager in gymnastic practice. On a 10-point scale, she had maintained a 2-3 (of 10 as baseline) level of pain, which was present prior to transplantation.

She was putting on her socks 46 days post transplantation when she heard a popping sound, and she developed sudden severe low back pain of 10/10. She was unable to stand or walk. Staying still and resting on her back relieved the pain; it was thought that the pain was due to severe muscle strain and spasm. She was admitted to the hospital and started on patient-controlled administration of pain medication. She was discharged 14 days later with prescribed Valium and oxycodone controlled-release.

She was readmitted with progressively worsening lethargy and confusion. She had a spinal MRI that showed compression fractures T5-L4. In an attempt to block her increasing and unrelenting back pain, she had an epidural catheter inserted. She received bupivacaine via the catheter. Although she became increasingly more alert and awake with decreased back pain, her mental status was consistent with delirium. The concern at this point was opioid toxicity or infection. Ten days later she was alert and oriented, and she could clearly state her symptoms; no infection was present. Her back pain was believed to be multifactorial but primarily related to moderate to severe steroid-induced myopathy that exacerbated myofascial pain and caused decreased ambulation and osteopenia. She was anorexic, possibly because of graft-versus-host disease (GVHD). She had plural and pericardial effusions and ascites. She had renal insufficiency probably caused by previous renal toxic medications. Upon discharge, much of the edema and insufficiency cleared.

A week later she was readmitted with anasarca, a 4-kg weight gain in 4 days, gut immobility, and renal insufficiency. She was in considerable pain, thought to be related to epidural catheter malpositioning. Shortly after admission, a narcotic antagonist was administered to reduce her gastrointestinal (GI) immobility. This increased her back pain and was discontinued, and her pain decreased. At this time, she had pneumonia due to cytomegalovirus (CMV). A thoracentesis was performed due to plural effusion, and 1.2 liters of fluid was removed.

A permanent epidural catheter was put in place. During the procedure, the patient had an acute onset of angioneurotic edema, which produced supraglottic airway obstruction. She was successfully intubated and ventilated. She was extubated 2 days later. Her pain continued despite placement of the new catheter.

Ms. C continued to deteriorate with significant pain and developed profound weakness, prerenal failure, dyspnea secondary to large pleural effusions, and progressive ascites. She became somnolent. The next day she was in respiratory distress and underwent dialysis, having 6 liters of excess fluid removed. This did not improve her condition, and all aggressive therapies were discontinued. A do-not-resuscitate order was written, and Ms. C died 14 hours later.

The ethical questions asked by the pain team and nursing team were with so much pain 2 months post transplantation until death 6 months later, why was there so much reluctance to treat the pain aggressively? In the future, how can we determine when pain has become a paramount problem and other treatment should take a secondary place to treatment of the patient's pain? In responding to symptom control in such a situation, how should we respond in an ethical manner?

Medical Indications

Ms. C, 27, has APL and is in apparent second complete remission. She has a history of presumed hepatic candidiasis with an apparent response to treatment. She was prepared for matched, unrelated donor peripheral stem cell transplantation. A majority of patients who relapse with APL die from their resistant disease. Recent studies have reported disease-free survival in 30%-40% of patients treated with bone marrow transplant.[1]

The two most significant risks in stem cell transplantations are, first, infection (viral, bacterial, or fungal because of the immunosuppressed condition of the patient prior to and during the transplant period until engraftment and new blood cells are produced to fight infections), and, second, GVHD, in which the donor's immune system cells attack the patient's tissues in the skin, liver, mouth, GI system, and other organs. Another significant risk is lung damage from the radiotherapy treatment.

In the process of stem cell transplantation, there are specific times pain control should be addressed. Appropriate timing and adequacy of pain control are essential for sufficient pain control. With ablative therapy prior to transplantation, mucositis is the most common painful complication. After transplantation, the next most common issue is pain from GVHD. Ms. C experienced mucositis. She did not experience pain from GVHD. However, she did have pain beyond what the transplantation team expected.

Patient Preference

Ms. C chose to enroll in a research protocol she believed had the best chance of cure for her leukemia.

The attending physician, study coordinator, Ms. B, and her husband reviewed the protocol, including the side effects. Because it was a phase I/II study, there was no guarantee that this would cure her, but there was a chance. All their questions were answered, and she signed an informed consent for treatment. She also enrolled in two other studies, one to evaluate different medication in the treatment of GVHD and the other in the prophylaxis of cytomegalovirus, a virus that is not an uncommon infection of transplant patients and can cause life-threatening infections. The same team reviewed the protocol with her, and her family answered all questions. She signed the informed consent and was enrolled.

Ms. C also discussed end-of-life issues and signed a consent not to perform heroic measures in the event there was no hope in survival. Ms. C's husband was given the power of attorney if, in the course of treatment and recovery, Ms. C could not make decisions for herself.

Informed consent is a communication from provider to patient as possible to make available as much information to the patient for an autonomous decision. This includes the acceptance by the patient of treatment after adequate discussion between provider and patient. The dialogue must include the type of intervention and its risks and benefits. Any other therapies and their benefits and risks should also be discussed. In this case, Ms. C was actively involved in the discussions about the treatment protocols. She was able to examine the details of the treatment studies with the attending physician and study coordinator. She expressed through her questions that she was appropriately concerned and understood the risks and benefits of the treatment studies.

Post transplantation, with her sudden severe low back pain of 10/10, a major concern voiced by Ms. C, her husband, and her family was control of Ms. C's back pain. The pain team developed a pain treatment plan that seemed to keep her pain at a level 5/10, but at times it was worse. Ms. C was again admitted with progressively worsening lethargy and confusion thought to be related to toxicity from her pain medications, although infection or recurrent disease could not be ruled out.

An MRI of her head showed mild white matter edema, for which inflammation is not a common cause, but no lesions. Her pain medications had been decreased with the thought that they had caused her lethargy and altered mental status. Her pain increased. Her continued preference was to treat her pain. An epidural catheter was placed in the thoracic spine region to attempt to block the chronic pain. This seemed to control her pain and decrease her agitation, although her mental status continued to wax and wane.

During one admission the attending physician thought she was intolerant of opioid pain medication. Ms. C was alert and oriented at that time and clearly identified her "excruciating" pain while sitting or standing. The pain team at this time attempted to control her pain with infusion of low-dose morphine into her epidural catheter. The team believed a long-term treatment of her back pain required a more permanent catheter placement. The team thought the pain was caused by moderate to severe steroid-induced myopathy that exacerbated myofascial pain, thus causing decreased ambulation and osteopenia. Ms. C was discharged from the hospital under some pain control. She was again admitted 10 days later for multiple issues including severe pain, gastric atony, and GVHD. The atony was treated with very low-dose Reglan because of severe somnolence in previous full-dose use and because Ms. C said she was "wiped out" by it. At this time, she also had anasarca and renal insufficiency, for which there was not a clear explanation. The concern was that her gut immotility was narcotic-induced, although she had been off all opioids for 1 week. In that week, she was in extreme pain and continued to request pain relief over other treatments. Opioid pain medication was again initiated. Ms. C continued to deteriorate and had developed a working diagnosis of CMV pneumonia.

Her pain was still an issue. She was taken to the operating room for a more permanent catheter placement. Ms. C developed an allergic response from medications about two thirds through the procedure, which required intubation and ventilation. She was extubated 2 days later. She continued on a downhill course. Her pain continued to be an issue with her and the family and the nursing staff. She became extremely lethargic and minimally responsive. Ms. C's husband requested the opportunity to discuss the prognosis and concern about further intervention therapy.

A family conference was held, which included Ms. C's husband, mother, sister, and grandparents. It also included the PA caring for Ms. C, the patient's ICU nurse, and the attending physician. Ms. C's course during the past few months was reviewed. Information regarding her critical condition was discussed and the fact that no further therapeutic options were available. The family then requested no further diagnostics be pursued and that comfort care be the goal. This decision was, as much as possible, a reflection of Ms. C's decision representing her values and desires. She had discussed with her husband that no extraordinary life-extending measures be taken if it would not change the outcome of her overall condition. A do-not-resuscitate order was written after the conference, and comfort care was initiated. Ms. C was placed on oxygen support and IV pain medication, and she died 14 hours later.

Quality of Life

Quality of life (QOL) assessment in the best situations is difficult. Objective tools for the provider to use are varied. Many times the subjective information from the patient who is suffering or impaired by disease or medical intervention to treat the condition is not fully appreciated or understood by the provider. Curtis and Patrick[2] discuss Wilson and Cleary's[3] conceptual model and the overlapping definitions and structure of QOL, health-related quality of life (HRQOL), health status, and functional status. They apply this model to the care of critically ill patients in the intensive care unit. The terms are defined as QOL, the broadest of the terms, which is holistic—the issues that are important to the patient's self-determination and self-satisfaction; HRQOL means the quality of life as it is affected by health or the subjective experience of the impact of health on life's quality; functional status is the ability to perform the tasks of daily living; and health status is the state of health in the present.

These are the terms that will be used to describe Ms. C's QOL during her course of diagnosis and treatment of her leukemia. Upon arriving at the outpatient department of the bone marrow transplant unit, her QOL was good. She had been employed and happily married. Her HRQOL at that time was good. However, her prognosis for the relapse of her APL was grim. Survival with untreated leukemia is very rarely documented. Her functional status on a Karnofsky Scale was 90: able to carry on activity with minor signs or symptoms. It was not 100 because of her back pain. The scale runs from 100 (normal; no symptom or signs of active disease) to 0 (death). Ms. C moved down the scale post transplantation. Although different providers may assign different values to the scale by patient behavior, the pain team agreed on specific behavior when evaluating their patients.

Ms. C's HRQOL, in all her discussions with nursing staff and other providers according to the data recorded by the providers, deteriorated after initial admission for back pain. Her Karnofsky rating dropped to a 50; she needed considerable assistance and frequent medical care. She needed assistance in walking and most activities of daily living. She recovered enough to be discharged to the outpatient service. When she was again admitted to the hospital with severe lethargy, she was in a state of confusion and again had considerable pain. Her Karnofsky score was 40. She was disabled and required special care. She was again discharged from the hospital, still needing considerable assistance from her husband and frequent visits to the outpatient department. Subsequently she was admitted to the hospital in very serious condition with a Karnofsky score of 30, severely disabled and requiring daily nursing care. A month later, she was very sick and in critical condition, requiring intensive care. This represents a Karnofsky score of 20; 3 weeks later she dropped to a Karnofsky score of 10. Moribund, the fatal process progressed rapidly, and the next day she died. As she moved down the scale, her ability to interact with her surroundings, communicate, enjoy the company of others, and utilize her mental faculties deteriorated.

The HRQOL for Ms. C declined rapidly after day 164 post transplantation. In each of the days until day 188, she suffered and was in moderate to extreme pain. Jonsen, Siegler, and Winslade[4] describe an objective QOL criterion as *restrictive quality of life* in a situation in which a person suffers a severe deficit of physical or mental health and if one's functional abilities depart from the normal range as stated by the person or observed by others. Ms. C certainly fit this description after day 164. The authors describe *minimal quality of life* as a situation in which one's physical condition has greatly deteriorated, the ability to communicate with others is severely restricted, and there is discomfort and pain. From day 180 Ms. C fit these criteria, although her pain and discomfort may well have placed her in this category much earlier.

Continued diagnostic tests, removal of opioid pain medication for 1 week to determine the origin of her gastric atony, and the use of opioid antagonists to determine the origin of lethargy, although reasonable methods of evaluation for diagnostic and potential treatment, significantly increased Ms. C's

suffering and pain and had a negative affect on her QOL. The struggle for the providers to assist Ms. C to maintain a reasonable HRQOL, cure her APL, treat the side effects of her transplant, and maintain quality clinical research was apparent throughout her course of therapy.

Contextual Features

Ms. C's APL was diagnosed in 1997, and she underwent traditional chemotherapy treatment and its toxic side effects. Her APL recurred in 1999, and she again underwent chemotherapy and obtained a complete remission. Statistically, after recurrence of APL, prognosis is poor. She elected to enroll in a clinical study for a peripheral stem cell transplant.

From the beginning of her transplantation course, she had back pain, which increased. The symptomatic treatment for pain was balanced with diagnostic and treatment issues. The nursing staff and the pain team's concerns for aggressive pain control did not appear to motivate the transplant treatment team or some of the consultants to undertake such therapy. The frustration of this was reflected by the transplant attending physician's concern at one point that "unfortunately this [pain] was not controlled by [present medication] alone...we are stuck with the problem of gut dysmotility if, in fact, the epidural administration of morphine is at the heart of this problem." Another note stated, "We were unable to remove the opioids from her without her developing significant pain."

In discussions with the social worker, Ms. C's husband and mother voiced concern about her pain and lethargy. The transplant team discussed with Ms. C and her husband the implication of the seriousness of the issues confronting her care. She had anasarca at this point in her hospital course. "I told her about a series of seven patients with anasarca associated with graft versus host disease....After the patient asked me how those patients did, I explained five of the seven died, thereby letting her and her husband know the severity of our current situation....I answered a few questions...and indicated to them we will continue to do everything possible to make her feel better." The situation had gotten worse. "We informed the family that if medical procedures proved to be inadequate to control [her condition] hemodialysis may be necessary....The family is eager to press along to do all appropriate and necessary intervention to...correct the problems....However, they do not want to continue if futile or no hope of recovery."

There did not appear to be a time when the transplant team and all the consultants (the pulmonary critical care team, pain team, nephrology department,

GI consultant, cardiology unit) plus the other teams of nursing and social work discussed the goals of treatment: when active treatment and diagnosis to palliative or symptom care should be offered. This could have provided a holistic approach for the patient and family.

Although not stated by any of the members of the transplant team or other members of the clinical teams, an underlying contextual feature in many clinical research trials is exemplified by a statement often made to the author of this chapter by his mentor in critical care transplant medicine: "Sometimes in cancer research you must push the envelope of traditional symptom care to view the research goal for future patients...."

Within this situation, the culture of critical medicine comes into play. Critical care medicine is focused on frequent review of body systems to evaluate the body system's ability to maintain life. Each body system tends to have a medical specialty, i.e., respiratory system a pulmonologist, cardiovascular system a cardiologist, kidney a nephrologist, and so on. Many times the critical care team attempts to coordinate this care. Pain and suffering are also evaluated. However, the struggle to keep the body systems functioning and supporting life tends to take priority.

Ms. C's mother shared with one of the staff members late in the hospital course, "Look at her. They have cured her leukemia but at what price?" Her anasarca had increased her weight from 100 to 140 pounds with edematous upper and lower extremities; when she was coherent, she was in pain.

Case Recommendations

Clinical research represents a unique modern conflict among physician-healer, physician-investigator, interprofessional patient care, and the patient's hope for cure. In cancer research, the goal is to improve care for future cancer patients. This is especially true in phase I and phase II clinical trials. Traditionally, phase I trials consider new agents for proper doses and the toxicities for each dose level, with little direct benefit to the patient. In phase II trials, levels of therapy are known. Toxicities are also known, and the maximum tolerable level of the therapy is known. This level of therapy is now administered and, with more patients receiving the maximum tolerable dose, high incidences of toxic side effects are expected.

Because Ms. C was enrolled in a phase I/II study, toxic side effects were expected. What appeared most frustrating to all the caregivers was that she had engrafted by day 12 post transplantation, and her graft never failed. However, her GVHD, kidney fail-

ure, steroid-induced myopathy and pain, and steroid-induced compression fractures were all in need of treatment. The question was the priority of treatment. The patient succumbed to the toxicities of her treatment. The ethical questions for the pain team and nursing team were: "In the future, how can we determine when pain has become a paramount problem and other treatment should take a secondary place? In responding to symptom control in such a situation, how could we respond most ethically?"

The following recommendations are made:

1. Early in the first admission, acknowledging the difficulty of having members of all the teams represented at a patient care meeting together, such a meeting is needed. The ethics committee may well ask for this meeting. The objective is to reassess the goal of therapy. Is now the time to move from aggressive active diagnosis and treatment therapies to more aggressive symptom management or to palliative therapy? Especially consider the tension between Ms. C's gastric atony and removal of opioid pain medication.
2. Have a psychiatric consultation to evaluate and possibly treat depression, considering the long course of pain and suffering. An antidepressant may enhance pain treatment therapies.
3. The third recommendation may not affect Ms. C directly, but it could help future patients in a situation of chronic unrelenting pain. In review of the research protocol, there is not a specific section that addresses pain and suffering. Any phase I or phase II cancer research protocol should include a section addressing treatment of pain and suffering that includes giving the consulting pain team and psychiatric staff priority in the treatment. This inclusion is especially needed in phase I and II studies that evaluate toxicities. Pain and suffering are frequently events in these studies.

Discussion of Pain and Suffering in Phase I and II Cancer Clinical Trials

It was anticipated in 2003 that there would be 1,368,030 new cancer cases and that 563,700 Americans would die of cancer, more than 1800 people a day. In the United States, 1 of every 4 deaths is from cancer. Since 1990, 18 million new cancer cases have been diagnosed.[5] Many of the patients expected to die of their cancer will enroll in phase I or II cancer research trials. Many of these patients will be suffering and in pain when they enroll.

Yet there appears to be little reference within these cancer research trials to the treatment of this pain and suffering or palliation for the patients enrolled in these trials. How should the ethical principles of non-maleficence and beneficence be applied to address the issues of pain, suffering, and palliation and incorporate their treatment as an integral part of phase I and II cancer clinical research trials?

Phase I and II cancer research trials involve the testing of new antitumor agents. The intention is to determine the toxicity and maximum tolerable dose of an agent. The trials enroll cancer patients who have failed traditional therapy.

Pain is a common problem with cancer patients. It is estimated that 80% of cancer patients are under-treated for their cancer pain.[6] This has been such a problem that the Department of Health and Human Services appointed a panel in 1993 to create guidelines for the management of cancer pain.[7]

Suffering is a multifaceted combination of negative experiences that people attempt to avoid or get away from. Cassell[8] describes suffering as "Person has many facets, and it is ignorance of them that actively contributes to patients' suffering. The understanding of the place of person in human illness requires rejection of historical dualism of mind and body." Lowey[9] describes the capacity to suffer as to "have primary worth." Suffering is experienced by the individual, but one needs community to express suffering.

Palliation is when the focus of treating pain and suffering in an incurable patient is primary and there is no curative goal.

Relieving pain and suffering has been the under-taking of medicine for centuries. Until the discovery and availability of antibiotics to the general population, the ability to use the word "cure" in the lexicon of medicine was rare. Physicians could easily describe the course of disease and give a fairly accurate prognosis. Alleviating pain with opioids was common. Suffering was appreciated and acknowledged by the patient as part of the disease process.

Nevertheless, what is suffering? Cassell[8,10] has pointed out that little attention is paid to suffering in medical education, research, or practice. The mind-body dichotomy in and of itself may be a cause of suffering as providers wrestle to relieve it. Suffering and fear are future-oriented. Suffering is loss of person. What make this individual a person? Personhood consists of a past from whence one has traveled. It includes life experiences, especially as they are considered in a medical situation. Person includes a cultural background with roles within family and community. Person has relationships with others and a relationship with self. Person has regular behaviors and daily routines. Person has a relationship with one's body and what it has done for and with one, what it is doing now, and when attacked by cancer

how it fails. To suffer, both a past and a perceived future are needed.

Person has a transcendent dimension. In Judaism, righteous suffers, and the best may suffer the worst. Nevertheless, pain and suffering are unwanted and should be prevented and treated. Asceticism is not encouraged and is in fact forbidden. In Christianity, suffering is a punishment for original sin. To suffer is to be with Christ. In Hinduism and Christian Science, suffering is illusionary and unreal. The goal of pain is to change thoughts and to see the world correctly.[11] An example of secular transcendence is patriotism: to suffer for one's country.

It may appear to be an overwhelming task to evaluate and treat suffering and how it affects patients. Given that genes of the human body have been mapped, this area of human need can be addressed. It appears overpowering for patients to suffer from and have no control over their pain. Often that pain feels as though it is never-ending. Providers who invalidate the patient's pain by telling the patient "it is psychological (therefore not real) or imaginary" can cause suffering.

Pain and suffering are often mentioned in the same breath, but they are distinct and separate. Continued pain can intensify suffering. If the source of pain can be identified and relieved, suffering can be decreased. Even if the person refuses pain medication, knowing the origin of the pain and that there is relief if needed may decrease the suffering.

Lowey[9] further defines suffering as individual and existential, unique to the person. Suffering within the individual happens in a community that defines the suffering itself. Suffering involves hurting, fearing loss, not understanding, often hopelessness, and powerlessness to change fearful events. Compassion is the feeling "inspired" by perceived or actual suffering by others. Without compassion, those who suffer lack understanding, and this creates a puzzle of logic for the field of bioethics.

In a medical setting, suffering is often associated with pain. Pain is a warning that something is wrong in the body and that action to address this must be taken. It is a noxious stimulus within the nervous system. To experience pain requires an intact neocortex, frontal lobe, and generally intact nervous system. Cassell explains suffering and pain in a skillfully short and succinct manner: "To feel pain requires different neurological structures than to experience suffering."[10]

In last 10 years, there have been strides in pain control, and each year more specific and targeted medications and other therapies come into the marketplace.[12-15] Guidelines, such as *Management of Cancer Pain* developed by the Department of Health and Human Services, provide a direction of care.[7]

Palliative care and symptom management[16] comprise concentrated, comprehensive, coordinated care for the relief of pain, symptoms, and suffering in terminal or incurable patients.[17] Two-thirds of terminally ill cancer patients suffer significant pain, depression, and other symptoms that often are managed inadequately.[15] One of the fundamental goals of medicine is the relief of pain and suffering. Emanuel expresses his concern about phase I trials that exclude pain relief interventions even though a fundamental goal of medicine is to relieve pain, suffering, and other symptoms.[16]

Phase I cancer research trials recruit patients who have failed all conventional cancer treatments.[18,19] The patients usually have a life expectancy of less than 3 to 4 months. These trials traditionally have had animal testing only, and this is the first human testing. The purpose of phase I trials is to determine the maximal safe dose (MSD) of an antitumor agent. This includes a qualitative toxicity profile, analyzing such side effects as nausea, vomiting, and hemorrhage. The trial will also develop a dose response profile that will include toxicological pharmacokinetic studies. *These trials anticipate a less than 5% response rate and offer no guarantee of benefit to patients enrolled.*[18]

Phase II cancer trials recruit patients with active measurable disease to determine whether the agent causes any significant antitumor activity by monitoring tumor regression, duration, and survival. In phase I studies, the MSD of the antitumor agent has been determined, but that does not mean the agent operates without toxicity or significant side effects. Phase II can involve new agents, analogs of established agents, or new ways of using established agents.

Patients are usually enrolled into trials by referral from community oncologists who have exhausted all other treatment options. When patients are enrolled, they are screened by history and physical examination and provided with a description of the trial, followed by a discussion of the clinical trial. They are then given an informed consent to sign, but are they truly informed?[15,20] Daugherty, Ratain, Grochowski, et al[21,22] conducted a study on 30 patients enrolled in phase I studies: 93% said they understood the informed consent; 33% were able to state the purpose of the trial; 85% decided to enroll for therapeutic benefit. No one identified altruism as a motivation for enrolling.

Emanuel has suggested seven ethical requirements for clinical trials. Trials must show:

• Social or scientific value
• Scientific validity
• Fair subject selection
• Favorable risk-benefit ratio
• Independent review
• Informed consent
• Respect for potential and enrolled subjects[23]

Within the concept of respect for potential and enrolled subjects, "the welfare of the subjects should be carefully monitored throughout the research project. If subjects experience adverse reactions, untoward events, or change in clinical status, they should be provided appropriate treatment and, when necessary, be removed from study."[23]

Cassell[24] discusses the history of the Belmont report and the loss of beneficence and autonomy as technology has moved to the forefront of medicine. Beneficence now serves as nostalgia more than current practice or modeled behavior.

Miller[25] presents his experience and concerns as a physician who enrolls patients into phase I cancer studies, which, by definition, are not meant to have therapeutic effect. Cancer patients in his experience persistently regarded the studies as therapeutic. Miller expressed the constant tension between science and medicine.

Daugherty and Siegler[20] in the gold standard oncology text, *Cancer: Principles and Practice of Oncology*, identify the ethical concerns in cancer clinical research trials, especially phase I and II, as follows:

• "One ought not to use others as a means to an end."
• "One should not allow harm to come to others."
• "The interest of an individual physician's patient should be placed above the interest of others."

As shown above, the application of phase I and phase II cancer clinical trials can create tremendous bioethical conflicts. One bioethical dilemma is enrolling cancer patients who may have 3 to 6 months to live into phase I trials and enrolling patients with measurable tumors into phase II trials. If these patients reflect the usual 80% of cancer patients, they are being undertreated for their pain and suffering. Nonmaleficence and beneficence are the ethical principles that are criteria in this predicament.

The principle of nonmaleficence[26] is the obligation not to inflict harm intentionally. "Morality is concerned with the harmfulness of harm for itself, not simply the responsibility of causing harm."[25] At its core, nonmaleficence stresses negative prohibitions of action, as in "not causing harm." This principle also provides the reasons for legal prohibition of certain forms of conduct. In its application, the principle of nonmaleficence must be obeyed impartially.

The principle of beneficence,[27] on the other hand, requires positive action that need not always be obeyed impartially. There is rarely if ever a legal consequence for failing to abide by these rules. These rules include refraining from causing harm, prevention from harm, and removal from harmful conditions. This principle implies a moral obligation to act for the benefit of others and to contribute to their welfare. Quality of life reflects the principle of beneficence. Quality of life includes physical mobility, freedom from pain and distress, the capacity to perform activities of daily living, and the ability to engage in social interactions. The principal of utility[27] is also encompassed by the principle of beneficence. Utility is often justified in medical research that is dangerous for humans if the benefit to society outweighs the danger to the individual.

The principle of autonomy has such primacy in American culture today that the encouragement of beneficence as a model in current medicine is difficult to find. Still, the obligation to abide by this principle does not make it cease to exist. It is a challenge that needs to be incorporated into everyday practice and research trials.

Phase I and II clinical trials enroll patients with significant cancer and, in the case of phase I trials, the patient probably has only a short time to live. This fact alone can cause suffering. The ethical principles of nonmaleficence not to inflict harm intentionally and of beneficence requiring the prevention of harm and removal from harmful conditions require physicians to look at and address the issues of pain and suffering of the patients in phase I and II cancer clinical trials.

The principles of autonomy and utility may argue against primacy of the treatment of pain and suffering. The autonomous patient with informed consent can decide to enter a phase I or II study and receive an antitumor agent and specific symptom treatments as provided by the research team. Utility allows for toxic therapies that will not provide the patient any

therapeutic value. This has been the traditional approach for new antitumor research.

Because the purpose of the trials is not only to identify toxicities but also to take patients to toxic levels, it would seem that the principle of beneficence would require a further explicit responsibility to incorporate palliative and pain care into the trials. Patients enrolled in phase I studies have only a few months to live and, because of the short life expectancy, palliative care would be the norm outside of a research setting. Why not explicitly integrate it within the study setting?

Palliative care therapies may interfere with the science of the study. Autonomy presents the problem of medical paternalism. Does a requirement for pain care and palliative care fall under that umbrella? What are the cost implications of required palliative care?

Patients with cancer who are enrolled in phase I and phase II clinical trials are usually suffering and in pain. The principles of beneficence and nonmaleficence require a response to this suffering and pain that can be presented at enrollment into the trials. Upon enrollment and after taking antitumor therapy and reaching a toxic level and/or failure, an explicit portion of the study to palliate and manage the pain should be set in motion. At times, the physician-scientist is at odds with him- or herself as a physician-provider. One way to ameliorate this dilemma is to incorporate into the studies points at which palliative care or pain teams are involved and are given the authority to establish treatment of pain and suffering as the primary goal.

"In a word, humanization of medicine will only occur when we allow the narratives of suffering together with the language of the sufferer to shape the care we deliver" (Rev. James Keenan SJ, PhD).[11]

Annotated Bibliography (Case 1)

1. Elkind D. Egocentrism in adolescence. Child Development, 1967;38:1025-1034.
2. The state of Native American youth health. University of Minnesota Adolescent Health Program Report. Minneapolis, MN: University of Minnesota Adolescent Health Program, 1996.
3. Trends in Indian health 1986-1996. Washington, DC: U.S. Department of Health and Human Services, Indian Health Service, 1997.
4. Stevens-Simon C. Providing effective reproductive health care and prescribing contraceptives for adolescents. Pediatric Review 1998;19:409-417.

   A review of the issues of unprotected sexual activity in adolescents. It presents ways for providers to participate in prevention that can affect the morbidities associated with high-risk sexual behavior in adolescents. Contraceptive technologies are presented with their benefits and risks for this age group.

5. Felice ME, Feinstein RA, Fisher MM, et al. Adolescent pregnancy: Current trends and issues 1998. Pediatrics 1999;103:516-520.

   This paper updates the reader on trends and issues on adolescent pregnancy, reviews the use of contraceptives, and provides startling data that 50% of adolescent pregnancies occur within the first 6 months of initial sexual intercourse. It also provides eight recommendations for addressing this issue of adolescent pregnancy, from abstention to involving the community in addressing the issue of teen pregnancy.

6. Fraser AM, Brockert JE, Ward RH. Association of young maternal age with adverse reproductive outcomes. New England Journal of Medicine 1995;332:1113-1117.

7. King NM, Cross AW. Children as decision makers: Guidelines for pediatricians. Journal of Pediatrics 1989;115:10-16.

   This provides guidelines for assessing and enhancing children's abilities to participate in health-care decision making. The article presents cases and discussion of the factors needed in assessing capacity, including reasoning, understanding, and voluntariness, in conjunction with the nature of the decision to be made.

8. Kuther TL. Medical-decision-making and minors: Issues of consent and assent. Adolescence 2003;38: 343-360.

9. Leikin SL. Minors' assent or dissent to medical treatment. Journal of Pediatrics 1983;102:169-176.

   The developmental concepts of illness are presented; characteristics of immaturity are discussed; issues of dissent from treatment are presented and explored; and the role of parents in consent is discussed.

10. Committee on Bioethics. Informed consent, parental permission and assent in pediatric practice. Pediatrics 1995;95:314-317.

    This paper discusses the idea of patient assent and parental permission. The formidable task of application and its shortcomings are described.

11. Sigman GS, O'Connor C. Exploration for physicians of the mature minor doctrine. Journal of Pediatrics 1991;119:520-525.

    This is a succinct paper on the mature minor doctrine from its origin to recent court cases.

12. Lebit LE. Compelled medical procedures involving minors and incompetents and misapplication of the substituted judgment doctrine. Journal of Law and Health 1992;7:107-130.

    This is a very detailed paper including the laws and theories of substituted judgment, informed consent, and misapplication of the substituted judgment doctrine and the development of a new standard.

13. Respect for autonomy. In Beauchamp TL, Childress JF, eds. Principles of Biomedical Ethics, 5th ed. New York: Oxford University Press, 2001:57-112.

14. Preferences of patients. In Jonsen AR, Siegler M, Winslade WJ, eds. Clinical Ethics: A Practical Approach to Ethical Decisions in Clinical Medicine, 5th ed. New York: McGraw-Hill, 2002:47-103.

15. Becker JL. Adolescent medicine. In Lemcke D, Pattison J, Marshall L, et al, eds. Primary Care of Women. Norwalk, CT: Appleton & Lange, 1997:15-24.

16. Respect for autonomy. In Beauchamp TL, Childress JF, eds. Principles of Biomedical Ethics, 5th ed. New York: Oxford University Press; 2001:57-112.

17. Ethics. In Reich WT, ed. Encyclopedia of Bioethics. New York: Free Press, 1978.

18. Culver CM, Gert B. Philosophy in Medicine: Conceptual and Ethical Issues in Medicine and Psychiatry. New York: Oxford University Press; 1982.

19. de Leon Siantz M. Children's rights and parental rights: A historical and legal/ethical analysis. J Child Adolesc Psychiatr Ment Health Nurs. 1988;1:14-17.

20. Sigman GS, O'Connor C. Exploration for physicians of the mature minor doctrine. Journal of Pediatrics 1991;119:520-525.

    This is a succinct paper on the mature minor doctrine from its origin to recent court cases. The court cases are examples of applied mature minor doctrine.

21. Hardwig J. What about the family? Hastings Center Report 1990;20:5-10.

    This report presents a theoretical rationale for including "family" in biomedical ethical analysis. This includes a fairly detailed criticism of present analysis, excluding family.

22. Nelson JL. Taking families seriously. Hastings Center Report 1992;22:6-12.

    This is an extensive discussion of the moral value of including "family" in medical decision making for a patient.

23. Foreman DM. The family rule: A framework for obtaining ethical consent for medical interventions from children. Journal of Medical Ethics 1999;25:491-500.

    This presents a proposal for a "family rule" that redefines informed consent for children so it should take place within a family unit and between parents and child (up to the age of 18).

24. Ross LF. Health care decision making by children: Is it in their best interest? Hastings Center Report 1997;27:41-45.

    A critical review of the American Academy of Pediatrics policy statement on informed consent, parental permission, and assent in pediatric practice. The commentary focuses on the moral and legal need for parents to facilitate their child's "long-term autonomy" without involvement of third parties (health-care providers or the state).

25. Oberman M. Minor rights and wrongs. Journal of Law and Medical Ethics 1996;24:127-138.

    This philosophical dialogue reviews the lack of laws that reflect the comprehensive theory of adolescent capacity. The issues of maturity and lack of a consistent assessment are thoroughly reviewed.

26. Alderson P. Commentary on the "family rule." Journal of Medical Ethics 1999;25:497-498.

27. Foreman DM. The family rule: A reply to Alderson. Journal of Medical Ethics 1999;25:499-500.

Annotated Bibliography (Case 2)

1. Servan-Schreiber D, Kolb NR, Tabas G. Somatizing patients, part I: Practical diagnosis. American Family Physician 2000;61:1073-1078.

   This is the first of a two-part series for primary care providers who diagnose and treat the somatizing patient. This paper provides an easy, straightforward approach and practice tips in diagnosing this prevalent and frustrating illness.

2. Spitzer RL, Williams JB, Kroenke K, et al. Utility of a new procedure for diagnosing mental disorders in primary care: The PRIME-MD 1000 study. Journal of the American Medical Association 1994;272:1749-1756.

3. Barsky AJ. A 37-year-old man with multiple somatic complaints. Journal of the American Medical Association 1997;278:673-679.

   This is a case presentation, with comments by and the insights of Dr. Barsky. He also answers questions about somatization in a fairly detailed manner.

4. Somatization disorder. In Tasman A, Kay J, Lieberman J. Psychiatry. Philadelphia: WB Saunders, 1997.

5. Servan-Schreiber D, Tabas G, Kolb NR. Somatizing patients, part II: Practical management. American Family Physician 2000;61:1423-1428, 1431-1432.

   This is the second in the series. This paper provides great insight into the empathetic treatment of illnesses that are frustrating for both provider and patient.

6. Stuart MR, Lieberman JA. The Fifteen-Minute Hour: Applied Psychotherapy for the Primary Care Physician, 2nd ed. Westport, CT: Praeger, 1993.

7. Somatoform and dissociative disorders. In Winokur G, Clayton P. Medical Basis of Psychiatry, 2nd ed. Philadelphia: WB Saunders, 1993.

8. Cloninger CR, Martin RL, Guze SB, et al. A prospective follow-up and family study of somatization in men and women. American Journal of Psychiatry 1986;143:873-878.

9. Respect for autonomy. In Beauchamp TL, Childress JF, eds. Principles of Biomedical Ethics, 5th ed. New York: Oxford University Press, 2001:57-112.

10. Justice. In Beauchamp TL, Childress JF, eds. Principles of Biomedical Ethics, 5th ed. New York: Oxford University Press, 2001:225-282.

11. Lawrence DM, Mattingly PH, Ludden JM. Trusting in the future: The distinct advantage of nonprofit HMOs. Milbank Quarterly 1997; 75:5-10.

    This article presents the positive aspects of nonprofit HMOs and speaks to the significant amount of research and analysis that have been done by these HMOs on outcomes for specific patient groups. The paper also points out how nonprofit HMOs have been at the forefront of public policy debates for the past 30 years.

12. Professional-patient relationships. In Beauchamp TL, Childress JF, eds. Principles of Biomedical Ethics, 5th ed. New York: Oxford University Press, 2001:283-336.

13. Pellegrino ED. Altruism, self-interest, and medical ethics. Journal of the American Medical Association 1987;258:1939-1940.

14. Orentlicher D. Managed care and the threat to patient-physician relationship. Trends in Health Care Law Ethics 1995;10:19-24.

15. Smith AJ. Avoiding the ethical pitfalls of managed care. Minnesota Medicine 1996;79:24-26.

    As president of the Minnesota Medical Association in 1996, Dr. Smith presents his perspective on the ethics of managed care in a succinct and readable format.

16. Christensen KT. Ethically important distinctions among managed care organizations. Journal of Law and Medical Ethics 1995;23:223–229.

17. Emanuel EJ, Dubler NN. Preserving the physician-patient relationship in the era of managed care. Journal of the American Medical Association 1995;273:323-329.

Annotated Bibliography (Case 3)

1. Substance-Related Disorders, 303.90; Alcohol Dependence. In Diagnostic and Statistical Manual of Mental Disorder (DSM-IV-TR), 4th ed. rev. Washington DC: American Psychiatric Association, 2000.

2. Diamond I, Jay CA. Alcoholism and alcohol abuse. In Goldman L, Bennett JC, eds. Cecil Textbook of Medicine. 21st ed. Philadelphia: WB Saunders; 2000:49-54.

3. Hanna EZ. Approach to the patient with alcohol abuse. In Gorroll AH, Mulley AG, eds. Primary Care Medicine, 4th ed. Philadelphia: Lippincott Williams & Wilkins, 2000:1169-1178.

   A great textbook, which includes this chapter on the approach to the alcohol abuse patient. The chapter gives insight on the assessment and how to interact with the patient suspected of abusing alcohol and guidelines for referrals and treatments for the primary care provider.

4. Walsh DC, Hingson RW, Merrigan DM, et al. A randomized trial of treatment options for alcohol-abusing workers. New England Journal of Medicine 1991;325:775-782.

   A specific job-related analysis of inpatient treatment of alcoholism; a well-supported data outcome study.

5. Weiss R. Inpatient treatment. In Galanter M, Kleber H, eds. Textbook of Substance Abuse Treatment, 3rd ed. Washington, DC: American Psychiatric Association; 2004.

   A great textbook on substance abuse. The text includes nature of addiction and various treatment modalities and addresses issues of special population and substance abuse.

6. Mee-Lee D, Shulman G, Fishman M, et al. Patient Placement Criteria for the Treatment of Psychoactive Substance Disorders, 2nd ed. Washington, DC: American Society of Addiction Medicine, 2001.

7. Bunn JY, Booth BM, Cook CA, et al. The relationship between mortality and intensity of inpatient alcoholism treatment. American Journal of Public Health 1994;84: 211-214.

   The authors review data from the Veterans Affairs database, comparing short-term and long-term inpatient treatment of alcoholic patients.

8. Simpson DD. The relation of time spent in drug abuse treatment to posttreatment outcome. American Journal of Psychiatry. 1979;136:1449-1453.

9. Hazelton LD, Sterns GL, Chisholm T. Decision-making capacity and alcohol abuse: Clinical and ethical considerations in personal care choices. General Hospital Psychiatry 2003;25:130-135.

   This paper discusses the conundrum of how to assess and address mandating a patient to stop destructive alcohol consumption. The authors also talk about the concept of personal care competence. The paper has a detailed discussion of competence and capacity.

10. Leo RJ. Competency and the capacity to make treatment decisions: A primer for primary care physicians. Primary Care Companion Journal of Clinical Psychiatry 1999;1:131-141.

11. Stuss DT. Biological and psychological development of executive functions. Brain and Cognition 1992;20:8-23.

12. Blume AW, Schmaling KA, Marlatt GB. Memory, executive cognitive function, and readiness to change drinking behavior. Addictive Behaviors 2006;30:301-314.

13. Nadler JD, Richardson ED, Malloy PF, et al. The ability of the Dementia Rating Scale to predict everyday functioning. Archives of Clinical Neuropsychology 1993;8:449-460.

14. Long, Hargrove, Winsley, et al. Senate Bill 5051, State of Washington, 57th Legislative Session, 2001 Regular Session.

This piece of legislation has had two hearings as of February 19, 2001; passed Washington State Senate, July 2001.

15. Respect for autonomy. In Beauchamp TL, Childress JF, eds. Principles of Biomedical Ethics, 5th ed. New York: Oxford University Press; 2001:57-112.

16. Schaler J. The case against alcoholism as a disease. In Shelton WN, Edwards RB, eds. Advances in Bioethics, vol. 3: Values, Ethics, and Alcoholism. Greenwich, CT: JAI Press, 1997.

This chapter argues against the medical model as the proper category for patient drinking excessive amounts of alcohol. The author challenges the use of the term "alcoholism" and addiction to alcohol from a diagnostic standard. It is well-written, challenging information, even if in a somewhat fuming style.

17. Jellinek EM. Phases of alcohol addiction. Quarterly Journal on the Study of Alcohol 1952;13:673-684.

18. Schaler J. Alcoholism as willful misconduct. Journal of the American Medical Association 1989;261: 864-865.

19. Reznick LA. Alcoholism and the medical model. In Shelton WN, Edwards RB, eds. Advances in Bioethics, vol. 3: Values, Ethics, and Alcoholism. Greenwich, CT: JAI Press, 1997.

The author discusses the origins and present-day issues of the medical model for diagnosing and treating alcoholism. He also responds to the issues of alcohol abuse as a willful behavior in the alcoholic patient.

20. Substance-Related Disorders, 303.90.

21. Hird S, McMillman R. Alcoholism and other forms of addiction. In Shelton WN, Edwards RB, eds. Advances in Bioethics, vol. 3: Values, Ethics, and Alcoholism. Greenwich, CT: JAI Press, 1997.

22. Stein MD, Cyr MG. Women and substance abuse. Medical Clinics of North America 1997;81:979-998.

This paper presents the issue of past neglect in research into alcoholism in women and the difference in secondary disease from alcohol abuse in women. The paper addresses the epidemiology, associated life experiences, and clinical consequences and treatment of substance abuse in women. It provides superb information and data on substance abuse and women.

23. Harris C, Mahowald M. Women and alcohol abuse. In Shelton WN, Edwards RB, eds. Advances in Bioethics, vol. 3: Values, Ethics, and Alcoholism. Greenwich, CT: JAI Press, 1997.

24. Wallace JM. The social ecology of addiction: Race, risk and resilience. Pediatrics 1999;103:1122-1127.

The author reviews the issues of racial differences in alcohol abuse and its relationship to the socioeconomic status of minorities. The author selectively reviews the literature on epidemiology, etiology, and consequences of alcohol abuse among white, black, and Hispanic adults and youth. This is a well-researched paper with excellent data and a challenge to providers and policy makers about alcohol abuse in minority communities.

25. U.S. Department of Health and Human Services. Drug use among racial/ethnic minorities. Washington, DC: NIH Publication No 95-3888; 1995.

26. Kandel D, Chen K, Warner LA, et al. Prevalence and demographic correlates of symptoms of last year dependence on alcohol, nicotine, marijuana, and cocaine in the US population. Drug and Alcohol Dependence 1997;44:11-29.

27. William DR, Collins C. US socioeconomic and racial differences in health: Patterns and explanations. Annual Review of Sociology 1995;21:349-386.

28. Wallace JM, Bachman JG. Explaining racial/ethnic differences in adolescent drug use: Impact of background and lifestyle. Social Problems 1991;38(3):333-340.

29. Shelton W. Justice and alcoholism. In Shelton WN, Edwards RB, eds. Advances in Bioethics, vol. 3: Values, Ethics, and Alcoholism. Greenwich, CT: JAI Press, 1997.

The author discusses the issues of justice and alcoholism and the responsibility of and to society. He also comments on other chapters of the text. This is a noteworthy analysis of the principle of justice in the context of alcohol abuse in the United States.

30. Strang DG, Molloy DW, Harrison C. Capacity to choose place of residence: Autonomy vs beneficence? Journal of Palliative Care 1998;14:25-29.

The author presents a case of a patient who has had a long-standing alcohol abuse problem and has difficulty caring for himself at home. He does not want to leave home, which creates the opportunity for dialogue to review and discuss the issues of autonomy and beneficence. An insightful paper expressing the challenges for health-care providers and patient refusal of treatment.

31. Justice. In Beauchamp TL, Childress JF, eds. Principles of Biomedical Ethics, 5th ed. New York: Oxford University Press; 2001:225-282.
32. Hanna EZ. Approach to the patient with alcohol abuse. In Gorroll AH, Mulley AG, eds. Primary Care Medicine, 4th ed. Philadelphia: Lippincott Williams & Wilkins, 2000:1169-1178.
33. Jonsen AR. Why has bioethics become so boring? Journal of Medicine and Philosophy 2000;25:689-699.

Annotated Bibliography (Case 4)

1. Felice ME, Feinstein RA, Fisher MM, et al. Adolescent pregnancy–current trends and issues 1998. Pediatrics 1999;103:516-520.

   This paper updates the reader on trends and issues on adolescent pregnancy, reviews the use of contraceptives, and provides startling data that 50% of adolescent pregnancies occur within the first 6 months of initial sexual intercourse. It also provides eight recommendations for addressing this topic, from abstention to involving the community in addressing teen pregnancy.

2. Fraser AM, Brockert JE, Ward RH. Association of young maternal age with adverse reproductive outcomes. New England Journal of Medicine 1995;332:1113-1117.
3. Kielich AM, Miller L. Cultural aspects of women's health care. Patient Care 1996;30:60-64.
4. Smith LS. Health of America's newcomers. Journal of Community Health Nursing 2001;18:53-68.

   This paper discusses issues for newcomers to America, both documented and undocumented. The paper reviews federal policy, court involvement with newcomers, health issues, and the high-risk health problem. Options for possible solutions for newcomer health care are addressed. This provides a new look at recent immigrants in a positive and encouraging manner.

5. Respect for autonomy. In Beauchamp TL, Childress JF, eds. Principles of Biomedical Ethics, 5th ed. New York: Oxford University Press; 2001:57-112.

   This is the newest updated version of this text. It has been rearranged to provide easier access to information. The presentation to the reader has changed also; it does not assume the reader has a graduate degree in philosophy. Although ethical theories are discussed in great detail, they are in the last few chapters of the book.

6. Summerfield D. The Mayas of Guatemala: Surviving terror. Lancet 1997;349:130.
7. Minkowski WL. Mayan Indian health in Guatemala. Western Journal of Medicine 1988;148:474-476.
8. Melville MB, Lykes MB. Guatemalan Indian children and the sociocultural effects of government-sponsored terrorism. Social Science and Medicine 1992;34:533-548.

   This is a rather frightening look into the 35 years of civil war aimed at the Mayan Indian population. This paper discusses the psychological effect of this civil war on children. Descriptions of their experiences were used to gather qualitative data for this long-term research project.

9. Lykes MB. Terror, silencing, and children: International, multidisciplinary collaboration with Guatemalan Maya communities. Social Science and Medicine 1994;38:543-552.
10. Monteith RS, Anderson JE, Pineda MA, et al. Contraceptive use and fertility in Guatemala. Studies in Family Planning 1985;16:279-288.
11. Berganza CE, Peyre CA, Aguilar G. Sexual attitudes and behavior of Guatemala teenagers: Considerations for prevention adolescent pregnancy. Adolescence 1989;24:327-337.
12. Glei DA, Goldman N. Understanding ethnic variations in pregnancy-related care in rural Guatemala. Ethnicity and Health 2000;5:5-22.

   This paper investigates the relatively low use of birth control in Guatemala. The study covers and compares issues such as social economic factors, accessibility to health services, and ethnic differences. The discussion points out midwives are the major contact for Guatemalan women, both Latina and Mayan Indian.

13. Ho J, Rao N, Tyree D. Should illegal immigrants be covered by Medicaid? Terry Sanford Institute of Public Policy, Duke University, Durham North Carolina. Available at duke.edu/ Accessed July 31, 2004.

14. Campbell P. Population Projections for States by Age, Sex, Race, and Hispanic Origin: 1995 to 2025. 1996 U.S. Bureau of the Census, Population Division, PPL-47. Available at census.gov/population/www/projections/ppl47.html Accessed August 15, 2004.

15. Ethno-Med. Collecting ethnographic data: The ethnographic interview page. Available at ethnomed.org/ Accessed August 15, 2004.

This site is a great resource for clinicians caring for multicultural patients; it provides practical information and provides resources for care. The links to other Web sites are invaluable.

16. National Health Law Program. Ensuring linguistic access in health care settings: Legal rights and responsibilities. Available at healthlaw.org/pubs/2003.linguisticaccess.html. Accessed August 15, 2004.

This Web site provides great information on the law governing non–English-speaking patients and the responsibilities of providers and health-care institutions in providing linguistic services to their patients. There are also suggestions on how to approach the issue with the institution.

17. Jecker NS, Carrese JA, Pearlman RA. Caring for patients in cross-cultural settings. Hastings Center Report 1995; 25:6-14.

This paper presents an approach to addressing ethical issues by providers and patients from different cultures. The approach changes the dynamic of provider to one of sometime student and the patient as teacher. The authors provide rationales for their three-step approach. The approach appears to be a practical way to learn and discuss cultural ethical issues. The three-step proposal takes time, however. If an ethical issue arises even in a busy clinic, this is one way to at least start the process of addressing cross-cultural ethical issues.

18. Carrese JA, Rhodes LA. Western bioethics on the Navajo reservation: Benefit or harm? Journal of the American Medical Association 1995;274:826-829.

Carrese and Rhodes provide a unique insight into perceptions of traditional Navajo culture. This paper provides the reader a chance to think about how a word can affect patients and their reality. This is a qualitative research project providing essential insights into a culture that can be used as a model as providers practice in a cross-cultural manner.

19. Buddhism, health, disease, and Thai culture. In Coward H, Ratanakul P. eds. A Cross-Cultural Dialogue on Health Care Ethics. Waterloo, Ontario, Canada: Wilfred Laurier University Press; 1999.

This book provides an opening to understanding some Eastern cultural principles. The authors contribute a scathing discussion of Western bioethics in their introduction. It will grab the reader's attention early.

20. Culhane-Pera KA, Vawter DE. A study of healthcare professionals' perspectives about cross-cultural ethical conflict involving a Hmong patient and her family. Journal of Clinical Ethics 1998;9:179-190.

21. Catherwood JF. An argument for intolerance. Journal of Medical Ethics 2000;26:427-431.

The author of this paper presents an ethical argument against multiculturalism. For readers who support multiculturalism and a cross-cultural ethic, this paper should be read to understand that not all ethicists or philosophers agree with a multicultural approach to ethical analysis.

Annotated Bibliography (Case 5)

1. Daugherty CK, Siegler M. Ethical issues in oncology and clinical trials. In DeVita VT, Hellman S, Rosenberg SA, eds. Cancer: Principles and Practice of Oncology, 6th ed. Philadelphia: Lippincott Williams & Wilkins; 2001:3119-3134.

2. Curtis JR, Patrick DL. The role of quality of life and health status in making decisions about withdrawing life-sustaining treatments in the ICU. In Curtis JR, Rubenfeld GD, eds. Managing Death in the ICU: The Transition From Cure to Comfort. New York: Oxford University Press; 2000:69-74.

This text reviews the issues of death in the ICU, addressing issues such as the concept of managing death in the ICU, the limit of life support in the ICU, practical skills in managing death in the ICU, and the societal issues: ethnicity, liability, and economics. This is the first text that tries to address what happens: how to approach disease treatment failure in the ICU. This text is useful for all providers working in an ICU and for students of all health professions.

3. Wilson IB, Cleary PD. Linking clinical variables with health-related quality of life: A conceptual model of patient outcomes. Journal of the American Medical Association 1995;273:59-65.

4. Jonsen AR, Siegler M, Winslade WJ, eds. Clinical Ethics: A Practical Approach to Ethical Decisions in Clinical Medicine, 5th ed. New York: McGraw-Hill; 2002.

5. Cancer Facts & Figures. American Cancer Society. Available at cancer.org/docroot/STT/stt_0.asp. Accessed August 15, 2004.

    This site offers a tremendous amount of reliable information for both patients and providers. This site has numerous valid links to other quality cancer resource Web sites.

6. Bonica JM. The Management of Pain. Philadelphia: Lea and Febiger; 1990.

    This is the classic text on pain; it provides information on basic pain pathways and transmission of pain and pain management.

7. Clinical Practice Guidelines: Management of Cancer Pain. Publication No 94-0592. Washington DC: Government Printing Office; 1994.

    The guidelines in this document provide basic and advanced approaches for pain management. This is a good resource.

8. Cassell EJ. The Nature of Suffering and the Goals of Medicine. New York: Oxford University Press; 1991.

    This is the modern classic text on pain and suffering. The author delves deeply into suffering. He addresses suffering from its nature and in chronic illness. He explores the depths of person and the measure of person. Cassell ends his book with a challenge to providers: "Face the suffering of your patients at their level and listen." It is a great text for those willing to move beyond the science of medicine and find and refine the art of medicine.

9. Lowey E. The role of suffering and community in clinical ethics. Journal of Clinical Ethics 1991;2:83-89.

    Lowey explores suffering "as that which makes us human and part of community." He proposes that the theory of suffering moves between a strongly autonomy-based ethic and a strongly beneficence- and social justice–based ethic. It is a very thoughtful discussion of suffering as it relates to community, the individual, and the provider.

10. Cassell E. The importance of understanding suffering for clinical ethics. Journal of Clinical Ethics 1991;2:81-82.

11. Keenan JF. The meaning of suffering: A Jewish perspective. In Pellegrino ED, Faden AI, eds. Jewish and Catholic Bioethics: An Ecumenical Dialogue. Washington DC: Georgetown University Press; 1999:83-95.

12. Mercadante S, Portenoy RK. Opioid poorly-responsive cancer pain, part 1: Clinical considerations. Journal of Pain and Symptom Management 2001;21:144-150.

13. Mercadante S, Portenoy RK. Opioid poorly-responsive cancer pain, Part 2: Basic mechanisms that could shift dose response for analgesia. Journal of Pain and Symptom Management 2001;21:255-264.

14. Edwards RB. Pain and the ethics of pain management. Social Science and Medicine 1984;18:515-523.

15. Khouzam RH. Chronic pain and its management in primary care. Southern Medical Journal 2000;93:946-952.

16. Emanuel EJ. Pain and symptom control: Patient rights and physician responsibilities. Hematology/Oncology Clinics of North America 1996;10:42-51.

17. Pellegrino ED. Emerging ethical issues in palliative care. Journal of the American Medical Association 1998;279:1521-1522.

18. Emanuel EJ. A phase I trial on the ethics of phase I trials. Journal of Clinical Oncology 1995;13:1049-1051.

19. Frei E. Clinical trials of antitumor agents: Experimental design and timeline considerations. Cancer Journal Scientific American 1997;3:127-136.

    The author presents the traditional venue of cancer clinical research trials and comments on the cost and excessive time from identification of a new antitumor agent until it is used in large trials. He argues for streamlining the process by combining phase I and II trials on a continuum. He argues that new antitumor agents are better targeted and will theoretically cause less toxicity and be more efficacious.

20. Daugherty CK, Siegler M. Ethical issues in oncology and clinical trials. In DeVita VT, Hellman S, Rosenberg SA, eds. Cancer: Principles and Practice of Oncology, 6th ed. Philadelphia: Lippincott Williams & Wilkins; 2001:3119-3134.

21. Daugherty CK, Ratain MJ, Siegler M. Pushing the envelope: Informed consent in phase I trials. Annals of Oncology 1995;6:321-323.

22. Daugherty C, Ratain MJ, Grochowski E, et al. Perceptions of cancer patients and their physicians involved in phase I trials. Journal of Clinical Oncology 1995;13:1062-1072.

23. Emanuel EJ, Wendler D, Grady C. What makes clinical research ethical? Journal of the American Medical Association 2000;283:2701-2711.

24. Cassell EJ. The principles of the Belmont report revisited: How have respect for persons, beneficence, and justice been applied to clinical medicine? Hastings Center Report 2000;30:12-21.

25. Miller M. Phase I cancer trials: A collusion of misunderstanding. Hastings Center Report 2000;30:34-43.

Miller presents a very personal journey as a director of phase I cancer studies recruiting patients into studies to a critic of the process. Miller provides suggestions to offer a more ethical approach to enrollment of patients into phase I trials and provides ongoing informed consent as new trial data are collected. Miller challenges the established science to humanize the process with information and dialogue with patients in a truthful manner.

26. Nonmaleficence. In Beauchamp TL, Childress JF, eds. Principles of Biomedical Ethics, 5th ed. New York: Oxford University Press; 2001:113-164.

27. Beneficence. In Beauchamp TL, Childress JF, eds. Principles of Biomedical Ethics, 5th ed. New York: Oxford University Press; 2001:165-224.

Thank you to all my colleagues at MEDEX Northwest who waited while I wrote and to my students and graduates who asked about the cases. Thank you for all the reviews and comments by the Department of Medical History and Ethics. Special thanks to Dr. Keren Wick, who always makes us look good with her compulsive editing style. Thank you to my personal editor Esther Herst.

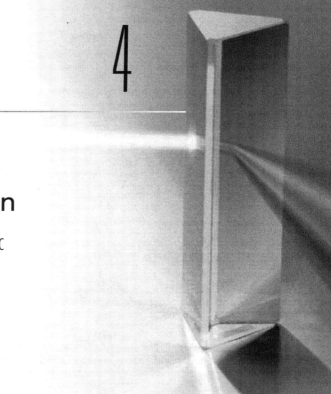

4

Ethics of Caring for a Diverse Population

Peter M. Stanford, MPH, PA-C

If we are to face up to race instead of whitewashing it, we must begin by acknowledging a fundamental reality: race is a relationship, not a set of characteristics that one can ascribe to one group or another.

Brown MK, Carnoy M, Currie E, et al. Whitewashing Race: The Myth of a Color-Blind Society[1]

CASE STUDY

"Patient Doe"*

911 Emergency receives a call at 9:30 on a Friday night. A resident in a large metropolitan neighborhood reports seeing a person lying face up on the sidewalk. In response to the call, police officers and a fire department unit arrive at the scene. A man is found sprawled near a dark alley. A small patch, about the size of a half dollar, of what appears to be blood is on the concrete under his head. He is disoriented, unable to give his name, and unsuccessful in his attempts to sit up. He is wearing a small watch and a wedding band. A large portable radio is found nearby. Although no wallet or identification is found, the officers believe no crime has been committed. As a result, the scene is not secured, and a preliminary investigation not initiated. Without identification, he is referred to thereafter as patient "John Doe" to those involved with the call.

Emergency Medical Technicians (EMTs) arrive on the scene. One is a basic EMT; the other had received advanced EMT training. The firemen describing Patient Doe's condition to the EMTs report "He's just drunk." Patient Doe is quickly assessed. There is now no verbal response to their questions or to painful stimuli. Patient Doe's eyes do not open spontaneously. During revival attempts, Patient Doe vomits but remains unresponsive. No sign or evidence of trauma is documented. The EMTs note the smell of alcohol (EtOH) on Patient Doe's breath and assess EtOH for possible intoxication. Patient Doe is assigned a Glasgow Coma Score of 6 and is designated Priority 3: Stable Patient. The patient is secured into the ambulance sitting upright on a cot rather than lying down on a backboard. A cervical collar is not affixed. Still unconscious and vomiting sporadically, the patient is transported to the Big

University Medical Center (BUMC) Emergency Department (ED). Because Patient Doe is deemed a low priority, the ambulance bypasses a closer hospital that also has a trauma center.

As typical for a Friday night, the BUMC ED is overburdened. Personnel in charge asked the Fire and Emergency Medical Services (EMS) on two occasions that night for permission to close the ED until nurses and physicians could catch up. Their requests were denied. Patient Doe arrived at the BUMC 1 hour after the initial EMS dispatch time and was the fifth patient brought by ambulance that evening assessed with alcohol intoxication.

The ambulance crew reports to ED admitting staff that they believe the patient had been drinking. With four other ambulances waiting to be checked-in, the triage nurse does not follow ED triage policy on treating an intoxicated patient and does not perform a neurological assessment; she just lists Patient Doe as intoxicated. Patient Doe is quickly assessed by a physician. The medical record does not mention head trauma. Intoxication is assumed, and no other explanations for Patient Doe's altered level of consciousness are investigated.

The evening charge nurse assigns Patient Doe to a holding area in a hallway to "sleep it off." No one is assigned to oversee Patient Doe's care. No order is given to check the patient's vital signs on a regular basis. Patient Doe is left unattended in the hallway. Over an hour later, a nurse finds the patient lying on the stretcher vomiting. Patient Doe is quickly re-evaluated and found to have a life-threatening brain injury that requires emergency neurosurgical intervention. Forty-six hours later, Patient John Doe was dead.

*Adapted from actual events.

QUESTIONS FOR DISCUSSION

1. Describe the developing situation.

2. What is your initial reaction, and what do you think about the situation, events, and activities that occurred before John Doe was transported to the hospital and after he arrived at the hospital?

3. What is most troubling about this situation as it developed?

4. Discuss Patient Doe's case in relationship to the following ethical concepts:
   a. Autonomy
   b. Beneficence
   c. Nonmaleficence
   d. Justice

5. Explain the extent to which each of the above ethical concepts was or was not practiced with Patient Doe.

6. Take a few minutes to ascribe the following attributes to Patient Doe. Explain your reasoning for each.
   a. Socioeconomic status
   b. Race/ethnicity
   c. Dress and physical appearance
   d. Age

7. Identify everyone involved in this case. Assume the role of each. Discuss what was done. Discuss what each character could have done differently.

8. List and discuss factors, such as discrimination, stereotyping, socioeconomic status, training, and gender bias, that may have influenced Patient Doe's care as demonstrated throughout the situation.

9. Indicate if you have experienced or observed any of the above events and how they may have influenced the care patients received.

10. Give examples where you have allowed any of the above factors to influence your interactions with a patient in your care.

11. Discuss the role the conditions in the ED played in affecting Patient Doe's care?

12. If Patient Doe had been a recognized, prominent politician or celebrity, would the attention and care he received been different? If so, discuss the ethical issues involved.

Bioethical Principles

Ethics is the science of morals. It represents the philosophical study of motivation, action, and ideas of right and wrong. Garvin describes ethics as a "critical study of standards for judging the rightness or wrongness of conduct."[2] The Physician Assistant (PA) Code of Ethics directs PAs to follow ethical guidelines when delivering care to patients. Simply put, it directs PAs to "do the right thing."[3] The following four bioethical principles; autonomy, beneficence, nonmaleficence, and justice, are discussed in relationship to the circumstances surrounding Patient Doe's case.

Autonomy

Autonomy means self-rule. Patients have the right to make autonomous decisions and choices. Health-care providers should respect these decisions and choices.[4] Applied to health care, autonomy charges practitioners and managed care organizations with a duty to respect the right of their patients or members to make decisions about the course of their care and treatment.[5]

Autonomy is an eloquent derivative of enlightened 18th-century philosophy. The Age of Enlightenment championed the ideal that the common people, just as any sovereign king, had an equal capacity to inquire, reason, make choices, and govern their own lives. Of this period of rebellious intellectual freedom and expression Jimack writes: "In the field of science Bacon, a contemporary of Montaigne, had spelled out an ambitious programme of enquiry, based on investigation and experiment instead of the acceptance of authority."[6]

Unenlightened medical practitioners, as did their regal counterparts, believed that only they knew what was best for those under their care. They failed to provide patients with appropriate information, treatment choices, or alternatives to consider. In this case study, by being unconscious, Patient Doe was unable to exercise autonomy over his care. Patient Doe had no advance directives, no family or friend present who could speak on his behalf. The loss of patient autonomy in emergency medicine presents both health-care professionals and patients with unique ethical problems. For the unconscious or incapacitated patient, legal and ethical authorities recognize a doctrine of implied consent: believing a reasonable person would consent to emergency treatment.[7,8] Without a family member or surrogate available to oversee treatment, intervening physicians (or PAs) are expected to act in the best interest of the patient.[9]

The actual protocol followed in such cases varies according to state laws and statutes and local rules and regulations. In some states, the physician's authority to act and subsequent decision making is guided by the type of medical decisions required; routine treatment, major medical treatment, or life-sustaining treatment. The attending physician may decide to render routine treatment, requiring no specific consent, or, if invasive treatment that carries potential risks is required, consult with a second physician.[10]

The Emergency Room as a Factor

However, as it turned out, patient consent was the least of Patient Doe's concerns. EDs have become overcrowded but are the primary portal to care for the insured and uninsured alike.[11] The American College of Emergency Physicians (ACEP) reports that people who cannot afford to pay for medical care and who have no health insurance often turn to EDs for treatment of conditions that have become acute because these people lack access to regular medical care. Emergency physicians see first-hand the consequences of a health-care system in which 40 million people are uninsured and millions more are underinsured. The nation's nearly 4000 hospital EDs are a portal for as many as 3 out of 4 uninsured patients admitted to U.S. hospitals.[12]

The ACEP describes a bleak picture of ED facilities, their medical staffs, and uninsured patients: The scarcity of primary care practitioners in inner cities and rural areas contributes to an increasing reliance on EDs. EDs are often the only source of medical care available at night, on weekends, and on holidays.[13]

The *Washington Post* cited an Institute of Medicine (IOM) report that assailed the conditions found in the nation's EDs: too often, busy EDs stabilize patients and then have to leave them lying on gurneys in hallways for 48 hours or more until a room becomes available and they can be admitted to the hospital. That is both a time of misery for the patient and less timely care and potentially poorer care, without the specialized equipment and expertise available to inpatients.[14]

In a busy urban ED, what kind of decisions would a *conscious* Patient Doe have to make in order to ensure the ED staff was cognizant of his actual injuries and receive more attentive care? What actions would need to be taken? According to the principle of autonomy, it would be appropriate for Patient Doe to be involved in his care, to speak up, and to correct any misconceptions concerning his circumstances. Patient Doe could have objected to being ignored, marginalized, or treated poorly, if those were his perceptions.

Through the doctrine of implied consent, an incapacitated patient like Patient Doe, unable to make autonomous decisions or address his or her treatment or care, confers autonomy to those providing care. Each provider—policeman, fireman, EMT, nurse, physician, and PA—carries the responsibility to attend to his or her portion of this conferred autonomy per role or specialty. The American Academy of Physician Assistants (AAPA) Guidelines for Ethical Conduct for PAs recognize this chain of custody and expects PAs to be equally aware and "morally bound to provide care in emergency situations and to arrange proper follow-up."[15]

In the case of unconscious Patient Doe, the absence of a family member or an assigned surrogate compels the medical team's members to not only "provide consent" to emergency treatment as needed but also to act as a guardian of Patient Doe's care. Each must facilitate the professionalism and attention a conscious Patient Doe would expect to receive: i.e.,

attentive and appropriate intervention by properly trained and qualified personnel.

What kind of care should an unconscious patient, believed to be intoxicated and without identification or proof of insurance, expect to receive? According to the principle of autonomy: the same care as an insured, sober, and conscious patient.

Beneficence

Beneficence means that PAs should act in patients' best interest. In certain cases, respecting patient autonomy and acting in their best interests may be difficult to balance,[16] particularly when a patient's choice is not congruent with a provider's treatment recommendations.[17]

Patients, conscious or otherwise, expect to receive, if not the best care, at least appropriate care. The medical profession's ethical expectation is that the provider acts as a guardian of the patient's best interests. Accordingly, PAs have an ethical obligation to see that each patient receives appropriate care.[18] Clinicians encounter patients who are in states of great stress and vulnerability, making them dependent on the clinician's skill and knowledge.[19] Often, this involves patients negotiating their way through, from the patient's point of view, an incredibly complex environment filled with endless, at times uncomfortable, invasive diagnostic tests and procedures, not to mention the patient's inherent feelings of loss of control and fears concerning life and death, disfigurement, permanent disability, or chronic pain. Cassell reminds health-care providers of the patient experience, particularly those who experience recurrent or chronic pain: what patients learn is how little tolerance other people have for their continued report of pain and how pain becomes less bearable the longer it continues; patients with recurrent pain even suffer in the absence of their pain, anticipating its return, as do people with severe, frequent migraine headaches who constantly worry whether another will reappear to ruin another important occasion.[20]

Acting in the patient's best interest implies, at the minimum, that clinicians be able to recognize situations (trauma: psychological, medical, environmental or social), that are dangerous to the patient's health and well-being. Individually or as part of a team, clinicians must accurately assess the patient's medical condition and amount of risk present, and intervene appropriately. This responsibility is heightened when a patient, as in Patient Doe's case, is unconscious, incapacitated, or at risk of being ignored or otherwise mistreated. Regardless of the circumstance of a busy practice or ED; of a patient's tardiness, attitude, or disposition, or of the clinician's conscious or unconscious bias, the same professional and ethical obligation remains: the provision of respectful, appropriate care.

In an overburdened ED, patients are in competition with each other for the same staff attention and resources. As in Patient Doe's case, the clinical decisions made for him were in competition with the clinical interests of other patients. The decisions that led to Patient Doe's failure to be treated according to hospital protocol suggest Patient Doe's best interests were not the primary driving force behind his care. Patient Doe, as with all patients entering the ED that night, was transferred into the care of the ED and seen first by a triage nurse. The responsibility of triage is to assess, evaluate, and manage the patient's clinical presentation in accordance with established ED protocols and patient care standards in order to facilitate efficient allocation of ED resources.

Triage derives from the French *trier,* meaning "to sort." In advanced triage, physicians may decide that some severely injured people should not receive care because they are unlikely to survive. The available care is then directed to those with some hope of survival. Clearly there are ethical implications to consider if treatment is intentionally withheld from those with a small chance of survival and given to others more likely to survive. Triage is generally reserved for situations involving mass casualties, although a variant of the concept is practiced in EDs as a strategy in response to increased demand.[21]

Was Patient Doe relegated to a hallway because his condition was assessed as unsalvageable? Was his condition appropriately assessed and determined to require only minimal attention? Was Patient Doe's assessment and assigned level of priority a cogent decision or the result of error, or was he ignored because he was assessed as being intoxicated? If any deficits in treatment were observed or recognized by a member of the medical staff, what prevented that person from speaking up and assertively intervening in Patient Doe's best interest?

Failure to address inappropriate or questionable patient care may be one of the first signs of professional burnout. A decreased ability to respond emotionally to patients and depersonalization (the inability to see a patient as a person) is associated with the stressors of the ED.[22,23] Cognitive biases influence individual and group behavior and decisions. Status quo bias explains how individuals accept and go along with established norms. Omission bias occurs when individuals or groups do not act although an alternative action or treatment in a clinical setting could offer a better clinical outcome.[24,25] Was the prevailing status quo bias in force at BUMC to wheel "drunks" over to the side and go see "real" patients? What compromised the accurate performance of routine clinical assessment in the

field and in the ED? Why did the ED staff fail to perform established protocols and investigate into other causes for the presenting symptoms in order to reduce the possibility of a misdiagnosis? Could the reason have been because of the patient's race, class, gender, or possibly appearance?

Nonmaleficence

Nonmaleficence means to do no harm, to impose no unnecessary or unacceptable burden on the patient.[26] Although a basic tenet of medical ethics, nonmaleficence gains special attention when balanced against health-care costs and limited resources or resources that are under pressure in a cost-containment world.[27,28] Diagnostic procedures and treatments are not without risk and risk-related costs. According to the IOM, at least 44,000 to 98,000 patient lives are lives lost each year due to preventable medical errors in hospitals, exceeding the deaths attributable to motor vehicle wrecks, breast cancer, and AIDS.[29] The cost of drug-related morbidity and mortality exceeded $177.4 billion in 2000.[30]

In Patient Doe's case, the risks of harm were not the result of a procedure or a reaction to a medication. Police officers responding to the call were unable to determine the circumstances or events that led to Patient Doe's lying helpless on the sidewalk. First responders were unable to assess an incapacitated patient and identify the extent of injuries and failed to take standard precautions for a possible head and/or neck injury. ED medical staff did not follow the established in-house protocols for patients believed to be intoxicated. Although there was no evidence of intentional harm to Patient Doe, discriminatory, biased, indifferent, or incompetent care leaves in its wake serious consequences. Emergency department clinicians are advised to avoid a diagnosis based only on behavior. They are encouraged to perform focused physical and neurological examinations on comatose patients.[31] Alcohol intoxication protocols generally require determination of blood or alcohol levels and serial observations of vital signs in addition to investigating and ruling out other possible causes to explain an unconscious patient's presenting condition.[32]

There was no documented evidence that severe head trauma was noted or included in the differential diagnosis to explain Patient Doe's condition. Other possibly life-threatening causes were not thoroughly investigated and ruled out. Hence, an unnecessary and inappropriate burden was placed on Patient Doe when it was incorrectly assessed and assumed, to tragic consequences, that his clinical presentation was due solely to alcohol intoxication. As a patient history was not possible given Patient Doe's comatose or semicomatose state, a brief but thorough physical examination consisting of close inspection, palpation, and a focused neurological assessment may have significantly changed the course and possibly the outcome of the case.

Justice

Justice means that patients in similar circumstances should receive similar care. Justice refers to the norms used for the fair distribution of society's resources, risks, and costs.[33] Norms are shared understandings about actions that are obligatory, permitted, or forbidden.[34] They are the standards against which people evaluate the appropriateness of their behavior.[35] Some are rational; others are affected by historical forces, tradition, institutions,[36] customs, and habits.[37] As social constructs, norms reflect prevailing social hierarchies. In social hierarchies, discrimination, prejudice, and stereotypes are practices utilized by individuals and groups to negotiate or maintain power and position, hence improved access to resources and a higher probability of survival.

Norms govern the distribution of social resources that flow though established social hierarchies. Who or what society values more will receive the most attention and access to social resources. Conversely, who or what society values less receives less of both. An individual's acceptance of inequality in hierarchies may be based on the belief that group hierarchies and competition for resources are inevitable.[38] Social hierarchies and norms guide individual and group members' behaviors until they are challenged, either interpersonally or structurally.[39]

The immediate and cumulative effect of these subtle and not so subtle norms—when they become exclusionary—is to form and reinforce "socially acceptable" negative stereotypes and discriminatory practices. In relationship to health care, they lead to the creation and support of a delivery system that by design contributes to disparities in access, distribution, and quality of health resources. Barry R. Bloom, PhD, Dean, Harvard School of Public Health, wrote in the foreword of "Health Disparities & the Body Politic: A Series of International Symposia" sponsored by the Harvard School of Public Health in 2005: "Perhaps most discouraging: despite enormous gains in quality of life stemming from advances in public health and medicine, disparities in health status, life expectancy, access to knowledge and medical technologies, and access to care have widened everywhere, both within and between countries."[40]

As an applied ethical principle, justice is obtained through maximizing the benefits and opportunities available to those at the lowest level of society by making the resources of society equally available to all. i.e., the "maximum" principle.[41] Accordingly, all

patients—rich or poor; insured or uninsured; those who suffer from injury or acute or chronic illnesses or who are at risk of developing a disease or medical condition; regardless of gender, ethnicity, belief, or lifestyle—should receive similar access to health-care services.

The Guidelines for Ethical Conduct for PAs identifies the role PAs are to play in addressing community health issues and encourages PAs to become involved in analyzing the conditions and behaviors that lead healthy citizens to becoming ill patients. In general, PAs should be committed to upholding and enhancing community values, be aware of the needs of the community, and use the knowledge and experience acquired as professionals to contribute to an improved community.[42]

In Patient Doe's case, the resources were available. Surrounded by potentially life-saving, state-of-the-art technology and highly trained medical professionals, the opportunity to render justice, i.e., equal care, presented itself. What went wrong? In the real world, the equal availability of resources is not always synonymous with the actual delivery or provision of those resources. Indifferent clinicians or other members of the health-care team can effectively sabotage the ethical promise of justice. In order for the ethical concept of justice to be realized, the resources available must be put into play. Caregivers must be motivated to act by a concern for the well-being of those they tend.[43]

Had Patient Doe's mental status not been impaired, he would certainly have asserted his need for immediate attention and prompt treatment. Had Patient Doe presented similarly impaired but been accompanied by a spouse, family member, or other surrogate, that person would have pressed for additional treatment or at least a heightened sense of urgency. The companion may also have been able to remain with Patient Doe in the hallway.

With no family member or surrogate present to act as an advocate and with a life possibly hanging in the balance, who will perform as an advocate? Who will hold those providing care accountable to their various medical oaths and professional codes of ethics? Without family or an appointed surrogate, BUMC and all the personnel involved in Patient Doe's treatment became, by serial default, Patient Doe's guardian and advocate, and they failed.

Some argue that the conceptual foundation of the ethic of justice is flawed and may lead to an unnecessary barrier between patient and provider. Clements (1996) writes: "The *ethic of justice* begins with an assumption of human *separateness*, so that in order to be obligated to others, we must in some sense consent to those obligations. Thus the ethic of justice emphasizes notions of *choice* and *will* in understanding our moral obligations. The *ethic of care* begins with an assumption of human *connectedness*, the result of which is that to a large extent we *recognize rather than choose* our obligations to others. In other words, the ethic of justice takes *freedom* as its starting point, while the ethic of care takes *obligation* as its starting point."[44]

It will never be known if an ethic of care as such would have significantly changed the outcome of Patient Doe's case. The family of Patient Doe would certainly have been more comforted to know that, despite succumbing to his injuries, he had been given the best of care rather than learning of the poor quality of care he actually received, which may have facilitated his demise.

Few health-care providers would intentionally practice stereotypical behavior (or comfortably admit doing so) that leads to poor patient outcomes. Ultimately, however, for ethical oaths to be more than well-meaning words, their tenets must be advocated and practiced by individuals, held in high esteem, recognized, and rewarded among peers within the profession. Every practitioner is vulnerable to conflict between the discriminatory internalized social customs or norms and their professional duty and obligation as a health-care provider. Recognizing this conflict, the AAPA Code of Ethics sets the appropriate standard: "Physician Assistants shall extend to each patient the full measure of their ability as dedicated, empathetic, health care providers, and shall assume responsibility for the skillful and proficient transactions of their professional duties."[45]

Health equity (justice) without application or advocacy does little good locally, nationally, or globally.[46] Epidemics and the threat of pandemics of infectious diseases should be reminders that while science has revolutionized medicine, a plan for ensuring equal access to care is needed. What affects one will at some point in time affect all. Excellence without equity presents as the chief human rights dilemma of health care in the 21st century.[47]

Becoming "Invisible"

On an early summer evening, without identification and unable to communicate, Patient John Doe entered a different world: a place where the stigma of stereotype defines attention (or lack of it) and the quality of care received. Patient Doe became, in the eyes of those providing care, "just another drunk," undeserving of concern and appropriate care. So labeled, for all intents and purposes, Patient Doe became invisible.

Invisibility is not a new American phenomenon. Ralph Ellison wrote in 1952 in the preface of *Invisible Man,* a novel in which an unnamed black man searches for his identity in a racist society: "I am an invisible man…when they approach me they see only my surroundings, themselves, or figments of their imagination—indeed, everything and anything except me."[48]

The "invisible" world Ellison wrote of was the segregation and oppression of black Americans, an entire race of people conveniently "not seen." Ellison's character, a young black male, sought to understand and survive in a society that burdened his everyday existence with racial discrimination, limited educational and job opportunities, poor housing, and limited access to health care. He existed in a society that offered no respect to his personhood and at any moment could imprison, strike out, injure, or kill him with near impunity.

In the five decades since publication of *Invisible Man,* the ranks of an "invisible nation" have swollen and changed. Their faces have additional hues. Their illnesses include HIV/AIDS, common and chronic diseases. Their languages represent a global and national economic diaspora. Their economic classes include the employed, "working poor," and the insured and underinsured. Their ages encompass the very young and the very old. Their communities are found in suburban cul de sacs and Appalachian hollows, rural western plains and southern bayous, and urban tenements and cardboard boxes under highways among Hollywood's rich and famous.

In August 2005 Hurricane Katrina washed through the American psyche and, in dramatic fashion, washed away, at least temporarily,[49] the "invisibility" of the poor. It allowed the United States and the world to see that poverty continues to touch millions of American lives. Katrina also reminded those following the events that "race still matters" as large numbers of poor and predominantly black New Orleans residents waited and waited and waited for slow incoming assistance and disaster relief.

Poverty and inequality in society continue, paradoxically, to feed and fatten the criminal justice and health-care systems with resulting crime and other costly social problems such as drug and alcohol abuse, homelessness, out-of-wedlock births, poor educational achievement, and domestic violence,[50,51] whose systemic cause and solutions are frequently disavowed and disinherited.[52] In other words, not only do the citizens of the invisible nation remain condemned to being invisible, the political, social, and economic disparities that contribute to their conditions remain equally invisible and largely unaddressed. The title for the invisible nation's national anthem may best be the oft quoted truism of French journalist and novelist Jean-Baptiste Alphonse Karr: *plus ça change, plus c'est la même chose*— "the more things change, the more they stay the same."[53]

The invisible nation has no discernible borders, requires no visa or passport. It easily accommodates transient visitors like Patient John Doe. In response to the civil rights movement of the 1960s and affirmative action of the 1970s, anyone, regardless of race, creed, class, or gender, can find himself suddenly relegated to citizenship in the invisible nation.

Changing Demographics/ Changing Challenges

In 2000 the U.S. Census Bureau reported that the white, non-Hispanic population accounted for 69.4%, a majority, of the total U.S. population. Also in 2000, the black population accounted for 12.7%, Hispanic 12.6%, Asian 3.8%, and all other races 2.5% of the population (Fig. 4.1).[54]

According to U.S. Census Bureau projections from 2000 to 2050, the white non-Hispanic population is projected to increase from 195.7 million to 210.3 million, representing an increase of 14.6 million, or 7%. By comprising just 50.1% of the total population,[55] white non-Hispanic Americans will be close to losing their status as the majority. During the same period, the Hispanic American population is projected to grow by 67 million, from 35.6 million to 102.6 million, an increase of 188%, becoming the largest American minority group, comprising 24.4% of the total population.[56]

Correspondingly, the African American population is projected to increase from 35.8 million to 61.4 million in 2050, an increase of about 26 million, or 71%, increasing their share of the country's population from 12.7% to 14%.[57] The Asian American population, currently the fastest growing segment, is projected to grow 213%, from 10.7 million to 33.4 million, doubling their percentage of the nation's population from 3.8% to 8% by 2050.[58]

The future of the United States will not be found on foreign battlefields. Great sacrifices, when necessary, guarantee and protect those principles and ideals proclaimed in the Preamble of the Constitution of the United States adopted in 1789: "We the people of the United States, in order to form a more perfect union, establish justice, insure domestic tranquility, provide for the common defense, promote the general welfare, and secure the blessings of liberty to ourselves and our posterity, do ordain and establish this Constitution for the United States of America."[59] The country's future was, however, clearly described in the opening of the executive summary of *Teaching Cultural Competence in Health Care: A Review of Current Concepts, Policies and Practices* from the Office of Minority Health, U.S. Department of Health and Human Services (DHHS), published in 2002: "With growing concerns about racial and ethnic disparities in health, and the need for health care systems to accommodate increasingly diverse patient populations, 'cultural competence' has become more and more a matter of national concern. Training physicians to care for diverse populations is essential."[60]

Health Disparities Among Minority Populations

African Americans, Hispanic Americans, Asian Americans/Pacific Islanders, and American Indians/ Alaska Natives, when compared with their white counterparts in the U.S. population, carry a disproportionate burden of suffering, morbidity, and mortality from illness and diseases, including cancer, cardiovascular disease and stroke, diabetes, and HIV/AIDS. Higher infant mortality rates and lower immunization rates further complicate the picture.[61] According to the Office of Minority Health, DHHS,[62] the causes of health disparities among minorities have been attributed to a variety of factors, including:

- Socioeconomic status, lack of access to quality health services, environmental hazards in homes and neighborhoods, and the scarcity of effective prevention programs tailored to the needs of specific communities[63]
- Shortages of health professionals in urban areas where minority populations are high[64]
- Patients' mistrust of the health-care system[65]
- Perceived discrimination[66]
- Poor communication between physicians and patients[67,68]
- Lack of cultural sensitivity and cultural competence of physicians and other health-care workers[69–71]

Some have argued that a direct link between racial and ethnic health disparities and the lack of culturally competent care has not been empirically demonstrated but agree that provision of culturally competent services can potentially improve health by increasing understanding between physicians and patients and potentially increasing patient adherence to treatment.[72] However, in its 2003 landmark report, entitled *Unequal Treatment: Confronting Racial and Ethnic Disparities in Health Care*, the IOM found that racial and ethnic disparities in health care do exist and that many sources, including health-care systems, health-care providers, patients, and utilization managers, are all contributors.[73] According to the Department of Human and Health Services, an increasingly large, consistent body of research indicates that racial and ethnic minorities are less likely to receive even routine medical procedures and experience a lower quality of health services.[74–76]

Research indicates that Native Americans, Asian Americans, African Americans, and Hispanic and Latino groups tend to underutilize health and mental health services.[77] Sue and Sue speculated that the underutilization of services is related to the cultural

Projected Population of the United States, by Race and Hispanic Origin: 2000 to 2050

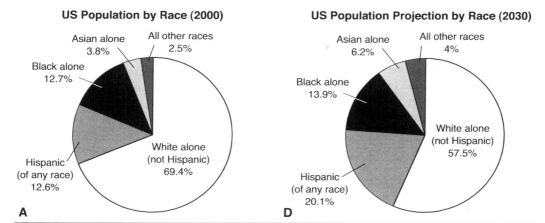

US Population by Race (2000)

Asian alone 3.8%
All other races 2.5%
Black alone 12.7%
White alone (not Hispanic) 69.4%
Hispanic (of any race) 12.6%

A

US Population Projection by Race (2030)

Asian alone 6.2%
All other races 4%
Black alone 13.9%
White alone (not Hispanic) 57.5%
Hispanic (of any race) 20.1%

D

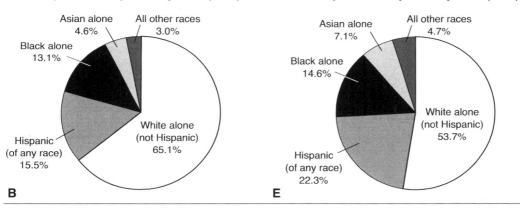

US Population Projection by Race (2010)

Asian alone 4.6%
All other races 3.0%
Black alone 13.1%
White alone (not Hispanic) 65.1%
Hispanic (of any race) 15.5%

B

US Population Projection by Race (2040)

Asian alone 7.1%
All other races 4.7%
Black alone 14.6%
White alone (not Hispanic) 53.7%
Hispanic (of any race) 22.3%

E

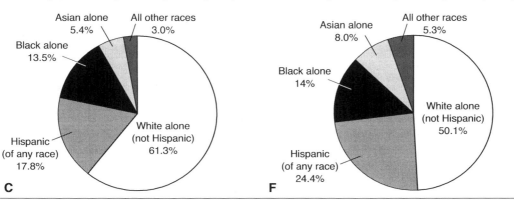

US Population Projection by Race (2020)

Asian alone 5.4%
All other races 3.0%
Black alone 13.5%
White alone (not Hispanic) 61.3%
Hispanic (of any race) 17.8%

C

US Population Projection by Race (2050)

Asian alone 8.0%
All other races 5.3%
Black alone 14%
White alone (not Hispanic) 50.1%
Hispanic (of any race) 24.4%

F

Percentages do not total 100%. Hispanic category includes data from Black, Asian, White, and all other races. While not encompassing the full matrix of race and Hispanic-origin categories, the race groups for which these interim population projections are available include: (1) White alone, (2) Black alone, (3) Asian alone, and (4) All other races alone and Two or more races. Other groups include: (1) Hispanic origin, (2) Hispanic White alone, (3) non-Hispanic origin, and (4) non-Hispanic White alone.

Figure 4.1 Projected population of the United States by race and Hispanic origin 2000 to 2050. (Modified from U.S. Census Bureau, 2004, U.S. interim projections by age, sex, race, and Hispanic origin. Accessed from census.gov/ipc/www/usinterimproj/)

insensitivity and inappropriateness of formalized services to culturally diverse groups.[78] Many African American and Latino patients reported perceiving racism in the health-care system and preferred a physician of their own race or ethnicity.[79] Self-reported surveys of perceived racial discrimination, in the longitudinal Coronary Artery Risk Development in Young Adults study in African American men and women, demonstrated such perception was statistically significantly associated with worse physical and mental health in both men and women, before and after adjustment for age, education, income, and skin color.[80] Johnson et al found racial and ethnic differences in patient perceptions of health-care system bias persisted even after controlling for demographics, source of care, and patient-physician communication variables.[81] Specifically, African Americans, Hispanics, and Asians were more likely than whites to perceive that they would have received better medical care had they belonged to a different racial or ethnic group and that medical staff judged them unfairly or treated them with disrespect based on race or ethnicity and how well they spoke English. Ma reported that Chinese Americans tend to avoid Western medicine unless their health problems are serious.[82] African American patients who believe that their provider has been disrespectful may not return to treatment, may try another provider, or may change their health-care plan.[83]

The reality is that racial and ethnic minority patients receive lower quality interpersonal care than white patients.[84] Patients feeling uncomfortable with the attitudes of medical staff and providers are presented with additional and unnecessary barriers to care, compounding other impediments such as cost and access. As a result, they may tend to put off seeking medical attention, wait longer, present sicker, and divulge less information to their health-care providers.

In response to these disparities, several major initiatives to improve the health of minority populations have been implemented by the DHHS. *Healthy People 2010* established a public health agenda, with the goals of eliminating health disparities and improving the overall health of all Americans by promoting health and preventing illness, disability, and premature death during the first decade of the 21st century.[85] The focus for disparity reduction is on six key areas shown to affect racial and ethnic groups differently at all life stages: infant mortality, diabetes, cardiovascular disease, cancer screening and management, HIV/AIDS, and child and adult immunizations.[86]

Increasing Health-Care Cost

In 2004 health care spending in the United States reached $1.9 trillion. By 2009 that figure is estimated to reach $2.9 trillion, or 16% of the gross domestic product, growing to 20% by 2015.[87] Future generations of taxpayers will be left with the burden and responsibility of paying the staggering health-care costs for an increasingly larger, albeit less healthy, portion of the population, if the health status of U.S. minority populations is not significantly improved.

Diversity Management: Cultural Competency

Opportunity 2000,[88] written in 1987 by the Hudson Institute for the Department of Labor, anticipated an increasingly diverse U.S. workforce by 2000. It described the aforementioned projected demographic changes, including a rise in the average age of the workforce and an increase in the number of women and minorities participating. In 1990 Dr. R. Roosevelt Thomas, Jr., developed the term "managing diversity" and developed training to sensitize and prepare workplaces for a more diverse environment.[89] According to the U.S. Government Accountability Office, diversity training can provide employees with an awareness of their differences—culture, background, education, language skills, personality, physical attributes, sexual orientation, and work role—and an understanding of how diverse perspectives and skills can improve organizational performance.[90] Similarly in patient care, providers must acquire and maintain the requisite knowledge and skills to provide attentive, quality care to diverse patient populations irrespective of their circumstance, background, education, language skills, personality, or sexual orientation.

Increased cultural competency among providers and health-care institutions has been identified as a potential strategy for improving quality and eliminating sociocultural barriers at the organizational, structural, and clinical levels, which have been identified as significant contributors to the disparities in health care.[91]

In *Teaching Cultural Competence In Health Care: A Review Of Current Concepts, Policies and Practices,*[92] cited at the beginning of this chapter, the Office of Minority Health reported efforts to develop national standards for Culturally and Linguistically Appropriate Services (CLAS) in Health Care.[93,94] It provided the following definitions: "Culturally Competent Care refers mainly to the family physician-patient relationship and the delivery of culturally competent care by individual physicians."

"Cultural and linguistic competence is a set of congruent behaviors, attitudes, and policies that come together in a system, agency, or among professionals that enables effective work in cross-cultural situations. (Linguistic minorities include people with limited English proficiency and low literacy skills as well as the hearing-impaired.)"

"Culture refers to integrated patterns of human behavior, which includes the language, thoughts, communications, actions, customs, beliefs, values, and institutions of racial, ethnic, religious, or social groups."

"Competence implies having the capacity to function effectively as an individual and an organization within the context of the cultural beliefs, behaviors, and needs presented by consumers and their communities."[95]

The report also emphasized: "It is important to point out that in our definition of cultural competence, the social groups influencing a person's culture and self-identity include not only race, ethnicity, and religion but also gender, sexual orientation, age, disability, and socioeconomic status."[96]

AAPA Ethics Guidelines recognize the importance of maintaining competence: "Physician Assistants shall strive to maintain and increase the quality of individual health care service through individual study and continuing education."[97]

Sadly, when the topic of cultural competence is raised, the eyes of students and seminar attendees, including minority members and others historically marginalized, immediately glaze over. The prevailing attitude is "I know about this stuff already." or "*I* don't need this stuff. *They* do." Addressing this type of denial, Alport writes: "But even conceding that honest ignorance and sheer habituation account for some of the denial, we must also grant that the deeper mechanism is often at work. We have previously seen that those who are deeply prejudiced are inclined to deny that they are prejudiced. Lacking personal insight, they are unable to take an objective view of conditions in their community. Even a citizen without prejudices of his own is likely to blind himself to injustices and tensions which, if acknowledged, could only upset the even tenor of his life."[98]

Gaining and Maintaining Cultural Competency

In order to maintain state licensure and national certification requirements, practicing PAs must accrue a minimum of 100 CME hours every 2 years.[99] If the goal is to maintain knowledge *and* clinical effectiveness, clinicians also must invest appropriate time learning how to relate to, understand, and provide care for a changing patient population. The challenge is to assess, identify, and confront any stereotypes and biases that, if unchecked, reduce their personal effectiveness or the effectiveness of their staff and practice as a whole. Once identified and named, such lapses are easier to address and expunge. Alternatively,

appropriate responses that adhere to the PA profession's ethical standards and strategies to maintain "due diligence" can be developed for situations that will present in the future.

Attention should be given to those activities that will increase cultural competence as well as clinical competence. Caution is urged for students or clinicians attempting to become more "sensitive." Seminars that portend to teach cultural competence or multiculturalism may inadvertently reinforce time-worn stereotypes and drastically oversimplify a much more complex challenge facing health-care providers. Knowing that ethnic group X reveres the Earth and that group Y believes in the balance of health forces within the body confers a novel but superficial awareness more likely to give a practitioner a false sense of being culturally competent. In his 1998 opening remarks entitled *How America Is Changing: The Impact of Demographics and Cultural Diversity on Health Care* at the National Conference on Quality Health Care for Culturally Diverse Populations, Harold L. Hodgkinson, Ph.D.,[100] observed: "There is a huge difference in how you treat people. This distinction is particularly important given the fact that the United States classifies individuals in pan-ethnic groups such as Asian or Hispanic. Particularly within health care settings, it is important to recognize the vast diversity present within these groupings....you can damage people by stereotypical attention to what people are supposed to behave like if they are Asian. There is a difference between an upper class Chinese with two college degrees who comes to the United States and a Hmong person who fled for his life from the Laos capital to the hills. Those two are simply very different cultures. So 'Asian' will not work... in a doctor's office."

Carrillo, Green, and Betancourt recognized the goal of cross-cultural training as related to continuing medical education is to help physicians improve their ability to understand, communicate with, and care for patients from diverse backgrounds.[101] Betancourt later suggested that a solution in improving practitioners' cultural competency lies in improving their ability to help patients understand those factors that affect their health. He explains: "Previous efforts in cultural competence have aimed to teach about the attitudes, values, beliefs, and behavior of certain groups. A more effective approach is to learn a practical framework to guide inquiry with individual patients about how social, cultural, or economic factors influence their [the patient's] health values, beliefs, and behaviors."[102]

Additionally, Betancourt advocates a patient-targeted practical approach: "At the end of the day, physicians need a practical set of tools and skills that will enable them to provide quality care to patients everywhere, from anywhere, with whatever differences in background that may exist, in what is likely to be a brief clinical encounter."[103]

However, improving practitioner cultural competency and removing barriers associated with health disparities does not begin with helping *the patient* understand how social, cultural, or economic factors influence their health values, beliefs, and behaviors. Improving practitioner cultural competency begins with *providers* understanding how social, cultural, and class and other factors influence formation of their health values, beliefs, and behaviors that affect and influence how they perceive, interact with, and subsequently treat or respond to their patients. Furthermore, having the "tools" associated with cultural competency does not necessarily mean those tool are used appropriately.

Much of the negative stereotyping, prejudice, and discrimination projected toward those who are different was assumed to be the result of ignorance or unfamiliarity. It was believed that learning about the attitudes, values, beliefs, and behaviors of people different from themselves would lead to a change in the beliefs and behaviors of providers. Similar to smokers who continue to smoke contrary to their provider's advice or after coronary events, knowledge does not necessarily change behavior.[104]

There are tools already available to practitioners: codes of ethics and caring about their patients. Understanding and applying the ethical codes of their respective health-related professions enables health service personnel, from patient care attendants to physicians and PAs alike, to optimize caring for their patients. A sincere personal commitment to maintaining an ethical practice, combined with an equal and genuine commitment to becoming culturally competent, should benefit the clinician-patient relationship and improve patient-related outcomes over time.

Cultural Competency: More Than Race and Ethnicity

Viewing cultural competence and the projected demographic changes of the U.S. population landscape and its inherent diversity only in terms of race and ethnicity drastically oversimplifies a much more complex challenge facing health-care providers. Ethnocentrism and racism are two of many potential barriers practitioners must resist and with which patients must contend. Within the rapidly changing and increasingly diverse population the potential exists for other negative stereotypes and resulting discrimination to manifest.

Bias and Stereotype Formation

Stereotypes are a conventional or formulaic conception or image of reality attributed or constructed by an individual or group of individuals. Stereotypes serve a cognitive function by reducing the complexity of the world and making it more manageable.[105] The ability to categorize people and circumstances quickly and to identify patterns is a fundamental quality, or cognitive process, of the human mind. All human decisions and judgments to some extent or another have reference to a stereotype.[106] This process is the foundation of stereotypes that underlie prejudice (attitude), bias (preference), and discriminatory practices (action).

Transference is a well-described phenomenon in psychotherapy and mental health counseling used to explain the unconscious tendency to assign to others positive or negative feelings and attitudes associated with significant persons in a patient's early life.[106] Transference describes a patient's transfer of such attitudes or feelings to a therapist. Countertransference is a transference reaction from the therapist to the patient, reflecting a reaction to the patient's behavior or the therapist own inner needs and conflicts.[108] From this perspective, the patient-physician relationship reveals its potential for acting as an unconscious mechanism through which inappropriate stereotyping is projected from the clinician toward the patient if the patient or any of his attributes or behaviors trigger these unconscious tendencies.[109,110]

Prejudices are preconceived judgments made without adequate evidence and are not easily alterable by presentation of contrary evidence. Prejudices prevent objective discussion or decision making of an issue or situation.[111] Ashmore and DelBoca conceptualized prejudice to be the expression of sociocultural norms, suggesting that individuals are basically motivated to seek approval and conformity to norms and established traditions.[112] In *The Nature of Prejudice*, Alport writes: "Few people know the real reason for their hatred of minority groups. The reasons they invent are merely rationalizations. This is the central thesis of all psychodynamic theories of prejudice. The scapegoat theory is one of this type. But there are others. When we say that prejudice covers up severe inferiority feelings; or that it gives security; or that it is bound up with repressed sexuality; or helps to relieve personal guilt feelings—we are in all cases talking in the realm of psychodynamics. In all these cases the sufferer is not aware of the psychological function that prejudice serves in his life."[113]

Crandall and Eshleman proposed a justification-suppression model that describes the process that leads to the expression of prejudice behavior or attitudes. They suggest that prejudices are not directly expressed but are restrained or "suppressed" by beliefs, values, and prevailing social norms. Prejudices are overtly expressed when a "justification," such as a significant emotion, event, ideology, or stereotype, acts as a trigger releasing the suppressed prejudices.[114] Whether prejudice is viewed as an expression of inner conflicts from unconscious drives that conflict with societal constraints or cognitive categorizations expressed in a social context, prejudice significantly influences behavior, which in turn influences the attention and care providers offer and the quality of care affected patients receive.

Health-care providers are not immune to stereotyping and subsequently projecting (countertransferring) their attitudes or feelings onto patients entrusted to their care. Examples of patients affected by common stereotypes include, but are not limited to, those who have limited or poor English fluency[115]; those who are obese[116,117]; those who are afflicted with disease[118] or are mentally ill[119]; those who are indigent, uneducated, or homeless[120]; those who are older or younger than the provider (ageism)[121]; and those who regularly experience overt or covert societal homophobia and gender inequities.[122,123] Any one stereotype alone or in combination with others further marginalizes the affected individuals or groups and affects the access, utilization, and quality of the care they receive.

Socially justified expressions of prejudice toward certain behaviors, diseases, or and illnesses are seen as acceptable by the society at large. Generally, these conditions or diseases are perceived to be a result of sexual promiscuity, smoking, drinking, use of drugs, etc. In the eyes of a judgmental society, all are seen as self-induced or acquired outside of accepted moral behaviors.[124] The conclusion in the minds of bias-prone individuals is that "those people" have poor morals and deserve what is coming to them. This attitude provides a codicil of righteousness to their inappropriate attitude, inattentiveness, and provision of second-class care.

One may assume that given Patient Doe's comatose or semicomatose condition, a patient would receive heightened attention and/or concern in a medical emergency situation. However, the exact opposite occurred. The stigma of alcoholism, real or otherwise, affected the care he received. Consciously or unconsciously, those responsible expressed a prejudice and turned a blind eye to Patient Doe's emergent situation.

Ethically Based and Culturally Competent Care

In the practice and application of law, the goal is to be "color-blind," i.e., to administer law in a fair and equal manner, without corruption, avarice, prejudice, or favor. The blindfolded "Lady of Justice" is iconic. Contemporary concepts of justice admonish legal professionals to be color-blind, not to discriminate or treat persons differently because of their skin color, religious beliefs, gender, or lifestyle choices. In con-trast, the practice of medicine is not based on rhetoric but rather on empiric reasoning and, increasingly, evidence-based outcomes requiring assessing differences and comparing outcomes.[125] The practice of medicine, unlike law, requires if not impels clinicians to discriminate. Practitioners must be aware of and notice variables such as race, gender, and eye color, which may have clinical significance for understanding and resolving the patient's presenting "chief complaint." Similarly, the response to treatment, health maintenance recommendations, and decisions of health-care providers and patients will vary from case to case, depending on the various circumstances. The ability to discriminate lies at the very heart of effective clinical reasoning and intervention.

Progress in mapping the human genome has led to advances in pharmacogenetics, which use a patient's genetic profile to optimize drug therapy. The role ethnicity plays in determining how well pharmacotherapeutic agents are metabolized has been increasingly appreciated.[126]

Discrimination as an Evaluative Tool

Satel reminds clinicians of their responsibility to use their discriminatory powers appropriately and responsibly: The public's health is best served by a balanced approach that considers race as a variable in both biomedical and social health research. In the debate over the proper place of race in scientific inquiry, the meaning of the human genome project has become a powerful Rorschach test. Deliberately ignoring race in biomedical research can lead to inferior or improper treatment.[127]

Each patient has a lifestyle, habits, beliefs, attitudes, health history, and genetic predisposition unique to him or her. Therefore, patients cannot be treated the same. Even when used in a figurative sense, "treating everybody the same" devalues individuals, strips them of their unique individual characteristics. Such an approach does not foster within a practitioner a deeper understanding of patients' beliefs or culture sufficient to develop and incorporate effective therapeutic interventions into health care. Such an approach does not make practitioners culturally competent nor does it reflect having a higher ethical standard. Unintentionally, it creates another stereotype: patients being "all the same" who can be treated all the same. Practitioners treating patients equally could easily find themselves with a waiting room full of patients, all on a beta blocker for hypertension, and wonder why not all of them are well controlled.

The quality and effectiveness of disease prevention and health promotion activities are dependent on understanding how a patient's gender, ethnicity, age, sexual orientation, and other variables influence and ultimately manifest as their "state of health." Researchers and practitioners in the medical and mental health communities realize that, when practicing among diverse groups of people, knowledge of gender and culture is important in evaluating health risks and must be incorporated into disease prevention and treatment regimens. In the preface to their *Handbook of Gender, Culture, and Health,* Eisler and Hersen cite the following examples: "...women, more than men, appear more vulnerable to depression, eating disorders, and sexual abuse. Men are more likely than women to show high cardiovascular reactivity to stress and suffer more coronary artery disease, and Black men suffer from more cardiovascular disease and hypertension than White men. Cultural homophobia can cause gay men and lesbians to receive lower quality health care than other groups. Native Americans have very high rates of diabetes due to the prevalence of obesity and high fat diets. Health risk behaviors such as smoking, alcohol and drug abuse, and unsafe sexual practices have been found to vary considerably among ethnic groups."[128]

Discrimination as a Detrimental Practice

When the ability to discern (discriminate) is no longer an evaluative skill or tool utilized in the *patient's* best interest, it becomes a detrimental practice leading to substandard care or poor patient outcomes. Clinicians are encouraged not to become superficially blind to their patient's differences nor gloss over their own stereotypes but rather to recognize these differences and learn how to incorporate them appropriately into effective intervention strategies. At the minimum, these changes may include providing patients with attentive face-to-face time, making literature available and posting in-clinic signs in the patient's language, assuring the availability of translators sensitive to the nuances of the language and the culture when needed, ensuring handicap accessibility, and incorporating nontraditional medical concepts and practices into the patient's care. Adding a health component to existing community organizations can help the clinician to gain familiarity with those involved, credibility and visibility, and access to hard-to-reach populations, particularly immigrant and refugee communities.[129]

Astute clinicians develop the ability to distinguish the difference between stereotypes and generalizations. Stereotypes subjectively categorize those affected as all alike, effectively rendering the patient's individual uniqueness invisible. Generalizations, on the other hand, indicate an objective awareness of cultural norms, serve as a starting point, and allow the clinician to factor in individual characteristics such as education, nationality, faith, and accultur-

ation.[130] Within their practice settings, health-care providers can use the CLAS recommendations[131] as a reference when assessing the services provided to their patients.

The PA oath of ethics encourages PAs to treat patients equally.[132] Equality lies in striving to provide professional, competent ethical care to all patients. PAs must tailor their approach to fit the relationship needs of the individual patient, i.e., whether the clinician is collaborative or prescriptive, how much personal information is shared,[133] or the amount of self-disclosure in the patient-provider relationship.[134] Effective PAs craft their ability to discriminate into a skill that builds bridges between themselves, patients, and communities of practice rather than create barriers.

Ethics is the practice of morals. It represents the philosophical study of motivation, action, and ideas of right and wrong. The PA Code of Ethics evens the playing field: rich or poor, gender or ethnicity notwithstanding. The Code of Ethics establishes the standard and expects equal application of its principles at all times.

Any discrimination; attitudes, behaviors, or decisions influenced by stereotype, prejudice, or bias motivated by ego or status (self-preservation) rather than the patient's best interests, are improperly motivated, inappropriate, and therefore unethical. When such attitudes manifest outside of the realm of thought into reality and become detrimental to a patient, the provider has become negligent. If not actually criminally negligent (letter of the law) by straying away from the standard of care, PAs can easily become ethically and morally negligent (spirit of the law). This ethical lapse is present whether or not the trespass ever comes to light.

The provision of competent, quality health care has in its foundation the provision of ethical care. The application of ethical behavior should not require knowledge about a different culture or group. However, becoming culturally competent does. For example, in many Islamic cultures, pointing the bottom of the foot or the sole of a shoe toward the face of an individual is considered disrespectful.[135] Knowing this offensive act does not in and of itself create a culturally competent or more ethical health-care provider. However, acknowledging and respectfully putting the knowledge into practice in the presence of Muslim patients is a step toward cultural competency. Ethical behavior is a professional obligation and the patient's expectation. Ethical behavior also implies the practitioner is competent in diverse settings, cultural and otherwise.

Health service providers learn ethical concepts from didactic exposure, personal experience, peer pressure, and role models. They learn to mediate their innate drive for self-preservation and shape it into the altruistic response of a professional capable of putting the needs of those in their care before their own. Otherwise, how does a first responder risk his or her own life by running into a burning building to rescue a stranger?—a behavior based on the ethical expectation of a chosen profession. In addition to the traditional patient medical history and a thorough physical examination, the provision of quality care requires a practitioner take the time to identify and nurture an understanding of the cultural, behavioral factors that have influenced and shaped the patient's health.[136] Not taking these factors into serious and deliberate consideration diminishes the attention, quality, treatment, and optimum outcomes expected by the patient and the profession.

The patient does not have the responsibility nor will always be able to present fully conscious, in good health, fluent in English, fashionably dressed, and gender-attractive. Patients do not have to meet the needs of the health-care provider. It is the professional duty and ethical responsibility of the PA (or other health-care provider) to meet the patient's need. Providers should periodically reflect and examine their individual attitudes, motivations, and practices accordingly and ask whom do they serve: themselves or the patient? Each must recognize and consciously leave inappropriate biases and attitudes outside of the examination room door before greeting the patient.

PAs are encouraged to maintain high ethical standards in their everyday clinical practices. This includes being aware and intervening when the attitudes, behaviors, or decisions of other providers put patients at risk. In Patient Doe's case, a single provider making sure the alcohol assessment or other clinical protocols were properly followed may have changed the tragic outcome. Similarly, voicing concern that hospital protocols are not being uniformly implemented may draw necessary attention and improve conformance quality, the extent to which guidelines, once developed, are correctly and consistently applied.[137] PAs must have the courage to stand up and "blow the whistle" rather than succumb to ethical illiteracy.[138]

Patient Doe and the "invisible nation" expect PAs and other health-care providers to strive to meet their ethical obligations to practice the highest standards and ideals of their chosen professions.

Summary

The PA Code of Ethics expects PA students to prepare for the challenges and responsibilities that lie ahead and that practicing PAs meet at the highest possible level of competence in addressing the needs of their patients and the community at large. Celebrity or notoriety, along with ethnicity, gender, and age or sexual preference, or other variances in the human condition (or its presentation), must not determine the amount of attention or quality of care a patient receives. Almost counterintuitive is the understanding that a practitioner does not have to be particularly socially aware or knowledgeable of health disparities in order to provide attentive, ethical care to diverse patient populations, although it may help. The only thing that should be color-blind or nondiscriminatory is the availability of ethical care in clinical practice.

It may not be possible for the human psyche to identify and designate every patient encounter or every clinical event with equal gravity, concern, or importance. However, it is reasonable to recognize and accept this small character flaw that may exist in those who choose careers in the healing arts.

Negative stereotype discrimination erodes and destroys the filaments of humanity that braid peoples and their communities together. Without these connections, individuals have difficulty acting beyond their innate sense of self-preservation, are unable to extend the benefits and privileges available in their fiercely protected group to other members of society. Health-care providers—students, practitioners, and institutions alike—must seriously assess their behaviors, policies, and responses that are likely based on stereotypes and, where warranted, be willing and motivated to make the necessary changes. Early and frequent instruction and facilitated clinical experiences that expose students to experiences outside of their preexisting norms of reference (communities of reference and origin) provide opportunities for them to critically compare and evaluate their attitudes and expectations in relationship to future professional standards, expectations, and obligations in order to identify areas of faulty logic and biases that may lie in relationship to their stereotypes and bias. [139]

The PA profession was specifically conceived and developed to address the maldistribution of primary health-care providers among medically underserved urban and rural populations.[140] The AAPA estimates that as of the beginning of 2006 there were 136 accredited programs with approximately 10,000 students enrolled and 58,665 PAs in clinical practice.[141] PA education has gained a reputation for innovative, patient, and community-oriented curricula that are progressive in teaching sensitive and necessary curricula in other emerging interdisciplinary fields.[142] PA programs are required by their accreditation agency, the Accreditation Standards for Physician Assistant Education (ARC-PA), to provide instruction in the issues of ethics and professionalism.[143] Health-care training programs must remain vigilant and maintain their efforts to implement contemporary curricula and experiential activities that instill the principles of ethical, professional, and cultural competencies for new graduates to build on.[144]

PAs must be vigilant in their professional practices. They must be able to self-reflect, confront, and correct the presence of inappropriate stereotyping and discriminatory practices within themselves and, appropriately, within institutions and among colleagues.[145,146] Once such practices are identified, PAs can form more tolerant attitudes from frequent participation or immersion in clinical and nonclinical activities that expose them to the conditions and communities of patients in the specific sociocultural or lifestyle situations with which they have difficulty.[147]

PAs and PA students must refrain from the societal pressures to conceptualize and pursue health care as just another profession—with good job prospects, an above-average income, a comfortable lifestyle, status, and benefits—while leaving behind the ethical foundation and moral imperatives that led to the conception of the profession.[148] In so doing individually, collectively, and as a profession, all that is truly important will have been left behind, invisible to the blinded eye.

Social and professional norms change when individual practitioners and the institutions they form no longer sanction formal and informal negative stereotyping and discrimination. As this change occurs, constituents of the invisible nation will be genuinely respected and cared for as constituent parts of a better United States that will be more responsive to their needs and less reactive to their differences. In such a country, Patient Doe would have had a greater chance of receiving appropriate and possibly life-saving attention and care. Distilled to the basics, or as students ask "What is the take-home message?," the question was answered in 1927 by Dr. Francis Peabody: "The secret of the care of the patient is in caring for the patient."[149]

CASE STUDY DISCUSSION

It was later determined Patient Doe, during an apparent robbery, had been struck on the head from behind. The medical examiner's report revealed extensive head trauma "with hemorrhaging and other injuries in critical regions of the brain, incompatible with life." A review of fire and EMS protocols governing clinical priority and transport decisions revealed that "a patient who is unconscious or who has a Glasgow Coma Score *less than 13* and does not respond to therapy should be designated as a priority 1, an unstable patient. Demonstrating altered mental status and assessed with a Glasgow Score of 6, Patient Doe had been assigned a priority 3.

The identity of Patient Doe remained unknown until his wife called the police to report her husband missing. He had been out for a walk after having dinner when he was assaulted and robbed. He had wine with his meal. Mr. Doe, a 63-year-old white male and prominent member of his community, was survived by his wife, family, and many friends.

If in the United States, a country historically so acutely sensitive to celebrity, class, caste, and race, an injured middle-class white male can so quickly and tragically become "invisible" because of stereotyping, what kind of care does this suggest for those permanently relegated to the invisible nation?

True change starts with respect. Patients want it. Practitioners want it. An exiled invisible nation wants it. Being respected means that one is recognized, that one exists in relation to someone else, that one is no longer invisible. Erich Fromm once observed: "To respect a person is not possible without knowing him; care and responsibility would be blind if they were not guided by knowledge. Knowledge would be empty if it were not motivated by concern. Knowledge...does not stay at the periphery, but penetrates to the core. It is possible only when I can transcend the concern for myself and see the other person in his own terms."[150]

The author would like to express appreciation to Carol V. Blake, PA-C, Clinical Coordinator, University of Maryland Eastern Shore Physician Assistant Department, for her contributions to writing this chapter.

References

1. Brown MK, Carnoy M, Currie E, et al. Whitewashing Race: The Myth of a Color-Blind Society. Berkeley: University of California Press, 2003.
2. Garvin, L. A Modern Introduction to Ethics. Cambridge, MA: Houghton Mifflin, 1953.
3. Lee S. Do the right thing. [Motion picture]. United States: 40 Acres and a Mule Filmworks, 1989.
4. American Academy of Physician Assistants. Guidelines for ethical conduct for the physician assistant profession. Adopted May 2000. Amended June 2004. Retrieved June 12, 2006, from aapa.org/gandp/ethical-guidelines.pdf

5. Biblo J, Christopher M, Johnson L, et al. Ethical Issues in Managed Care: Guidelines for Clinicians and Recommendations to Accrediting Organizations. Kansas City, MO: Midwest Bioethics Center, 1995.
6. Jimack P. The French Enlightenment I: Science, materialism and determinism. In Brown S. ed. British Philosophy and the Age of Enlightenment. New York: Routledge, 1996; 228-248.
7. World Medical Association Declaration on the Rights of the Patient. Adopted by the 34th World Medical Assembly, Lisbon, Portugal, September/October 1981, and amended by the 47th WMA General Assembly, Bali, Indonesia, September 1995, and editorially revised at the 171st Council Session, Santiago, Chile, October 2005. Retrieved June 17, 2006, from wma.net/e/policy/l4.htm
8. Iserson KV, Sanders AB, eds. Ethics in Emergency Medicine, 2nd ed. Tucson, AZ: Galen Press, 1995.
9. Lo B. Resolving Ethical Dilemmas: A Guide for Clinicians, 2nd ed. Philadelphia: Lippincott Williams & Wilkins, 2000.
10. Moreno JD. Who's to choose: Surrogate decision-making in New York State. The Hastings Center Report 1993;23:5-11.
11. Trzeciak S, Rivers E. Emergency department overcrowding in the United States: An emerging threat to patient safety and public health. Emergency Medicine Journal 2003;20:402-405.
12. American College of Emergency Physicians Web site. Retrieved June 17, 2006, from acep.org/webportal/PatientsConsumers/critissues/CostsofEmergencyCare/default.htm.
13. Ibid.
14. Neergaard L. Probe says U.S. emergency care in trouble. The Associated Press. Retrieved June 19, 2006, from washingtonpost.com/wpdyn/content/article/2006/06/14/AR2006061400925.html
15. See Reference 4.
16. Ibid.
17. Carrese JA. Refusal of care: Patients' well-being and physicians' ethical obligations: "But doctor, I want to go home." Journal of the American Medical Association 2006;296:691-695.
18. See Reference 4.
19. Hall MA, Berenson RA. Ethical practice in managed care: As dose of realism. Annals of Internal Medicine 1998;128:395-402.
20. Cassell EJ. The Nature of Suffering and the Goals of Medicine, 2nd ed. New York: Oxford University Press, 2004; 35.
21. Schneider S, Zwemer F, Doniger A, et al. A decade of emergency department overcrowding. Academic Emergency Medicine 2001;8:1044-1050.
22. Bell RB, Davison M, Sefcik DA. First survey: Measuring burnout in emergency medicine physician assistants. Journal of the American Association of Physician Assistants 2002;3:40-55.
23. Goldberg R, Boss RW, Chan L, et al. Burnout and its correlates in emergency physicians: Four years' experience with a wellness booth. Academic Emergency Medicine 1996:1156-1164.
24. Samuelson W, Zeckhauser R. Status quo bias in decision making. Journal of Risk and Uncertainty 1988;1:7-59.
25. Aberegg SK, Haponik EF, Terry PB. Omission bias and decision making in pulmonary and critical care medicine. Chest 2005;128:1497-1505.
26. See Reference 4.
27. See Reference 5.
28. Gervais KG, Priester R, Vawter DE, et al, eds. A Casebook. Washington, DC: Georgetown University Press, 1999.
29. Kohn L, Corrigan J. Donaldson M, eds. To Err Is Human: Building a Safer Health System. Committee on Quality of Health Care in America. Institute of Medicine, Washington, DC: National Academy Press, 2000.
30. Ernst FR, Grizzle AJ. Drug-related morbidity and mortality: Updating the cost-of-illness model. Journal of the American Pharmaceutical Association 2001;41:192-199.
31. Stevens RD, Bhardwaj A. Approach to the comatose patient. Critical Care Medicine 2006:31-41.
32. Yost DA. Acute care for alcohol intoxication. Postgraduate Medicine 2002;112:14-26.
33. See Reference 4.
34. Crawford S, Ostrom E. A grammar of institutions. American Political Science Review 1995;89:582-600. Cited by Ostrom, E. Collective action and the evolution of social norms. Journal of Economic Perspectives 2000;14:157-158.
35. Raven H, Rubin J. Social Psychology: People in Groups. New York: Wiley, 1976.

36. Wildavksy A. Choosing preferences by constructing institutions: A cultural theory of preference formation. American Political Science Review 1987;81:3-22. Cited by Etzioni A. Social norms: Internalization, persuasion, and history. Law & Society Review 2000;34:173.
37. Etzioni A. Social norms: Internalization, persuasion, and history. Law & Society Review 2000;34:157-178.
38. Pratto F, Sidanius J. Stallworth L, et al. Social dominance orientation: A personality variable predicting social and political attitudes. Journal of Personality and Social Psychology 1994:741-763. Cited by Colella A, Dipboye R, eds. Discrimination at Work: The Psychological and Organizational Bases. Mahwah, NJ: Lawrence Erlbaum Associates, 2005; 439.
39. Bettenhausen K, Murnighan J. The Development of an intragroup norm and the effects of interpersonal and structural challenges. Administrative Science Quarterly 1991;36:20-35.
40. Bloom B. Foreword. In Health disparities & the body politic. A series of international symposia at Harvard School of Public Health. Boston, Massachusetts, 2005. Retrieved June 16, 2006. Available at hsph.harvard.edu/disparities/book/HealthDisparities.pdf
41. Rawls J. A Theory of Justice. Boston: The Belknap Press of Harvard University, 1971.
42. See Reference 4.
43. Abel E, Nelson M, eds. Circles of Care: Work and Identity in Women's Lives. Albany, New York: State University of New York Press, 1990.
44. Clement, G. Care, Autonomy, and Justice: Feminism and the Ethic of Care. Boulder, CO: Westview Press, 1996; 13.
45. See Reference 4.
46. Pogge T. Responsibilities for poverty-related ill health. Ethics and International Affairs 2002;16:71-79.
47. Farmer P. The major infectious diseases in the world: To treat or not to treat? New England Journal of Medicine 2001;345: 208-210. Cited by Dwyer J. Illegal immigrants, health care and social responsibility. Hastings Center Report 2004;34.
48. Ellison R. Invisible Man, 2nd ed. New York: Vintage, 1995.
49. Fletcher R. Bush's poverty talk is now all but silent, aiding poor was brief priority after Katrina. Washington Post, July 20, 2006. Retrieved July 29, 2006, from washingtonpost.com/wp-dyn/content/article/2006/07/19/AR2006071901735.html
50. Rodgers HR. American Poverty in a New Era of Reform. Armonk, NY: ME Sharpe, 2000.
51. Bridges GS, Myers MA, eds. Inequality, Crime, and Social Control. Boulder, CO: Westview Press, 1994.
52. Barak G, ed. Crime and Crime Control: A Global View. Westport, CT: Greenwood Press, 2000.
53. Karr JBA. Love To Know 1911 Online Encyclopedia. Accessed: June 12, 2006, at 1.1911encyclopedia.org/k/ka/karr_jean_baptiste_alphonse.htm
54. U.S. Census Bureau. More diversity, slower growth: Census Bureau projects tripling of Hispanic and Asian populations in 50 years; non-Hispanic whites may drop to half of total population. U.S. Census Bureau Press Release March 18, 2004. Retrieved June 19, 2006, from census.gov/Press-Release/www/releases/archives/population/001720.html
55. Ibid.
56. Ibid.
57. Ibid.
58. Ibid.
59. Preamble of the United States Constitution. Retrieved June 13, 2006, from law.cornell.edu/constitution/constitution.preamble.html
60. U.S. Department of Health and Human Services, Office of Minority Health. Teaching cultural competence in health care: A review of current concepts, policies and practices. Retrieved June 13, 2006, at omhrc.gov/assets/pdf/checked/em01garcia1.pdf
61. U.S. Department of Health and Human Services, Office of Minority Health. Minority health disparities at a glance. Retrieved June 13, 2006, from omhrc.gov/templates/content.aspx?ID=2139
62. American Institutes for Research. Teaching cultural competence in health care: A review of current concepts, policies and practices, 2002. Report prepared for the Office of Minority Health. Washington, DC: Author.
63. Satcher D. Commentary: Our commitment to eliminate racial and ethnic disparities [electronic version]. Yale Journal of Health Policy, Law and Ethics 2001:1-14.
64. American Medical Student Association. Diversity in medicine: What is the Problem? 2001. Retrieved August 6, 2006, from amsa.org/div/
65. Coleman-Miller B. A physician's perspective on minority health. Health Care Financing and Review 2000;21:45-56.

66. Kreiger N. Embodying inequality: A review of concepts, measures, and methods for studying health consequences of discrimination. International Journal of Health Services 1999;29:295-352.

67. Vermeire E, Hearnshaw H, Van Royen P, et al. Patient adherence to treatment: Three decades of research: A comprehensive review. Journal of Clinical Pharmacy and Therapeutics 2001;26:331-342.

68. Woloshin S, Bickell NA, et al. Language barriers in medicine in the United States. Journal of the American Medical Association 1995;273:724-728.

69. Rutledge EO. The struggle for equality in healthcare continues. Journal of Healthcare Management. 2001;46:313-326.

70. Geiger HJ. Racial stereotyping and medicine: The need for cultural competence. Canadian Medical Association Journal 2001;164;1699-1701.

71. Canto JG, Allison JJ, Kiefe CI, et al. Relation of race and sex to the use of reperfusion therapy in Medicare beneficiaries with acute myocardial infarction. New England Journal of Medicine 2000;342:1094-1100.

72. Vermeire E, Hearnshaw H, Van Royen P, et al. Patient adherence to treatment: Three decades of research: A comprehensive review. Journal of Clinical Pharmacy and Therapeutics 2001;265:331-342.

73. Smedley BD, Stith AY, Nelson AR, eds. Unequal treatment: Confronting racial and ethnic disparities in health care. 2003. Institute of Medicine. Washington, DC. Available for purchase at iom.edu/CMS/3740/4475.aspx

74. Geiger HJ. Racial stereotyping and medicine: The need for cultural competence. Canadian Medical Association Journal 2001;164:1699-1701.

75. Lillie-Blanton M, Martinez RM, Salganicoff A. Site of medical care: Do racial and ethnic difference persist? [Electronic version]. Yale Journal of Health Policy, Law and Ethics 2001;15-32.

76. Rutledge EO. The struggle for equality in healthcare continues. Journal of Healthcare Management 2001; 46:313-326.

77. U.S. Department of Health and Human Services. Mental health: Culture, race, and ethnicity: A supplement to Mental Health: A Report of the Surgeon General. Rockville, MD, 2001.

78. Sue D, Sue D. Counseling the Culturally Different, 3rd ed. New York: John Wiley & Sons, 1999.

79. Chen FM, Fryer GE Jr, Phillips RL Jr, et al. Patients' beliefs about racism, preferences for physician race, and satisfaction with care. Annals of Family Medicine 2005;3:138-143.

80. Borrell LN, Kiefe CI, Williams DR, et al. Self-reported health, perceived racial discrimination, and skin color in African Americans in the CARDIA study. Social Science and Medicine 2006;63:1415-1427.

81. Johnson RL, Saha S, Arbelaez JJ, et al. Racial and ethnic differences in patient perceptions of bias and cultural competence in health care. Journal of General Internal Medicine 2004;19:101-110.

82. Ma GX. Between two worlds: The use of traditional and Western health services by Chinese immigrants. Journal of Community Health 1999;24:421-437.

83. Copeland VC, Scholle SH, Binko J. Patient satisfaction: African American women's views of the patient-doctor relationship. Journal of Health and Social Policy 2000;17:35-48. Cited by Copeland VC. African Americans: Disparities in health care access and utilization. Health and Social Work 2005;30:265-270.

84. Cooper LA, Beach MC, Johnson RL, et al. Delving below the surface: Understanding how race and ethnicity influence relationships in health care. Journal of General Internal Medicine 2006;21:S21-27.

85. Healthy People 2010: Understanding and Improving Health, 2nd ed. Retrieved July 01, 2006, from healthypeople.gov/Document/html/uih/uih_1.htm

86. Ibid.

87. Borger C, et al. Health spending projections through 2015: Changes on the horizon. Health Affairs 2006;25:61-73.

88. U.S. Department of Labor. Opportunity 2000: Creating affirmative action strategies for a changing workforce. Washington, DC: U.S. Government Printing Office, 1988.

89. Thomas R Jr. From affirmative action to affirming diversity. Harvard Business Review 1990;68.

90. United States Government Accountability Office Report to the Ranking Minority Member, Committee on Homeland Security and Governmental Affairs, U.S. Senate. January 2005 diversity management expert-identified leading practices and agency examples. Found at gao.gov/new.items/d0590.pdf

91. Betancourt JR, Green AR, Carrillo JE, et al. Defining cultural competence: A practical framework for addressing racial/ethnic disparities in health and health care. Public Health Report 2003;118:293-302.

92. See Reference 62.

93. Office of Minority Health to develop national standards for culturally and linguistically appropriate services (CLAS) in Health Care. Retrieved July 13, 2006, from hsag.com/culture_matters/CLAS_Standards_Sheet.pdf.

94. U.S. Government Printing Office. Federal Register, vol 65, no 247. December 22, 2000. Retrieved July 29, 2006 from healthlaw.org/library.cfm?fa=download&resourceID=61086&appView=folder&print

95. Cross T, Bazron B, Dennis K, et al. Towards a culturally competent system of care: A monograph on effective services for minority children who are severely emotionally disturbed. Washington, DC: National Technical Assistance Center for Children's Mental Health, Georgetown University Child Development Center, 1989.

96. See Reference 94.

97. See Reference 4.

98. Allport GW. The Nature of Prejudice. Reading, MA: Addison-Wesley, 1979; 503.

99. National Commission on Certification of Physician Assistants (NCCPA) certification requirements. Retrieved June 13, 2006, from hnccpa.net/CME_requirements.aspx

100. Hodgkinson HL. How America is changing: the impact of demographics and cultural diversity on health care. Retrieved June 13, 2006, from http://www.diversityrx.org/CCCONF/98/summary02.html#_Toc 473954736

101. Carrillo JE, Green AR, Betancourt JR. Cross-cultural primary care: A patient-based approach. Annals of Internal Medicine 1999;30:829-834.

102. Betancourt JR. Cultural competence and medical education: Many names, many perspectives, one goal. Academic Medicine 2006;81:499-501.

103. Ibid.

104. Kmietowicz Z. More than half of smokers go on smoking after coronary events. British Medical Journal 2005;331:862.

105. Duckitt J. The Social Psychology of Prejudice. Westport, CT: Praeger Publishers, 1994.

106. Biernat M, Kobrynowicz D, Weber DL. Stereotypes and shifting standards: Some paradoxical effects of cognitive load. Journal of Applied Social Psychology 2003;33:2060-2079.

107. Zinn WM. Transference phenomena in medical practice: Being whom the patient needs. Annals of Internal Medicine 1990;113:293-298.

108. Ibid.

109. Tyson RL. Countertransference evolution in theory and practice. Journal of the American Psychoanalytic Association 1986;34:251-274.

110. Gabbard GO. A contemporary psychoanalytic model of countertransference. Journal of Clinical Psychology 2001;57:983-991.

111. Definition of prejudice. Retrieved June 20, 2006, from honelook.com/?w=prejudice&ls=a

112. Ashmore R, DelBoca F. Conceptual approaches to stereotypes and stereotyping. In Hamilton D, ed. Cognitive Processes in Stereotyping and Intergroup Behavior. Hillsdale, NJ: Erlbaum, 1981.

113. See Reference 98.

114. Crandall C, Eshleman A. A justification-suppression of the expression and experience of prejudice. Psychological Bulletin 2003;129:414-446.

115. Fiscella K, Franks P, Doescher MP, et al. Disparities in health care by race, ethnicity, and language among the insured: Findings from a national sample. Medical Care 2002;40:52-59.

116. Blaine B, Williams Z. Belief in the controllability of weight and attributions to prejudice among heavy-weight women. Sex Roles: A Journal of Research 2004;51:79-84.

117. Carr D, Friedman MA. Is obesity stigmatizing? Body weight, perceived discrimination, and psychological well-being in the United States. Journal of Health and Social Behavior 2005;46:244-259.

118. Duffy L. Suffering, shame, and silence: The stigma of HIV/AIDS. Journal of the Association of Nurses AIDS Care 2005;16:13-20.

119. Crisp A, Gelder M. Stigmatisation of people with mental illnesses. British Journal of Psychiatry 2000;177:4-7.

120. Masson N, Lester H. The attitudes of medical students towards homeless people: Does medical school make a difference? Medical Education 2003;37:869-872.

121. Grant LD. Effects of ageism on individual and health care providers' responses to healthy aging. Health and Social Work 1996;21:9-15.

122. Bonvicini KA, Perlin MJ. The same but different: clinician-patient communication with gay and lesbian patients. Patient Education Counseling 2003;51:115-122.

123. Saulnier CF. Deciding who to see: Lesbians discuss their preferences in health and mental health care providers. Social Work 2002;47:355-365.

124. Goffman E. Stigma: Notes on the Management of Spoiled Identity. London: Penguin, 1990. Cited by Mason T, Carlisle C, Watkins C, et al, eds. Stigma and Social Exclusion in Healthcare. London: Routledge, 2001.

125. Evidence-Based Medicine Working Group. Evidence-based medicine: A new approach to teaching the practice of medicine. Journal of the American Medical Association 1992;268:2420-2425.

126. Carey L. The role of pharmacogenetics in future practice. Journal of the American Association of Physician Assistants 2004;17:31-47.

127. Satel S. Medicine's race problem—Hoover Institution policy review online, no. 110. December 2001. Retrieved June 12, 2006, from policyreview.org/DEC01/satel.html.

128. Eisler RM, Hersen M, eds. Handbook of Gender, Culture, and Health. Mahwah, NJ: Lawrence Erlbaum Associates, 2000.

129. Jones L, Khamphakdy-Brown S, Klevens C, et al. The empowerment program: An application of an outreach program for refugee and immigrant women. Journal of Mental Health Counseling 2006;28:38-48.

130. Juckett G. Cross-cultural medicine. American Family Physician 2005;72:2267-2274.

131. See Reference 93.

132. See Reference 4.

133. Zinn WM. Transference phenomena in medical practice: Being whom the patient needs. Annals of Internal Medicine 1990;113:293-298.

134. Psychopathology Committee of the Group for the Advancement of Psychiatry. Reexamination of therapist self-disclosure. Psychiatric Services 2001;52:1489-1493.

135. San Francisco Department of Public Health, Environmental Health Section. Enviro-Times newsletter. Retrieved June 13, 2006, from http://www.sfdph.org/eh/enviro%5Ftimes/series/cdpiw%5Fpart1.htm

136. Martin J, Nakayama T. Intercultural communication in contexts. Mountainview, CA: Mayfield Publishing, 1997. Cited by Toale MC, McCroskey JC. Ethnocentrism and trait communication apprehension as predictors of interethnic communication apprehension and use of relational maintenance strategies in interethnic communication. Communication Quarterly 2001;49:70-83.

137. Kedikoglou1 S, Syrigos K, Skalkidis Y, et al. Implementing clinical protocols in oncology: Quality gaps and the learning curve phenomenon. European Journal of Public Health 2005;15:368-371.

138. Deasy J. Sound of the whistle-blower above the noise. Journal of the American Association of Physician Assistants 2001;2:53.

139. Sheldon J. Addressing stereotypes and ageism in a life span development course. Teaching of Psychology 1998;25:291-293.

140. Hooker RS, Cawley JF. Physician Assistants in American Medicine. New York: Churchill Livingstone, 1997.

141. American Academy of Physician Assistants. Facts at a glance. Retrieved July 25, 2006 from aapa.org/glance.html

142. See Reference 140.

143. The Accreditation Review Commission on Education for the Physician Assistant (ARC-PA). The standards. Retrieved June 14, 2006, from arc-pa.org/Standards/finalcopy92605.pdf

144. Cruess R, Cruess S. Teaching professionalism: General principles. Medical Teacher 2006;28:205-208.

145. Murray-Garcia JL, Harrell S, Garcia JA, et al. Self-reflection in multicultural training: Be careful what you ask for. Academic Medicine 2005; 80:694-701.

146. Fincher C, Williams JE, MacLean V, et al. Racial disparities in coronary heart disease: A sociological view of the medical literature on physician bias. Ethnic Disease 2004;14:360-371.

147. Arredondo P, Arciniega G. Strategies and techniques for counselor training based on the multicultural counseling competencies. Journal of Multicultural Counseling and Development 2001;29:263-268.

148. Marsh F, Yarborough M. Medicine and Money: A Study of the Role of Beneficence in Health Care Cost Containment. Greenwood Press: New York, 1990.

149. Peabody FW. The care of the patient. Journal of the American Medical Association 1927; 88:877-882.

150. Fromm E. The Art of Loving. Harper & Row, New York, 1956.

5

Religious Ethical Considerations

Danny L. Franke, PhD

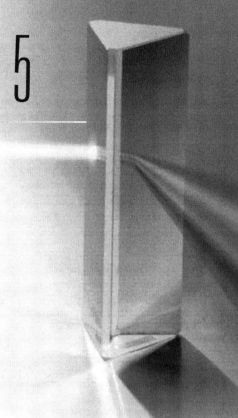

Ethics is about values. Ethical dilemmas come about routinely because values come into conflict with each other. One major source of values is that of religious and spiritual convictions, beliefs, and practices. Many times in the practice of medicine there is no apparent conflict between values promoted by medicine and values promoted by religion. However, at other times, these two sources of values come into conflict, and it becomes evident in the clinical setting. This chapter seeks to identify some of these values and analyze the ethical dilemmas.

Moral philosophy, or ethics, operates in the realm of philosophical inquiry and analysis. Logical reasoning is the method for solving ethical dilemmas. Moral philosophy does not rely on emotions, superstition, or chance as a means of arriving at some normative answer to a dilemma. The logically stronger relationship between premises and conclusion means a more forceful argument as to what should be done. Proofs in ethics are of the nature as described by James Rachels: "So we can support our judgments with good reasons, and we can provide explanations of why those reasons matter. If we can do all this, and for an encore show that no comparable case can be made on the other side, what more in the way of 'proof' could anyone want? It is nonsense to say, in the face of all this, that ethical judgments can be nothing more than 'mere opinions.'"[1]

Process of Arriving at Values

There is a four-step procedure necessary for analyzing the values in our lives. It is a logical and at times a difficult but necessary procedure if we are to fully appreciate the role of values in life.

The first step is to identify key values. This involves the simple yet necessary response of realizing what they are. It may be useful to make a list, write them down, record them in some manner for later reflection.

The second step is to understand those key values. Understanding is not the same as identifying. This step requires a search for the sources of values. It involves looking into why we hold any particular values as a value. Why are they important? Why should I keep them?

Third is the step to articulate key values. It is a higher level of thinking that requires both an understanding and expression of what we hold as important. This involves communication of our values to ourselves, to others, and to society at large.

Fourth is the step to promote values; that is, to influence society and others (such as family, neighbors, or coworkers) by way of these values. For

physician assistants (PAs), one might think of the influence of values in the work environment and with patients.

To go from step one to step four involves a high level of reasoning along the way. It involves reflection and analysis instead of the all-too-usual illogical desire to influence others without knowing why one holds the particular values oneself. Step four is the normal desire to seek to share and influence others with that which we hold as having value. It is a thoughtful reflection and sharing of what one sees as important. Professional relationships between physicians and PAs ought to include this approach. Professional relationships between PAs and patients ought to include this as well. Such is part of good medicine.

Identification of Key Values

There are some key values in medicine as well as some key values in religion that are worth mentioning. In no way is this meant to be an exhaustive list, but rather a beginning for the purpose of discussion.

One key value in medicine is the principle of nonmaleficence. Nonmaleficence is understood as an obligation to not intentionally inflict harm. This is often reduced to the phrase "Do no harm." Another key value is the principle of beneficence. This value states to contribute to the welfare of others, or "Do good."

The principle of justice is often thought of as a value in medicine. However justice is defined, it always entails a sense of fairness. And, of course, the principle of autonomy is a major value for medicine. Autonomy captures the sense of respect for human beings as individuals worthy of respect.

There are many more principles or values in medicine. Confidentiality and truth telling are two such examples. These are principles involved in everyday clinical medicine; they reflect core values such as privacy and trust. These two principles are crucial to PA/patient relationships because privacy and trust are crucial to meaningful relationships.

One key value in most religions is that of respect for life. "Life" here includes both human and nonhuman life. How we treat each other and other nonhuman living beings reflects the values concerning respect for life. Most religions also have some value thought of in terms of sacrifice for life. Out of an ultimate respect for life comes a notion of the value of a sacrifice of life for others.

The idea of freedom to worship or being allowed to practice one's religious convictions becomes a value in religion. The opportunity and ability to freely practice what one believes is of great value. For many, the opportunity of serving others is a religious value held dear as a living practice of the religious ideal or conviction of beliefs.

Finally, peace and justice are often identified as religious values. Peace is a complex value that often entails far more than the mere lack of conflict. It is a positive value that entails a sense of wholeness for the individual and community. Justice again entails a sense of fairness, although there are a variety of theories of how this is to be accomplished.

A few points are worth mentioning concerning values in medicine and religion. First, many of these values overlap into other areas. That is, values in medicine are not just values for medicine, and values in religion are not just values for religion.

Second, we usually think of all of these values as relevant and important but not absolute. We can identify and articulate why they are important and ought to be respected under usual circumstances. Yet we can also examine conditions whereby some particular value must be put aside for purposes of a higher value. Even the value of life itself is sometimes thought worthy of sacrifice for a greater good or cause (value). Whether the values are autonomy, confidentiality, or life, they are not absolute in the sense that nothing else or any other value can ever justifiably override them.

Finally, values may be subject to change over time, but the values listed here are core values that have stood the test of time. Perhaps it is more the degree of intensity accorded certain values that changes over time rather than the values themselves.

Relationship Between PAs and Physicians

The professional relationship and working arrangements among PAs and physicians can be very different from one clinical setting to another. A PA may be more closely supervised by the physician in charge, depending on such issues as type of care provided (general or specific), type of facility in which the care is provided (public/private, clinic/hospital), patient load, and number of available employees or health-care practitioners. Management styles of physicians vary as do management styles in other professions.

What is clear is that there is a professional relationship in which both PAs and physicians are understood as unique health-care professions with a goal and direction. While both professions are similar in many ways, they are different in significant ways.

In a letter in 1993 from AAPA President William H. Marquart to John L. Clowe, MD, President of the American Medical Association, Marquart wrote:

"Physician assistants do not seek independent practice, direct reimbursement from third party payers, or federal preemption of state practice acts....All actions affirm positions held by the profession since its inception 25 years ago: that PAs practice with physician supervision and that third party coverage of PA services should be paid to the PA's employer...."[2]

"PAs originated from a concept developed by physicians—the need for an assistant who could assume physician-type responsibility and extend their usefulness. As a result of this concept, a close working relationship with physicians has held PAs in good stead. Therefore it is not surprising that PAs and their physician employers agree about the degree of supervision and autonomy, and physicians report that the quality of their lives have [sic] improved as a result of hiring a PA."[3]

It becomes clear that the professional relationship between PAs and physicians is one of varying amounts of professional autonomy for the PA. The same is probably the case concerning professional values, both medical and religious. Although this is a very important issue in the practical application of medicine, it may not always be a point of discussion in the job interview. To the extent there is agreement on these issues, there is a smoother working relationship. To the extent that there is disagreement on these issues, it probably interferes with a good working relationship. Therefore, these values are worth discussion at the beginning of the professional relationship.

Application in Three Key Areas

Consent and Refusal of Treatment: Key Area Number One

What Informed Consent Is About

Medicine is based on the premise that patients need to be fully informed and to consent before treatment takes place. Informed consent implies the patient is competent, the information has been disclosed, the information has been understood, and the patient voluntarily authorizes consent or refusal of treatment. Emergency situations are cases in which consent is assumed. Being fully informed and consenting voluntarily are crucial to good medicine, clinically and morally.

One of the primary points of tension in clinical medicine occurs when the patient refuses to consent to treatment that the PA or physician believes is the treatment option of choice. There can be any number of reasons whereby this disagreement takes place. This chapter focuses on conflicts of values in religion and medicine.

Case 5.1
Refusal of Blood Transfusion in Child

"Daniel is a nine-year-old boy being treated for acute lymphocytic leukemia (ALL). It has become apparent that he will require platelet transfusions in order to prevent serious hemorrhage. His hemoglobin is dangerously low and he will also require red cell transfusions. Daniel's parents are practicing Jehovah's Witnesses. While they have consented to his treatment to date and very much want their son to pull through this, they are now hesitant to agree to the needed transfusions because this would violate their strongly held religious convictions. Daniel's doctors insist that the transfusions are critical and that they will obtain a court order if necessary so that this critical intervention will not be withheld from their patient."[4]

Case 5.2
Refusal of Blood Transfusion in Adult

"Debra is a 45-year-old multiparous woman who has been healthy all her life. She delivered a healthy 8-pound infant, her fourth child, but shortly afterward she developed severe postpartum hemorrhage and hypertension. Her blood pressure normalized when intravenous saline was given, but the bleeding continued. Her hematocrit is now dangerously low at 18 percent (hemoglobin 6.0 grams per deciliter). Immediate blood transfusions are medically indicated, and it is likely that the bleeding will continue unless surgery is performed.

Before this time, Debra had identified herself as a Jehovah's Witness. She has always been capable of making her own decisions and had stated previously that because of her religious beliefs, she could not receive blood transfusions under any circumstances. The obstetrician explains to Debra and her husband that her life is in danger and he 'cannot be responsible' if his 'hands are tied' by this prohibition against transfusing blood. Debra's husband says that they are aware that there are alternatives to blood transfusions and he hopes the doctor is aware of them."[4]

Case 5.3
Refusal of Hemodialysis

"A 31-year-old Hispanic woman, a wife and mother of two children ages three and five, telephoned the Hemodialysis Center on Friday morning. 'I won't be coming in for my run this afternoon,' she told the nurse and then her physician. 'I have decided to seek healing through faith alone.' A nationally known faith healer would be at her church Sunday, and it was time for her to put her life and future into God's hands. Yes, she continued, her husband and she had discussed her decision. 'He supports me and believes in God's power to heal my kidneys.'"[5]

Conflict of Values

It is not necessarily the case that values in medicine and religion must be in conflict with one another. In the majority of cases, they are values that support each other. But for the purpose of dealing with ethical dilemmas, it is appropriate to examine when the values are in conflict with each other.

As described in the case of the refusal for a blood transfusion, there is a clear example of values in conflict. On the one hand, there are the religious values identified with the practice of refusing a blood transfusion on religious grounds. The autonomy of the religious believer in this case is at stake. The freedom to practice one's religious convictions, even when it may result in death, is at the core of the patient's choice. It is not a case of a patient making a decision for another, nor is it a case of the patient being a minor or incompetent. Therefore, the patient's wishes ought to be respected as a result of the patient's religious values.

In the United States, we pay a tremendous respect to religious freedom. We grant a very wide berth to being able to live out one's religious convictions and practices as long as they do not harm another nonconsenting individual. This is the case even when the religious values may result in harm to self, or when the religious values are such that they are held by a small minority within the larger pluralistic religious community. A key part of this is that life in a free country is most meaningful when one is free to practice religious values or convictions.

This, of course, is not absolute. If one is coerced by way of being forced into holding a certain religious value, it is not a free choice. This at times is a difficult decision for courts to arrive at. Also, the freedom is not absolute in that it does not extend beyond oneself to that of forcing one's religious values on another. However, religious values, even when unpopular or dangerous to self, are respected as being at the heart of what it means to be a citizen in the United States. On the other hand, the value from medicine clearly identified in this case is the principle of beneficence. The desire to do good is at the heart of medical practice. In this case, the doing of good is clearly identified as providing a blood transfusion to a patient in need. The loss or lack of blood, to a serious enough extent, can be replenished only by a blood transfusion. There is not enough time for the body here to naturally replenish itself. And current technology does not afford the luxury of artificial means of the blood supply (although this also might be rejected in similar such cases).

Providing a blood transfusion is not seen by the medical team as particularly invasive. So the disappointment on the part of the medical team in not being able to provide a rather common service, especially in the midst of the possible loss of life, is a problematic scenario. One might argue from the perspective of the values of medicine that overriding the patient's religious values is morally acceptable due to the severity of the situation. In such a case, one might argue that the doing of good is an ultimate good (saving life) with a minimum exertion (not an invasive or risky procedure).

So there is a clashing of values. In this particular case and others like it, religious values are in conflict with medical values. The purpose of values in medicine is to enhance the quality and length of life. In this case, however, it is certain religious values that give life its ultimate meaning. Therefore, to extend the length of that life might actually disrupt or destroy the quality or meaning of that life in this case. The best procedure might be to step back and examine the bigger picture. This means respecting values of religion as giving ultimate value to life and then respecting the values of medicine to extend that life, but only within the perimeters of the religious values themselves. In other words, medicine helps one to live life but life as one chooses to live it within the realm of religious convictions and values.

To deny ultimate meaning to life for the extension of a period of time is to misappropriate the key ranking of values in this instance. The tension between the key values in medicine and religion is real in this case. The conversation between the two sets of values needs to be continued as a way of providing the best medical care possible for patients.

Role of the PA

The normal procedure involves a PA offering a treatment plan and the patient readily accepting such a plan. Actually, this may not be all that usual. It is more and more the case that patients are informed about issues before seeing their health-care practitioner due to the voluminous material readily available through television, print media, and the Internet. Therefore, it is probably the case that patients come into contact with the PA with a plan of treatment already in mind. The last 20 years or more have seen an expansion in the understanding and respect for the autonomy of the patient. The more acceptable professional relationship today is a kind of partnership, or shared responsibility, between the patient and the PA. This, of course, comes with the realization that a patient may at any time decide to refuse treatment rather than consent to treatment. When a significant reason for the refusal of treatment is based on religious convictions, one has a classic conflict of values between religion and medicine.

What, then, is the role of the PA in such conflicts? First, the PA must keep in mind the respect for the autonomy of a competent patient. Perhaps it is most difficult to offer good professional advice, only to have it rejected. But the practitioner of medicine under routine conditions must always be prepared for just this sort of possibility. PAs need to realize that patients come with a variety of agendas and options. When religious values are added, it will be no surprise that some patients will refuse some treatment option based on religious understandings. This ought not to be taken personally by the PA. Rather, this can be a positive opportunity for personal and professional growth and maturity.

Second, the PA must be aware of his or her own prejudices concerning competency. Just because a patient does not agree with a health-care provider does not make the patient incompetent. When religious values are part of the analysis and the religious values of the patient are quite different from those of the PA, it is easy to assume the patient's decision is one of an incompetent person. The PA may need to pursue advice from those more familiar with the religious values in question.

Third, the PA, while being professionally respectful of the patient's religious values, is also entitled to some level of provider autonomy. That is, the PA ought not to be coerced or forced to do what he or she understands to be in direct violation of his or her own religious values. At times this may be resolved by having a discussion with the patient. At other times it may entail helping to secure a different health-care provider for the patient. At most, where options are limited, it may require a third party to help the two work through the conflict. But there needs to be a respect for the religious values of the PA while at the same time not resulting in coercion or manipulation of the patient.

Healing and Curing: Expectations in Medicine: Key Area Number Two

What Healing and Curing Are About

The goal of medicine is to restore one to good health. There are many dimensions to such a goal. Sometimes this involves a change in lifestyle (diet, exercise, work environment, etc.). At other times it involves an interaction that is more direct by way of invasiveness (surgery, treatment, etc.). Of course, good health cannot always be restored or restored completely. At that point, a goal may be to provide for the best quality of life possible. When medicine is involved at the end of life, the goals may be different again. Then, helping one to be comfortable, as free of pain as possible, and providing for a dignified transition from life to death may also be worthy goals of medicine.

In the midst of these goals, patients and PAs have expectations. When the expectations between them are the same, the practice of medicine runs smoothly. When the expectations differ, problems can arise for the patient and PA alike. One of those areas where there can be different expectations is in the area of healing and curing.

For the sake of this discussion, "curing" refers to the absence of some particular disease or illness; the primary cause has been eliminated. "Healing," on the other hand, is a term that is more holistic in its application and refers to an overall look at life, an evaluation of where the patient is in the midst of life and health and an approach to whatever the patient's condition might be that is healthy and positive, including restoration of peace in the midst of chaos. In such a use of these terms, it is possible for a patient to be cured but not healed or healed but not cured.

For one to be cured but not healed would be a scenario in which the patient no longer has the illness or disease. Yet the patient's lifestyle or outlook on life has not changed for the better; there has been no learning experience; and there may even be unhealthy and/or destructive aspects continuing in the patient's life. For one to be healed but not cured would be a scenario in which the patient continues to have the illness or disease, but the patient's lifestyle or outlook on life has changed for the better, there has been a learning experience, and there is a renewed attitude toward the goals in continuing to live. While this patient may die

from the illness or disease or continuously suffer from the side effects, the patient has adjusted in such a way that he or she has a healthy holistic and peaceful approach to whatever life remains. Such a patient learns to adapt and to make the most of the life that exists.

There is a difference here that is relevant to medicine, and for many patients religion plays an important role in this distinction between healing and curing. Religion offers both hope and a meaning and purpose to the lives of countless people. Religion can offer that which medicine per se cannot.

To discuss a level of quality of life may be a medical issue. But to measure what it is that gives quality to life is beyond medicine itself. Therefore, a quality-of-life discussion in medicine is aimed at to what extent the patient is able to physically pursue that which gives life quality and meaning. That can be radically different from one patient to another. Thus, the frustration for the PA may come from two directions. The PA may believe the patient has much to commend in his or her life, whereas the patient may not agree. Or the patient may feel positive, and the PA may have a hard time agreeing. The clinical conflict may come from either direction.

In the book entitled *Realized Religion,* the relationship between religion and health is examined. A conclusion is that religion "is generally good for human health because it promotes a healthy lifestyle, opposes self-indulgent and self-destructive behavior, encourages moral behavior, provides vital social support and an ethical value system, establishes an interpretative framework to understand the complexities of life and human existence, and promotes spiritual growth, which generally assists believers in overcoming the stresses and vicissitudes of living. Furthermore, religion provides access to a divine force (God) who has the perceived power (sovereignty) to influence human events (transcendence) and who hears requests (prayers) that are health promoting if not healing."[6]

There can also be a negative aspect to religion and medicine. The study concluded "that scientific evidence supports the contention that religion is good for human health, and when individuals misunderstand religion or misuse religion in the service of their own emotional, psychological, or spiritual pathologies, it is not religion per se that is pathological, but rather the abuse of religion that is sick, harmful, and sometimes evil."[6]

It is often the case that "faith healing" has been distinguished from a more scientific and modern medical approach of "curing illness and disease." Quoting from *Realized Religion,* faith healing has generally been regarded as the "remnant of primitive or peasant, old country traditions, or as characteristic of uneducated, lower class persons who cannot afford modern 'scientific' medical treatment."[6] Yet while this may have been the case at a certain time in history, it does not appear to work as a neat distinction in contemporary times. We live in a time of both science and religion as major players in health care and medicine. As a WebMD article states, "People confronting illness often turn to religion for help, and there are increasing claims that those with strong religious beliefs are better able to recover from sickness and enjoy better overall health."[7] Such is not limited to primitive, undereducated, and lower-class patients. The same article points out that Susan Sered of Harvard Divinity School says "it is probably not possible to accurately measure the impact of religions on health using clinical studies." But she adds that such studies "do have merit in showing the benefits of a holistic approach to good health."[7]

Another article notes that the leader of the hospice movement, Cicely Saunders, was a deeply religious woman and that the founding spirit of St. Christopher's hospice was Christian. "The goal of hospice was not proselytizing or evangelism. One of the principles of St. Christopher's was 'that dying people must find peace and be found by God, quietly, in their own way, without being in any way subjected to pressure from others, however well-meant.' Staff were welcome who did not share Christian faith. They were expected to join in making hospice a place of healing for patients, families, and staff."[8]

It is this conflict between curing and healing that is at the heart of both complementary and conflicting values in medicine. Western medicine is more directed toward cure by virtue of the objective scientific approach to medicine. However, this is slowly changing in that the influence of religion is being examined more and more in medical training today. For many patients, the scientific approach works fine until it no longer works; that is, until patients dealing with illness and disease become more focused on an overall sense of healing or holistic health in the absence of cure.

Conflict of Values

Quality-of-life issues related to healing and curing can result in a conflict of values. When the PA is motivated by curing and the patient is motivated by healing, there can be a conflict of values. Beauchamp and Childress rightly note that "slogans such as 'quality of life' sometimes are more misleading than illuminating and thus need careful analysis." They point out that "some writers propose that we reject moral judgments about quality of life and rely exclusively on medical indications for treatment decisions." The problem they allude to is that it is "impossible to determine what will benefit a patient without presupposing some quality-of-life standard and some conception of the life the patient will live after a medical intervention."[10]

CASE STUDY

Case 5.4
Differences in the Family

"Jimmy T is an 11-year-old boy who suffers from lymphoma. The oncologist has indicated that without chemotherapy Jimmy is likely to die within six months. She has also indicated that chemotherapy provides an effective cure in only 20 percent of cases like Jimmy's; in most of the cases, chemotherapy provides at best an additional three-month to six-month extension of life. Jimmy is also compromised by an incurable neurological disease. This disease will eventually make it impossible for him to walk, talk, use his hands effectively, or control his excretory functions. Already his speech is slurred, and he cannot hold a pencil. Even without the lymphoma,

the prognosis for him because of the neurological disease is death by the age of 18. Jimmy has been raised in a strong religious environment, and his belief in God has been an important comforting factor for him. After having the facts fully explained to him, he has accepted his situation and the inevitability of his death at a young age. He says that he does not want the chemotherapy and that he is ready to 'go to God.' His parents, however, cannot reconcile themselves to losing Jimmy. They override Jimmy's decision and tell the oncologist to proceed with the chemotherapy."[9]

One attempt to measure quality of life is by way of quality-adjusted life years (QALYs). "The basic idea of quality-adjusted life years or QALYs is that 'if an extra year of healthy (i.e., good quality) life-expectancy is worth one, then an extra year of unhealthy (i.e., poor quality) life-expectancy must be worth less than one (for why otherwise do people seek to be healthy?).' QALYs represent trade-offs between quality and quantity of life, and thus can be used to measure the net health effectiveness of programs or activities. QALYs represent an attempt to bring the two dimensions of length of life and quality of life into a single framework of evaluation."[10]

The question becomes one of how to determine quality of life. "Analysts often start with rough measures such as physical mobility, freedom from pain and distress, and the capacity to perform the activities of daily life and to engage in social interactions. Quality of life thus may appear to be one way to talk about the ingredients of a good life. However, this description renders the notion so amorphous and so variable as to be unusable in health policy and health care."[10] The problem is that these are terms and concepts that have meaning to the patient. Yet what is meaningful from another perspective is whether there is a procedure or medicine that will give a longer life to the patient. When such exists, the PA may believe it is his or her duty to engage in such procedures or practices.

Again, a classic conflict of values arises between patient autonomy on the one hand (no more intervention on some level) and beneficence on the other hand. Perhaps the patient wants to shift to a health-care plan more in line with palatable care. Perhaps the PA is still interested in a far more aggressive and/or invasive plan of treatment. If the patient's religious values gives him or her a sense of wholeness and healing, even when there is no cure and end of life seems close, there can be a tremendous struggle between the patient and PA. There need not necessarily be a conflict, but there may be different motivations for the values of each party.

Perhaps a difficult clinical decision to arrive at is whether the patient is merely depressed or has given up hope. How much the PA ought to influence the patient is difficult to arrive at with certainty and accuracy. There is a place for the PA to provide hope, as long as it is not a false hope or unfairly encouraging the patient with unrealistic results. There is also the possibility that the patient might arrive at a sense of healing and have a more realistic outlook toward the situation involving his or her care. The tool involved in such an analysis may be communication. The analysis itself is not an easy one and goes somewhat beyond the scope of this chapter. Suffice to say that a conflict of values between patient and PA may arrive at this distinction between healing and curing, thus leading to an ethical dilemma.

Role of the PA

"To the extent possible, a treatment course that is acceptable to the patient and provider alike should be negotiated. It is first necessary to discover the common goals that are sought by the patient and the physician and to settle on mutually acceptable strategies to attain these goals." One of the common goals in such sound advice is that of religious values. But religious values are extremely diverse, and there are few guarantees of commonality. Even within the same religion or a branch within the same religion, there are many interpretations and varieties of values. There are certainly some broad agreements, but the details render a variety of approaches. Therefore, one cannot rely on this mutually acceptable strategy taking place.

Perhaps the key is found in an exploration of virtues perceived to be held by those practicing medicine; in particular, the virtue of compassion. According to Beauchamp and Childress, "the virtue of compassion is a trait combining an attitude of active regard for another's welfare with an imaginative awareness and emotional response of deep sympathy, tenderness, and discomfort at the other person's (or animal's) misfortune or suffering."[10] Furthermore, "compassion need not be restricted to other's pain, suffering, disability, and misery, but in health care these conditions are the typical sources of compassionate responses." This expression of compassion can make a critical moral difference. "People feel reassured and cared for by a person of compassion. The emotional tone displayed in the interaction is part of the assistance rendered."[10]

Compassion, when properly displayed, is an appropriate (even desirable) virtue for a PA to demonstrate toward the patient. An appreciation for the patient's religious values may be a key part of the understanding and demonstration of compassion. To understand patients' misfortune or suffering is to also understand their goals and meaning for their lives, especially in light of their religious values. Likewise, when their religious values help them to achieve a sense of healing or wholeness, in the midst of illness and disease, this too requires a kind of compassion. The PA must be ready to sympathize and empathize without being required to accept the same religious values for his or her own life. The virtue of compassion will not eliminate all conflicts of value between the patient and PA. It is, however, a significant start. To begin in an attitude of compassion is to at least be open to the possibility of arriving at a mutually agreed upon plan of care for the patient.

In a world of conflicts concerning expectations in medicine, compassion is a good place to begin. It can also be a good virtue for the patient to exhibit toward the PA when they struggle with the lack of a cure for the illness or disease. It certainly has been and can be the case that the patient can teach the PA. It can never be the case that everyone can be cured. It is an optimistic, but worthwhile, goal that all might be healed. Such healing when demonstrated between the patient and PA is a most meaningful experience in medicine.

Prayer and Other Religious Practices: Key Area Number Three

What Prayer Is About

One of the major practices of all religions is prayer. At the heart of the monotheistic religions (Judaism, Christianity, and Islam) prayer is communication with God. Prayer as petition concerning health and illness is central to religion. The place of prayer in medicine is of much debate and discussion these days. The relationship between prayer and health has been a major research topic for the last 20 years. Such research has focused on brain activity, immune response, effects on the heart and blood pressure, and times of recovery.

Yet "in spite of an obvious and widespread enthusiasm for prayer among Americans, even the few researchers and critics who are cordial to investigating prayer scientifically feel that there is little hard evidence to support its effectiveness in healing."[11] As a physician, Dossey goes on to address why he has such an interest in prayer. "The most practical reason to examine prayer in healing is simply that, at least some of the time, it works." Furthermore, "the evidence is simply overwhelming that prayer functions at a distance to change physical processes in a variety of organisms, from bacteria to humans."[12]

Dossey continues, "'Prayer' comes from the Latin precarius, 'obtained by begging,' and precari, 'to entreat'—to ask earnestly, beseech, implore. This suggests two of the commonest forms of prayer—petition, asking something for one's self, and intercession, asking something for others. There also are prayers of confession, the repentance of wrongdoing and the asking of forgiveness; lamentation, crying in distress and asking for vindication; adoration, giving honor and praise; invocation, summoning the presence of the Almighty; and thanksgiving, offering gratitude. But like the 108 names for the Ganges in Hinduism, the classic function of prayer can seem endless; theologian Richard J. Foster describes twenty-one separate categories."[12] Prayer is an act of great meaning for most people practicing religion, and it is an activity that can at times cause a conflict in values between the patient and PA.

Conflict of Values

The values of autonomy of the patient (and patient families) again conflict with beneficence on the part of the PA. Religion is not just a set of beliefs but a set of practices as well. To practice what one believes is to live out one's religion. As long as that practice does not harm other nonconsenting adults, it is a practice held in high regard in the United States. To be able to live out one's religious convictions, both those acceptable to most of society and those considered more rare, is part of what makes life meaningful. In the United States, this is a constitutionally protected right. Of course, there are public debates, discussions, and judicial interpretations of where to draw the line. Yet as religion and its practice affect medicine, great respect is given to the religious practice of patients. Even when the decision to do so may conflict with standard medical procedures, there is a respect for religious values.

Prayer is not the only such practice that can lead to a conflict of values. Yet prayer, and the many varieties of what prayer means, is a practice that often leads to conflicts when seen as an addition to or even as an alternative to standard medical practice. And prayer seems to be a part of every religion. Although it occurs in many forms and varieties, prayer is one thing all patients can feel they can exercise in their lives as a religious practice.

Role of the PA

Many questions are raised by the relationship between prayer and medicine. An article in the *New England Journal of Medicine* begins with the fact that polls indicate that the U.S. population is highly religious, that most people believe in the healing power of prayer and the capacity of faith to aid in the recovery from disease. Furthermore, it noted that 77% of hospitalized patients wanted physicians to consider their spiritual needs.[15]

One major question is whether a PA ought to pray with the patient. Dr. Koenig of Duke University Medical Center supports such an option. He notes that "the majority of patients in most studies—as many as 78 percent—indicate that they would like their physicians to pray with them, especially if they are religious and if they are in a situation of high stress. Many patients, however, are afraid to ask their doctors because they are afraid such a request would offend the doctor."[15] Dr. Koenig suggests that physicians take a brief spiritual history and find out what the patient might desire. The patient could then be informed that if this is their desire the physician would pray with them. No coercion need be applied but merely a sensible approach to this topic.

Another researcher points out that "physicians must walk a fine line between sympathetic and re-

Case 5.5
Conflict Between Pain Relief and Voodoo Practice[9]

"Marie F, a 40-year-old Haitian immigrant, is hospitalized with terminal lung cancer. Initially, the nurse responsible for Marie's care complied with her (competent) request for pain medication. Then Marie's brother, Jean, arrived from another city and found his sister delirious and mumbling incomprehensibly (as patients often do under a heavy dose of pain medication). In accordance with the voodoo religion of his family's culture, Jean took Marie's behavior to suggest the presence of evil spirits in her body; if not exorcised, he thought, the spirits would bring harm to their entire family. Upon learning that Marie's delirious mumbling occurred after she was given pain medication, Jean demanded that the medication be discontinued, explaining, 'The medicine brought the spirits into her, so we need to stop the medicine to get the spirits out!' At this point, the nurse feels conflicted between honoring Marie's request for pain control measures and respecting her family's religion."

Case 5.6
Conflict Between Prayer and Fetal Therapy[13]

"Amniocentesis reveals that Rachel's fetus has a rare metabolic disease. According to her doctor, there is a new form of genetic therapy available in which a gene can be introduced that will override the defective gene so the fetus will begin producing the missing enzyme. The therapy has been shown to be effective in more than 60 percent of cases. Without the therapy, the doctor informs her, the child will in all likelihood be born seriously mentally retarded. However, as a Christian Scientist, Rachel is opposed to surgical intervention as well as genetic tampering. She refuses to give permission for the surgery and instead decides to pray for the baby's well-being. The hospital decides to take the case to court."

Case 5.7
Conflict Between Care and Hindu Practice[5]

"A Hindu woman was scheduled for surgery at a Catholic hospital. Prior to her arrival, a male relative appeared asking to see her room so that he could 'cleanse' it. The staff assured him that the room was perfectly clean. He said, 'No, a ritual is needed to cleanse the room of evil spirits.' He was promptly and forcibly ejected from the hospital."

Case 5.8
Conflict Between Emergency Surgery and Prayer[14]

"A 28-year-old man is brought to the ER by his wife and family. A diagnosis of acute appendicitis is made and emergency surgery is recommended. The wife and family, however, insist that their minister first sees the patient. The minister is out of town and cannot be reached for at least 24 hours. The family objects to the hospital chaplain seeing the patient and requests that the physician and nurses join them in holding hands in a prayer circle for healing."

spectful attention to patients and the experience of undue influence over them."[16] She suggests that the discussion begin with asking about sources of support and important concerns affecting the medical care to be provided.

Raising concerns about praying with the patient causing harm rather than being of a benefit to the patient is Dr. Sloan of Columbia University Medical Center. "If physicians spend their limited time with patients engaging in spiritual inquiries, they will have even less time to address depression, smoking cessation, weight control or diabetes self-care—factors that are demonstrably related to disease. In this way, bringing religious matters into clinical medicine will deprive patients of adequate medical care."[18]

Of major concern to Dr. Sloan is the problem of manipulation and coercion. "When physicians make claims about the benefits of religious activities, patients can feel manipulated or even coerced into engaging in religious behaviors that are not their own, merely to avoid displeasing their doctors." Furthermore, "asserting that such activities (religious) promote health can lead patients who do poorly to question their religious devotion and to express guilt and remorse over their supposed religious failures."[18]

Both Doctors Koenig and Sloan make credible points. Perhaps the real issue is time spent with the patient. In a rushed practice of medicine, where the patient is neither asked nor given the opportunity to express the values in their life, the medical treatment is not the treatment of a person but rather of an identification number. A patient for whom prayer is meaningful may appreciate sharing that information with the PA. To the extent that there is a sense of comfort in sharing in such a practice, the patient would welcome it. In the end, it is quality time (and not necessarily a lot) that is experienced together.

Obviously, some PAs will be more comfortable with such a request than others. As all people have different agendas, this includes PAs and other healthcare practitioners. When the desire appears to be there, outspoken or not, on the part of the patient, and when it is not part of an agenda to force the PA's religious beliefs on the patient, and when the setting is such that timing is appropriate, it is not wrong for the PA to pray with a patient; nor is it wrong for a PA to refuse a request to pray with a patient when these conditions are not present. Even then, however, the PA can turn down the request for personal reasons without manipulating the patient or hurting the patient's feelings. Respect can be shown even when participation is not appropriate.

Another question concerns what kind of prayer to say, given the diverse religious and cultural spectrum in the United States today. A patient's request for prayer may be radically different from the prayer they might receive. More so than at any other time in history, the presence of a variety of religions and religious expressions surface in all parts of the country, not just the urban centers of population. There are, of course, still relationships between PAs and patients in which an understanding of each other's religious values are known. But this is changing rapidly. In fact, in many clinical settings, there is little or no personal relationship or knowledge of each other between PA and patient.

As this becomes more the case and as ideas and concepts such as religion and spirituality take on a variety of meanings in a pluralistic society, this second question becomes ever more appropriate. What prayer to offer while being sensitive to religious values is a real issue. When in doubt, honesty is always the best answer. The PA ought not to assume his or her

prayer would be the prayer of the patient. Therefore, communication with the patient, open discussion of values and goals in their lives concerning their medical care, and respect and dignity for the patient are all crucial for a meaningful patient/PA relationship. What is becoming evident in the research is that prayer and religion are being openly discussed as meaningful for many patients. What is meant by prayer, religion, and spirituality is becoming an ever broader concept. That which is meaningful to patients and their health care cannot help but be meaningful on a professional level for the PA.

Conclusion

There are two major points to make in conclusion. The first involves the fact that some cases involved adults as patients, and some involved children as patients. Religious values are to be understood as the values held by autonomous agents. Children certainly hold meaningful religious values. They can be very meaningful in the lives of children of all ages and quite often are maintained as values for their lives into adulthood. However, as regards conflict of values between medicine and religion, adults are the real autonomous agents.

Whether philosophically or legally, children as minors are not considered autonomous agents, unless granted such status by the judicial system. Of course, the seriousness of the conflict may play a role as to how deeply a child's religious values are respected when in conflict with the values of medicine. Surely in the most serious of cases, a child's religious values may be overridden for the values of medicine. "The American Academy of Pediatrics (AAP) recognizes that religion plays a major role in the lives of many children and adults in the United States and is aware that some in the United States believe prayer and other spiritual practices can substitute for medical treatment of ill or injured children." However, it is the position of the AAP that "constitutional guarantees of freedom of religion do not permit children to be harmed through religious practices, nor do they allow religion to be a valid legal defense when an individual harms or neglects a child."[19]

The AAP makes four recommendations that call for all those entrusted with the care of children to:

1. Show sensitivity to and flexibility toward the religious beliefs and practices of families
2. Support legislation that ensures that all parents who deny their children medical care likely to prevent death or substantial harm or suffering are held legally accountable
3. Support the repeal of religious exemption laws

4. Work with other child advocacy organizations and agencies and religious institutions to develop coordinated and concerted public and professional action to educate state officials, health-care professionals, and the public about parents' legal obligations to obtain any necessary medical care for their children[18]

In addition, some aspects of the relationship between PAs and their supervisory physicians unique to values in religion and medicine need to be addressed.

The PA is committed to practicing medicine with physician supervision. Kohlhepp articulates the value of supervision. "Supervision benefits PAs because the supervising physician is, by definition, readily available to consult, supply advice, and assume the care of patients who require physician care. In their turn, physicians benefit from the supervisory role. They can be certain that patients seen by the health care team are managed in a manner consistent with the physician's preferences. The team approach allows the physician to focus attention and energy on the most complex and critical problems, while those patients and tasks that can be handled by the PA are directed to the PA's care."[20]

Kohlhepp notes that the Institute of Medicine, in an attempt to focus attention on the importance of improving the quality of health care available, was advancing a campaign of "Cooperation Among Clinicians." This is what the PA/physician relationship is about. "Among the multiple dimensions of the unique relationship between PAs and physicians is an association built on mutual respect and trust, where the PA provides quality, physician-directed care. Grounded in similarities in medical reasoning, the uniqueness of the physician-PA team leads to effective delegation, appropriate consultation, and efficient patient care."[20]

But what about grounded in similarities in religious values? Is there a mutual respect and trust concerning religious values? Perhaps more important than these questions are the following: When are these issues discussed or addressed by PAs and physicians? When is the appropriate time for a discussion of religious values? Communication is the key to any successful professional relationship. Yet for a variety of reasons (lack of time, lack of interest, personal space, ignorance, irrelevance, fear of the unknown or prejudice), religion may never be discussed until the unfortunate situation where there is a conflict of values between the patient and the PA.

This ought to be a topic for consideration at the very beginning of communication. Just as other values are important to the patient/PA/physician relationship, so too may religious values be. The primary topics at the time of employment interviews are probably geared more toward time management and work ethic. However, as conflicts of values lead to ethical dilemmas, more discussion ought to be addressed in this area as well during the interview process. And as values in religion and medicine come in conflict in the clinical setting and cause ethical dilemmas for health-care practitioners, this too ought to be a relevant topic for discussion during the interview process. If professional supervision is to be successful, there needs to be a methodology in advance for when there is a conflict in values.

When illness and disease threaten the health and possibly the life of an individual, that person is likely to come to the PA with both physical symptoms and spiritual issues in mind. "An article in the *Journal of Religion and Health* claims that through these two channels, medicine and religion, humans grapple with common issues of infirmity, suffering, loneliness, despair, and death, while searching for hope, meaning, and personal value in the crisis of illness."[21]

When religion and medicine work together, the patient has an expansion of resources to provide for success. Healing can truly take place even if curing is not an option. And healing can certainly take place even when curing is also taking place. The patient who has access to values from both medicine and religion has a full arsenal to combat illness and disease. It is unfortunate that there are times when the values of medicine and the values of religion come into conflict. When this happens, ethical dilemmas arise in the clinical setting. This chapter has sought to explore a few possibilities for solving such dilemmas. The future is bright with the prospect of PAs and other health-care practitioners being better prepared for just such ethical dilemmas. The goal is not to expect to eliminate all ethical dilemmas of this nature but rather to help patients and health-care providers alike work through such dilemmas toward more meaningful results.

References

1. Rachels J. The Elements of Moral Philosophy. New York: McGraw-Hill Publishers, 2000;43.
2. Ballweg RA, Stolberg S, Sullivan E. Physician Assistant: A Guide to Clinical Practice, 3rd ed. Philadelphia: WB Saunders, 2003.
3. Hooker RS, Cawley JF. Physician Assistants in American Medicine, 2nd ed. Churchill Livingstone Publishers, 2003;195.

4. Ahronheim JC, Moreno JD, Zuckerman C. Ethics in Clinical Practice, 2nd ed. Aspen Publishers, 2000;99, 453.
5. Dugan DO. Faith is part of the solution. Park Ridge, Ill.: The Park Ridge Center Bulletin, 1997;2.
6. Chamberlain TJ, Hall CA. Realized Religion. West Conshohocken, Pa: Templeton Foundation Press, 2000;19, 23, 66.
7. Boyles S. Is religion good medicine? Accessed March 13, 2002 at webmd.com/content/article/19/1689_52014.htm
8. Giblin MJ. Care of the dying. Park Ridge, Ill.: The Park Ridge Center Bulletin, 2001;4.
9. Mappes TA, Degrazia D. Biomedical Ethics, 5th ed. New York: McGraw-Hill Publishers, 2001;686, 691.
10. Beauchamp TL, Childress JF. Principles of Biomedical Ethics, 4th ed. New York: Oxford University Press, 1994;215–216, 308–309,310, 466–467.
11. Jonson A, Siegler M, Winslade W. Clinical Ethics: A Practical Approach to Ethical Decisions in Clinical Medicine, 5th ed. New York: McGraw-Hill Publishers, 2002.
12. Dossey L. Healing Words. San Francisco: Harper, 1993;1–2, 5.
13. Brannigan MC, Boss JA. Healthcare Ethics in a Diverse Society. Mountain View, Calif.: Mayfield Publishing Company, 2001;247.
14. Sloan RP, et al. Spirituality/Medicine Interface Conference. Southern Medical Association, Professional Development Planner, vol. 3, April 2006.
15. Should physicians prescribe religious activities? New England Journal of Medicine 2000;342.
16. Koenig HG. Separating fact from fiction. Science & Theology News, 2006.
17. Saylor F. Doctors debate wisdom of mixing medicine and faith. Science & Theology News, 2003.
18. Sloan R. Medicine and prayer don't mix. Science & Theology News, 2006.
19. Committee on Bioethics, American Academy of Pediatrics. Religious objections to medical care. Pediatrics 1997;99:279–281.
20. Kohlhepp W. Contemorary concepts of physician supervision. Journal of the American Academy of Physician Assistants 2003;16:48–51.
21. University of Washington School of Medicine Web site. Spirituality and medicine.

Ethical Decisions
Near the End of Life

Moira Fordyce, MD, MB, ChB, FRCP Edin, AGSF

Ethical Dilemma: When to Prolong Life

Emma Jones is a 73-year-old woman recently admitted to a nursing home. Two weeks ago she suffered a severe hemorrhagic stroke, which resulted in a left hemiplegia, aphasia, and difficulty swallowing. She was in the hospital for just over a week, made little progress with rehabilitation, and has been discharged to the nursing home for further rehabilitation.

She lived alone before the stroke and was independent in all activities of daily living. A widow for 10 years, her only relative is a granddaughter, Sarah, who lives with her husband and two children in another town, more than 100 miles away.

Mrs. Jones is able to respond to questions only with a nod or shake of her head. You are not sure how much she understands.

You meet with her granddaughter and learn that she is devoted to Mrs. Jones, who brought her up after her parents were killed in an automobile accident when she was 4 years old. Sarah is very upset about her grandmother's poor condition and lack of progress.

Unfortunately over the next 2 weeks, Mrs. Jones continues to deteriorate and does not eat, and the nursing home staff ask for a family conference. Staff members want a feeding tube inserted so that she can receive nourishment. At the family conference, Sarah is vehement that her grandmother would not wish this. She states that she has had many conversations with her and that having a stroke is what her grandmother dreaded most: Mrs. Jones cared for her stroke-disabled husband for 3 years until he died. Mrs. Jones told Sarah on many occasions that if she were ever unable to care for herself, she would prefer not to live. Unfortunately she does not have a living will, nor does she have written advance directives for health care. The nursing home staff is sympathetic, but the director of nursing wants a feeding tube inserted. When you approach Mrs. Jones to try to find out what she would wish, all she does is shake her head, then cries. Sarah insists that nothing be done to "force feed" her grandmother, that she should be given hospice care and be allowed to die peacefully.

QUESTIONS FOR DISCUSSION

1. How would you address the principle of patient autonomy in this case?

2. Could the granddaughter be seen as an agent for her grandmother under the rationale of substituted judgment?

3. How would you apply the principles of beneficence and nonmaleficence in this case, balancing Mrs. Jones' reported wishes, Sarah's commitment to honor them, and the strong views of the director of nursing and the nursing home staff?

4. What are the risks and benefits of the different kinds of tube feeding?

5. Is it ever justifiable to have a trial of such an intervention for a clearly defined, limited period to discover if the patient responds and improves?

6. If the care setting were different—for example, if the patient were still in the acute hospital or had been discharged home—how would this affect these decisions?

7. What other help might you seek to resolve these difficult issues optimally?

Clinical Medical Ethics

Clinical medical ethics is medical ethics in practice, which attempts to identify, analyze, and resolve moral and ethical dilemmas that arise in patient care. The only certainty in life is that we will die. Just as each life is unique, so is each death. At this solemn time, a number of important ethical issues can arise, which will be addressed in this chapter. Those of us who have worked with dying patients know that the greatest good that can be achieved for the dying is bodily comfort and peace of mind. How to make this happen requires knowledge, thought, collaboration with other health professionals and, most of all, good communication with, and genuine compassion for, the patient and caregivers.

My Perspective

I am a clinician who has cared for patients of all ages near the end of life, over a practice span of almost 40 years, the first 14 in Great Britain and the remainder in the United States. I have discussed the issues addressed in this chapter many times with family, friends, colleagues, ethicists, and various religious persons. I have given much thought to them over my life and will continue to do so.

As well as reviewing the principles involved, I share strategies my colleagues and I have developed in dealing with ethical issues and the results of some of my experiences in end-of-life care over the years. I hope they will help you work through the many ethical and moral dilemmas that will arise in daily patient care, especially at this sensitive time.

Denial of Death

All ethical decisions near the end of life are influenced by the reality of death. Death is inevitable. Although it is true that the longer we live the closer to death we move, death can come at any age. Yet many people in this fast-paced, information-drenched, high technology age seem to deny this. They behave as if death is optional and refuse to think about it, much less discuss it and what medical care they will want near the end of life if unable to speak for themselves due to illness or injury. Fortunately, this is beginning to change.

The Terri Schiavo case (see below) caught the attention of the nation and has made many people more willing to think in terms of advance directives (also see below). At a recent senior health fair attended by 400 persons, the majority of them older adults, the station with information about living wills and durable power of attorney for health care (DPAHC) was mobbed. The statement is repeated again and again "I don't want what happened to Terry to happen to me!" This tragic case impressed everyone who followed it and is raising awareness of the importance of advance health-care planning at any age.

More than 75% of Americans die in institutions, too many of them suffering until the end, with unpleasant symptoms poorly managed. This leaves the survivors feeling sad, often angry and confused. Is this the way dying should be, they wonder? The dignified, peaceful death at home, surrounded by family and friends, is now not common. This is a loss for both the patient and the caregivers for many reasons. The patient lacks the comfort and reassurance of his or her familiar surroundings, and the caregivers are deprived of seeing a "natural death" in the home. This affects the caregivers' attitude toward their own dying and death and can leave them fearful and worried. On the

other hand, there are cultural groups that do not wish a death in the home—some believe it is bad luck; others fear that unhappy spirits will remain in the house, so they want the dying person moved elsewhere.

Dying in this society can be complex, with ethical decisions often involving not only the patient but also family and other caregivers, physicians and other health professionals, and even politicians. It is the health professional's moral and ethical duty to have the knowledge required to give high quality care to the dying person, to be able to help with difficult decisions, and to ensure that the death is as good as it can be for all concerned.

Along with denial of death comes a loss of grieving rituals in many groups. This is a backward step, because grieving can be part of the healing process, helping the survivors to gradually return to more normal life while allowing them to have their loss acknowledged. Not allowing survivors to express their grief can isolate them.

Stages of Grieving

The health professional needs to learn about the grieving process in order to understand what the patient and caregivers are going through after receiving a fatal diagnosis. The patient is grieving before death; the survivors are grieving both before and after death, and this can influence the medical and ethical decision making that may be needed. Elizabeth Kübler-Ross[1] described five stages in this process:

1. **Denial**
   - "No, it cannot be me! They've made a mistake."
   - "The diagnosis is wrong!" This can lead to a frantic search for confirmation.
   - "It can't be fatal, there must be a cure!" This can lead to time and money spent on "miracle cures" and open the door for quacks and medical charlatans.
   - This stage is usually temporary, and the patient moves on to one of the following.
2. **Anger**
   - "Why me?" "How can God do this to me? How can He let this happen?"
   - "It's the doctor's fault. He/she should have made the diagnosis sooner."
   - It is important that the health professional not take the patient's anger personally but stay calm and try to understand why he or she is angry.
3. **Bargaining**
   - "Just let me live until…and I'll build a shrine, donate money, make a pilgrimage…."
   - Most bargains are made with God, include a deadline, and are usually kept secret. This stage tends to be short.

4. **Depression**

 • Sadness, loss of interest, and withdrawal occur. There are two types of depression that the terminal patient can experience. The first is reactive depression to the diagnosis, its effect on his or her life, and other worries about survivors. The second develops in anticipation of pending losses and death. With patience, love, and understanding, both kinds of depression can be helped.

5. **Acceptance**

 • The patients who reach this fifth stage are fortunate. They can put their affairs in order, talk with family and friends, forgive and be forgiven for real or imagined transgressions, and can approach death with calmness and dignity. Great comfort can be obtained from acceptance, and it can start the healing of the wounds we all give each other in our journey through life.
 Acceptance by the dying person can make grieving and recovery easier for the survivors.

The five stages are not necessarily experienced in the above order, and the patient and caregivers can move from one to the other in either direction. The length of time in a stage varies from person to person, and not all stages are experienced, but it is still a useful framework to help understand the feelings during and after a fatal diagnosis is made and after death occurs.

What Is a "Good Death"?

Most people's immediate response to this is "pain free." The fear of uncontrolled pain looms large, with good reason. Many people die in institutions, and care of the terminal patient in most hospitals and nursing homes is far below a reasonable standard. Most physicians in the United States are not good at caring for the patient nearing death and have not learned how to control pain and other symptoms effectively. The reasons for this are often due to fear and lack of information.

 For example, lack of information about:

• How to assess, prevent, and manage pain
• How to manage pain medications
• The great number of medications available to prevent and manage pain and other unpleasant symptoms
• How the patient's anticipation of pain, feelings of being ignored, and anxiety need to be addressed to have the best results

 For example, fear about:

• Overdosing the patient
• Prescribing narcotics—"the Drug Enforcement Administration will get me!"

• Medication side effects
• The patient becoming addicted to the narcotic
• The narcotic becoming less effective

 Physicians may deny that the patient is suffering or have a punitive attitude toward the patient—"Learn to live with it!"

 It is medically and ethically indefensible to let any patient die in pain, especially considering the large armamentarium of medications available. There are small steps being taken to raise the awareness of physicians about this important area; for example, the requirement in California that all physicians have at least 12 hours of continuing medical education in pain management to obtain or renew their medical license. But the 12 hours are spread over 5 years! There is no similar requirement for physician assistants.

 Patients vary in how and where they would like to die. Some want to be fully conscious and aware right to the end; others want to slip into unconsciousness, then die quietly. Some wish to die suddenly on a golf course; others want to die in their sleep. Many people wish to die in a familiar place surrounded by family and friends, if given a choice; others may wish to die alone, usually to spare the caregivers' feelings. This unfortunately can backfire, as the survivors may be extremely distressed that their relative died alone. They might even blame themselves for not being more attentive. Whatever can be done to preserve dignity and respect for the patient and give peace of mind to the survivors will ease the sadness of this final event.

Care Near The End of Life

High-quality care until death is the medical and ethical right of every patient but unfortunately is not common. The denial of death and pursuit of acute care contribute to this. The main focus of Western medicine is on hospital care, whereas the majority of sickness care is given outside the hospital setting. Too many health professionals are culpably unaware about the basics of symptom control in the dying patient and have never considered the many aspects of suffering, of which pain is only one.

 Care of the terminal patient ideally should involve a team of experienced health professionals who will work closely with patient, family, and friends. This is a multifaceted endeavor, with interactions among the following[2]:

• The illness and its effects
• The effect of old age in elderly patients
• Mental problems such as depression and anxiety
• Fear of being disregarded and not valued
• Fear of uncontrolled pain

- Feelings of loss—status, job, self-esteem
- Feelings of being too ugly to look at or touch
- Financial concerns
- Relationships with caregivers and friends

No one person can deal effectively with all the issues that can arise; that is why an experienced team is needed for optimal care. The hospice or home care nurse is the key person, closely linked with a medical social worker. A physician is the medical director of the team and must be available at all times for consultation, to visit, and prescribe for the patient. (In this author's practice, four physicians experienced in end-of-life care shared calls so that someone was available all the time.) Other valuable team members are rehabilitation therapists (they can do much to make the patient comfortable, teach the caregivers gentle exercises, make the home safer), a pharmacist, and a dietitian. Other experts, for example a psychiatrist and/or geriatrician, can be consulted as needed. Volunteers, with the patient's permission, can also contribute a great deal to day-to-day care and family support. If the patient is religious, a member of the clergy of the particular faith, although not usually a member of the team, can provide counsel and spiritual comfort to patient and caregivers and often can give helpful insights to the team.

If the physician involved believes he or she cannot do this difficult work or has no experience with end-of-life care, then the physician has the moral and ethical duty to involve experienced health professionals to optimize the care.

Some terminally ill patients fear hospice care because they think that all medications and other therapies will be stopped immediately and they will just be allowed to die. This is far from the truth—any medication that is making the patient feel better will be continued, and good control of unpleasant symptoms will allow the patient to relax and experience a better quality of life, for however long this might be.

Know Thyself!

To be of maximum help to your patients when it comes to complex ethical problems near the end of life, you must think about your own attitudes toward dying and death. Ask yourself the following questions:

1. How do you regard your own death? Do you realize you, too, will die some day?
2. What events have occurred in your life that might influence your attitudes to death and dying now?
   - Death of a family member
   - Death of a pet
   - Death of a close friend
   - Death of a patient

- Serious illness (an imminent death)
- A long illness, such as Alzheimer's dementia (a prolonged death)
- Suicide? (Devastating in its effects on those left—sorrow, anger, guilt—"Could I have prevented it?")

3. Have you thought about how to give bad news with maximum compassion? where to meet with the patient and caregivers? A quiet place with minimal noise and interruptions is best. Not over the telephone, unless the persons involved are a long distance away.
4. Have you, or a family member, been given bad news in a particularly brutal way, for example, abruptly, over the telephone? If so, how did this make you feel?
5. Have you thought about what questions the patient and family might ask you? Questions that are frequently asked are:
   - What will it be like?
   - Will the patient go into a coma?
   - Will it be painful?
   - How long does the patient have?

   It is important to know the signs of approaching death and be able to talk with the patient and caregivers about this.
6. Have you thought about the pros and cons of issues such as tube feeding, use of intravenous therapy, use of antibiotics, transfer to hospital, do not resuscitate orders?
7. Will you be able to take time with family members? Consider HALT—do not do a sensitive interview if you are:
   - **H**ungry
   - **A**ngry
   - **L**ate for another event
   - **T**ired

   This is an ideal to aim for, but in fact you will often have to do your best under difficult circumstances.
8. Do you consider listening to the patient an active or passive activity? Do you think listening confers benefit, or should you fill the time available giving advice?
9. What words will you use to give bad news, to discuss the possible prognosis?
10. Should you show empathy for the patient, or stay detached and analytical?
11. Do you believe that if you become emotionally involved in the case you will be less able to help the patient?
12. Are you comfortable interacting with the patient and one or more family members at the same time?
13. Do you believe you should be able to answer every question you will be asked?

14. Are you comfortable working with end-of-life team members? Do you welcome comments from them?
15. Have you considered having a team member with you at the patient interview?
16. Do you know enough about symptom management to be able to discuss this with the patient and caregivers?
17. Are you willing to consult an expert in symptom management as needed?
18. Do you consider death is always a defeat?
19. Do you have a sense of failure or guilt after a patient dies?
20. Do you believe you should make some contact with the survivors after the patient's death?

In the author's practice, we sent a letter to the caregivers after a death, commenting about the patient and praising them for the care they gave him or her. It finished by saying "Keep in touch with us and let us know if we can help in any way." The responses we got to this simple act showed how much it touched the caregivers. It allowed the survivors to keep in touch with us, ask questions, and resolve doubts that could have festered. We then followed up with physician/nurse telephone calls as needed.

Complex Decisions

Decisions near the end of life can be clear and simple, but many are not. The complex ones can involve legal, financial, medical, cultural, religious, and social aspects, as well as ethical issues. Even politics has become involved in some difficult cases. Not all problems can be solved; some must be let go but reviewed continuously as the situation changes.

Only 20% to 25% of the population dies suddenly. The rest die more slowly. It is important to remember that as every person and situation is unique, dying and death are full of ambiguities. One complicating factor is the "illusion of choice." Death is not optional. The choices that can be made relate to the manner of dying—Where will it be? What treatments will we allow? What kind of symptom control will we have? Even, in some cases, when will it happen?

If the patient is of sound mind and can make his or her wishes known, this is helpful. However, if he or she is not able to do this, a large family with divergent opinions can make arriving at consensus difficult. The better you know your patient, the caregivers, and the patient's culture, the better you can help them. Detailed evaluation of your patient and caregivers at the first few visits pays richly thereafter and can even save time subsequently (health-care professionals are often driven by time constraints). More than one visit

might be needed; remember, at the first encounter the patient evaluates you and decides whether to trust you at this unique time of life.

No matter how strong your own personal convictions, you must never impose them on the person nearing death. Neither preach nor proselytize; neither try to convince nor convert. If the patient has a religious belief, even if you do not share it, support it, and use it to help. Should the patient's belief take a guilty or punitive form (for example, if the patient believes the disease is a punishment for past misdeeds), then with the patient's permission, try to find a religious professional with experience in end-of-life care to help, counsel, and comfort. Such a person can help the patient make difficult decisions.

General Ethical Principles

Following is a discussion of clinical medical ethics as applied to the special patient care issues near the end of life. It is important to realize that some of these principles can be in conflict. The example usually given is effective pain medication tending to shorten life. More often than not, good pain management actually prolongs life: the patient, no longer anxious and dreading pain, can relax, talk with family and friends and put his or her affairs in order. Even in the cases when life is shortened, the quality of the final days is greatly improved by good symptom control. It is the patient's right to have quality care at all times.

Competent professional judgment and a trusting relationship between patient and physician are of the greatest importance in reaching optimal decisions and converting dilemmas into choices. Involvement of other end-of-life team members can also contribute to resolving many of the ethical problems that can arise.

Following is the author's own ethical framework, which is discussed in the following sections:

- Autonomy
- Responsibility
- Decision-making capacity
- Beneficence
- Nonmaleficence
- Truth telling
- Confidentiality
- Trust
- Informed consent
- Justice: resource allocation

Autonomy

Each individual has the right, at any time, to accept or refuse any form of medical treatment or testing. Therapy can be refused, even if it might prolong life.

This means that treatments that are proving futile near the end of life can be withdrawn.

The person approaching death must be listened to, treated with respect, and made to feel that, although dying, he or she is still of value. In cultures that place individuality above all else, the patient remaining in control, if possible until death, can be considered paramount. Other cultures favor a group decision, in which the whole family is involved. It is important that health professionals get to know the customs of the groups with which they work and learn how to incorporate beliefs of others into patient management. If someone other than the patient is the main decision maker, the health professional must aim at achieving a balance between listening to the wishes of this surrogate and protecting the patient if his or her wishes differ from those of the surrogate. In this situation, the wishes of the patient should be followed. This can be difficult in some cases and needs time for discussion and considerable experience on the part of the health professionals involved.

Always ask the patient if other family members may be contacted. Do not make assumptions about this. Even within a seemingly close family, confidentiality must be respected. Ask if there is a key person in the family who can communicate with all the others. Ask also if there is someone who should not be given information.

If the patient is not of sound mind, try to identify a key family member with whom to communicate and/or respected authority figures in the community whom the patient might wish to play a part.

There are several groups that are at high risk of having their autonomy compromised or even disregarded. Special care must be taken with them at all times but especially near the end of life. They are:

- The elderly, especially if also poor
- The disabled, whether physically and/or mentally impaired
- The poor; those lacking health insurance do badly in every aspect of preventive health, sickness, or end of life care
- The homeless
- Residents in skilled nursing facilities (SNF)

Many people are in an SNF because they have no one to care for them or their caregivers live so far away that they have no advocates.

Patients with cognitive impairment tend to be disregarded when it comes to determining their wishes, but in the early to middle stages of dementia, an experienced health professional can obtain useful information from them. Even if they seem unable to express their wishes, they must still be treated with respect, and efforts must made to find out their needs. There are special considerations when the cognitively

impaired patient nears life's end. The question of what is futile care in this situation needs to be considered (see below on Futile Care and Nutrition and Hydration).

Following the principle of respect for autonomy, treatment must not be instigated *against* the wishes of a competent patient. This includes life-prolonging and life-sustaining treatment. It follows that withholding or withdrawing this kind of treatment is ethically justified if that is the wish of the competent patient.

The autonomy of the health-care team must also be respected. The team cannot be forced to administer procedures or treatments when it is clear that the harms outweigh any benefits or there are no benefits. A physician's medical and ethical duty is always to strive to heal, if possible, and relieve suffering but not to prolong life, or the act of dying, at all costs. There comes a time when a patient must be allowed to die. At this time, a physician has no legal or moral duty to prescribe procedures or treatments that simply prolong the process of dying. In practice, good communication and open discussion among the patient, caregivers, and health professionals almost always result in satisfactory resolution of such dilemmas that may have arisen (also see below on Futile Care).

Responsibility

It is the health professional's responsibility to be competent, stay up to date with medical advances, and behave in a courteous manner to patients and caregivers at all times. The time before death is especially sensitive for the patient and caregivers, and competence, compassion, and courtesy will go a long way toward comforting them. The patient has a responsibility to try to follow a regimen that has been agreed upon.

Decision-Making Capacity

"Incompetent" is a legal term that implies an absolute and unchanging condition. "Decision-making capacity" means the ability to choose, having considered the pros and cons, and understood the possible consequences of actions. In some patients, it may be partial and vary over time as their mental condition changes. The concept of a sliding scale for making a decision is useful. More understanding would be needed in deciding whether to undertake a serious procedure with possible high risks than for a common, low risk procedure.

In California the terms "incompetent" and "lacking capacity" are interchangeable. Ethical dilemmas can arise if the patient near the end of life lacks decision-making capacity and has not left clear indications of the treatments he or she would choose or refuse. In such cases, proxy decisions can be made: an individual other than the patient can decide on treatments. This can be a family member, a trusted friend, or a court-appointed conservator in the case of a person who has no one. In consultation with caregivers, if there are any, and the patient's attending physician, the standard requires the proxy to act in the best medical interests of the patient. Such shared decision making can prevent the proxy feeling that he or she alone is deciding whether the patient will live or die and might avoid futile treatments that only prolong dying.

If the patient has expressed wishes before losing capacity, the proxy decision maker should follow them rather than decide what to do. This is called "substituted judgment" because the proxy is substituting the patient's prior wishes about treatments for his or her own. The proxy's duty in this instance is not to decide what to do but to ensure the patient's wishes are carried out.

Beneficence

The health professional must act in a way that is in the patient's best interest but is not obliged to provide a treatment so that the harm outweighs the benefit, even if a competent patient requests it. Near the end of life, the issues that arise most often are the pros and cons of artificial nutrition and hydration when the patient is no longer able to take in fluid and food by mouth.

Conflicts can arise with other ethical principles. For example, a medication that controls symptoms well that has undesirable side effects conflicts with "do no harm." Each case must be considered on its merits.

Nonmaleficence

Primum non nocere: "first do no harm." Unfortunately, "harm" can be part of a beneficial package, and each case needs to addressed individually to see if the benefits are sufficiently great to outweigh the risks. The risk-benefit analysis is a useful concept in clinical practice and can help with difficult ethical decisions. It can be summed up as follows:

- A high-risk (serious) condition with reasonable likelihood of cure can justify use of a high-risk procedure or treatment with significant side effects.
- It would be hard to justify using a high-risk therapy for a low-risk condition (unlikely to harm the patient) that will run its course without treatment and without residual effects.

In a person nearing death, close scrutiny is essential before a painful or dangerous or high-risk procedure is undertaken. Questions such as the following must be considered:

- What will be the benefit to the patient?
- What harm might result?
- Will it restore any significant amount of function to the person?
- Will it make the time left to the individual more pleasant or comfortable?
- What is the dollar cost? This is a valid question in these days of rapidly escalating medical costs.

Truth Telling

Tell the truth, the whole truth. Is this always, without exception, the moral and ethical thing to do? Is it always in the best interests of the patient?

Most clinicians in the United States believe that patient and caregivers should be given information about the patient's condition, even when the news is bad. Not all cultural groups agree with this approach, and it is important to know the customs and views of the group with whom you are dealing. Is there a key person in the family or the group who should be consulted at times like this? Does the patient *want* to know the whole truth? What if the patient does not want one or more family members told the diagnosis? Such situations can arise; each one has unique features, needs careful consideration, and even consultation with experts in end of life care.

I always answered my patient's questions honestly but tailored what I said to the patient's understanding. I ended each interview by saying "Do you have any other questions for me?" and "If you think of anything else that troubles you, make a note of it and we'll talk at my next visit." My hospice patients and their caregivers were also encouraged to telephone my office or the physician or hospice nurse on call, at any time, if they had concerns.

Confidentiality

The health professional/patient relationship allows the health professional to have access to the most intimate fears, confidences, and actions of the patient. Confidentiality must be maintained, not just on paper, but also while discussing the case or corresponding with other members of the health-care team. If in doubt, always ask the patient, if competent, or the principal caregiver, if the patient is not.

Trust

Trust is the most important aspect of every health professional/patient relationship. With trust, the patient, caregivers, and other team members all benefit, and treatment outcomes are improved. Without trust, the likelihood of success in medical, therapeutic, or ethical areas is reduced, and the patient does less well generally.

"Sensitivity, understanding, and respect are essential to building trust. Trust is a vital determinant of treatment adherence, and, ultimately, may be more important to therapeutic outcome than any procedure or medication."[2]

Patients, and particularly caregivers, are hypersensitive in the sad time leading up to death. What the health professional does and says and how it is said will be long remembered for better or ill. Poorly chosen words or an irritable gesture can damage the fragile trust that has been created.

The important ethical decisions that might arise at this time need this trusting relationship, and the patient and family must believe that their health-care provider will at all times answer their questions and help them to make the best decision. It is the duty of the truly caring health professional to do more than merely give patient and caregivers a menu of options from which to choose. Advice must be given about the risks and benefits of each therapy or procedure, and recommendations must be made to help people make the best choice. If the health professional does not feel competent to do this well, he or she must consult with someone who does.

Informed Consent

In clinical practice, full disclosure of every pro and con of any procedure or treatment can be difficult. Even if all the known facts can be told, if they are not clearly expressed, they might not be fully understood. Even when explanations are crystal clear, most people remember only a fraction of what they have been told. The health-care practitioner should make a well-considered judgment about what, when, and how to tell the patient. Also, not every person wants full disclosure. In the case of a fatal diagnosis in some cultures, the family wishes to be told, not the patient, and the patient might agree with this.

Throughout my years of practice, I have shared information with my patients, then asked them if they had any questions. Irrespective of the background or culture, I always answered the questions as honestly and clearly as I could. I have had a small number of patients who did not want to hear a fatal diagnosis, and an even smaller number who died still in complete denial of the reality of their condition. This makes it difficult to deal with ethical treatment dilemmas that might arise near the end of life, but forcing patients to listen to information they do not wish to hear can destroy whatever trust has built up. I have known patients to be told a fatal diagnosis in the clearest possible terms, but if they did not wish to hear it, they were still able to block it out of their mind completely. Those who know the patient well might be able to help in difficult situations like this.

Justice: Resource Allocation

Just because a procedure or treatment exists does not mean it should be used. Equitable allocation of resources is a reasonable approach. This can function at the health professional/patient level near the end of life with regard to futile care and also regarding the just use of society's resources. For example, a patient with advanced, widely disseminated cancer of the prostate goes into renal failure. To offer dialysis in such a case would not be ethical, unless there were exceptional circumstances, because of the burdens of the dialysis treatment itself, the likely poor quality of the life prolonged, and the costs and constraints of renal dialysis resources.

These 10 items can be used as a framework within which to address the complex ethical and moral dilemmas that can arise near life's end. No one principle consistently overrides the other, and conflicts among them often occur. Rules and guidelines cannot be rigidly enforced because no two situations are alike, each person is unique, and so is each dying and death.

Advance Directives and Intensity of Treatment Near the End of Life

Federal legislation called the Patient Self-Determination Act became law in the United States in December 1991. According to this law, institutions such as hospitals, nursing homes, home health agencies, hospices, and health maintenance organizations that are reimbursed by Medicare, Medicaid, or both, are required to inform patients about their rights to make health-care decisions and about advance directives for care should the patients become too sick or injured to speak for themselves. As technology in medicine continues to advance, it becomes more important for individuals to make well-considered decisions about the amount of medical intervention they want applied in the case of incapacitation from illness or injury, especially near the end of life. With the technology now available, some patients who have died can be resuscitated and kept alive indefinitely with severe, irreversible brain damage, either in coma, or in a persistent vegetative state (PVS).

"Individuals in such a state have lost their thinking abilities and awareness of their surroundings, but retain non-cognitive function and normal sleep patterns. Even though those in a persistent vegetative state lose their higher brain functions, other key functions such as breathing and circulation remain relatively intact. Spontaneous movements may occur, and the eyes may open in response to external stimuli. They may even occasionally grimace, cry, or laugh. Although individuals in a persistent vegetative state may appear somewhat normal, they do not speak and they are unable to respond to commands."[3]

People in a PVS have no voluntary or purposeful movement; no ability to communicate; no ability to chew or swallow; must be fed via nasogastric, gastrostomy, or jejunostomy tubes; and have no control over bowel and bladder. They require total heavy care. PVS is a tragedy for the survivors as well as the patient. Most sufferers never recover, so there is no resolution, and the family cannot mourn and then move on to continue with their life. Many PVS patients end up in nursing homes at great expense, which can wipe out a family's finances. The very few who remain at home are maintained there at considerable cost to the family and society. A case that illustrates these points is that of Theresa Marie Schiavo.

The Terri Schiavo Case: Problems in Decision Making When Survivors Disagree

Theresa Marie "Terri" Schiavo (December 3, 1963–March 31, 2005) was a woman from St. Petersburg, Florida, whose medical and family circumstances and attendant legal battles fueled intense media attention and led to several high-profile court decisions and involvement by politicians and interest groups. When she was 26 years old in 1990, Schiavo collapsed in her home and experienced respiratory and cardiac arrest. She remained in a coma for 10 weeks. Within 3 years, she was diagnosed as being in a PVS.

In 1998, when it became legal to do so, Terri's husband and guardian, Michael Schiavo, petitioned the courts to remove her gastric feeding tube. Terri's parents, Robert and Mary Schindler, opposed this. The courts found that Terri was in a PVS and that she would not have wished to be kept alive. In 2003, the matter began to receive national attention.

By March 2005, the Schiavo case included 14 appeals and numerous motions, petitions, and hearings in the Florida courts; five suits in federal district court; Florida legislation struck down by the Supreme Court of Florida; a subpoena by a congressional committee in an attempt to qualify Schiavo for witness protection; federal legislation (Palm Sunday Compromise); and four denials of *certiorari* from the Supreme Court of the United States.

Despite intervention by the other branches, the courts continued to hold that Terri Schiavo was in a PVS, and would want to cease life support. Her feed-

ing tube was removed a third and final time on March 18, 2005. She died 13 days later at a Pinellas Park, Florida, hospice on March 31, 2005, at the age of 41.

Brain Autopsy Result

Examination of Terri Schiavo's nervous system revealed extensive injury. Her brain weighed only half that expected for a female of her age, height, and weight. Microscopic examination revealed extensive damage to nearly all brain regions, including the cerebral cortex, thalami, basal ganglia, hippocampus, cerebellum, and midbrain. The changes in her brain were of the type seen in patients who enter a PVS following cardiac arrest. Throughout the cerebral cortex, the large pyramidal neurons that comprise some 70% of cortical cells—critical to the functioning of the cortex—were completely lost. There was marked damage to important relay circuits deep in the brain (thalami), another common pathological finding in cases of PVS. The damage was, in the words of Dr. Jon Thogmartin, "irreversible, and no amount of therapy or treatment would have regenerated the massive loss of neurons."[3]

Dr. Stephen J. Nelson, PA, cautioned that "[n]europathologic examination alone of the decedent's brain—or any brain for that matter—cannot prove or disprove a diagnosis of persistent vegetative state or minimally conscious state. The vegetative state is a behaviorally defined syndrome of complete unawareness to self and to environment that occurs in a person who nevertheless experiences wakefulness. In other words, PVS is a clinical diagnosis. Ancillary investigations, such as CT scans, MRI, EEGs, and lately fMRI and PET scanning, may only provide support for the clinical impression—as might the pathologic findings, after death. In the case of Terri Schiavo, seven of the eight neurologists who examined her in her last years stated that she met the clinical criteria for PVS; the serial CT scans, EEGs, the one MRI, and finally the autopsy findings, were consistent with that diagnosis."

This tragic case highlights several medical ethical dilemmas. Is an intervention that will allow death justified? Who should be the chief decision maker? How good is proxy or substitute judgment? Not least it emphasizes the importance of advance directives.

If there is no clue what an individual wants if he or she is in a state similar to that of Terri Schiavo, it can mean years of conflict and misery for the survivors. Over the years, many different views were expressed. Those at one end of the spectrum say that because the person in a PVS is not alive in any meaningful sense, the right to life does not exist, and all support systems can ethically be withdrawn. The opposite view is that PVS sufferers are alive, and life must be preserved at all times, no matter what the cost.

Advance Directive, Living Will, Durable Power of Attorney

If a patient is unable to communicate, an advance directive can authorize the physician to provide, withhold, or withdraw life-prolonging procedures. Another individual can be designated to make medical decisions on the patient's behalf if necessary, and he or she can designate anatomical donations after death. Because not all possible situations can be covered and written down, good communication and trust between health professionals and family is key.

Two ways that an incapacitated individual can make his or her wishes known is to have prepared in advance a **living will** or, better, a **durable power of attorney for health care (DPAHC)**.

A **living will** is a written directive to family members and health professionals that generally states the person's wishes about the use of extraordinary measures to prolong life in the event of terminal illness or coma when there is no hope of improvement. If the wish expressed is that no extraordinary measures be used, all comfort and supportive care would be given.

A **DPAHC** is a document that gives authority to another adult to make decisions about medical treatments and procedures if the person named in the DPAHC becomes incapacitated and unable to do so. A DPAHC is generally preferable to a living will; it is clearer, more uniform, and more widely accepted. Anyone of sound mind who is at least 18 years of age can fill out such a form. A lawyer is not needed to make it legal. Many hospitals and medical societies can provide copies of a standard form. The agent (surrogate) named on the DPAHC is not permitted to agree to certain treatments, including commitment to a mental hospital, electric shock treatment, or psychosurgery (an operation to change personality). The DPAHC does not allow the surrogate to make financial decisions; it is for health care only.

The person making a DPAHC must talk with the chosen agent and family members to be sure that the wishes expressed in it are clearly understood. The physician should also be informed. A backup person or persons should be named in case the chosen agent is not available.

Copies of this document should be given to the chosen representatives, other family members, the lawyer, and the attending physician. The original should be kept in a safe place along with other important documents.

The DPAHC form can also be used to record treatments the individual wishes and does not wish to be carried out, without naming an agent. This will not have the same legal standing as the full DPAHC because no agent is named, but it is still a valuable indication of the person's wishes.

The DPAHC remains in effect indefinitely unless the form used has a stated time limit, in some cases 7 years. A different period can be specified. It can be changed or revoked at any time by the person making it, as long as the revised wishes can be communicated.

Many people execute this document because they have seen dying inappropriately prolonged in a family member and do not wish this to happen to them. The Terri Schiavo case has made many people aware of the importance of advance planning. It takes time to think, discuss, get the whole packet together, make copies and give them to everyone involved, and talk to people about medical wishes, but the effort is worthwhile. It has to be done only once and then updated as needed.

The interventions near the end of life that can be addressed in such documents are:

• Cardiopulmonary resuscitation
• Nutrition and hydration
• Antibiotics
• Intravenous therapy, including blood transfusion
• Respirators
• Renal dialysis
• Transfer to hospital

Cardiopulmonary Resuscitation (CPR)
If the patient is of sound mind but has not given instructions about CPR, this must be discussed and the wishes documented. Physicians who are uncomfortable discussing this with their patients may end up giving them printed information about it but without discussion and the opportunity for the patient to ask questions and have them answered. When I introduced the topic to my patients, I made it clear I was talking about attempts to bring a person back after death (in the case of sudden cardiac arrest in a person who is not terminal, all measures would be taken to save him or her). Many studies now confirm that the results of CPR in terminal patients, nearing death due to illness or old age, are not successful. In the few cases where the heart does start again, the patient does not live long before dying again. Also, in the late stages of a condition like Alzheimer's dementia, for which there is as yet no cure, CPR in the event of death is not justified because if the patient dies and is brought back, further deterioration is certain. It can take several discussions to help the family accept this.

It is important to have clear do-not-resuscitate orders recorded and known by all those involved with the patient, including the family.

Nutrition and Hydration Near the End of Life
Patients nearing the end of life go through several stages as their condition deteriorates. A pivotal one is when total care is needed, and the patient has to be fed. Appetite diminishes as death approaches, and intake of food decreases. This is a normal part of the

dying process, is not unpleasant for the patient, and allowing it to happen should not be considered "giving up" or killing the patient—the disease is doing that. If the patient is dying fairly rapidly from, for example, widely disseminated terminal cancer, it is easier to accept that appetite will be poor and that nourishment will not confer any benefit. In the case of a patient in late-stage Alzheimer's dementia who is dying more slowly, the decision whether to tube-feed can be more difficult. In this case, the questions are: does extending the duration of life simply ensure further deterioration and increasing dependence? where there is no possibility of cure or even improvement, is it ethical to make the person survive longer just to become more disabled?

Individuals, cultures, and religions have different answers to these difficult questions. Some individuals and groups want everything done, right to the end, irrespective of the consequences. Others prefer to leave life with few interventions but want all comfort and supportive care for themselves and their caregivers.

Dehydration, or loss of body water, is part of the normal dying process, except in cases of sudden death. *Near the end of life* can mean the last few days or hours prior to the death of the patient. In this context, issues such as artificial nutrition and hydration become irrelevant; comfort care and support for the patient and caregivers are paramount. However, if *near the end of life* is defined as the last several weeks or months of life in a terminally ill patient, the question of whether dehydration should be allowed to occur merits closer examination.

Reasons for Dehydration Near the End of Life
Dehydration in the dying occurs for the following reasons:

- Diminished function occurs in the period before death, whether or not it is accompanied by decreased nutrition or dehydration.[4] This in turn contributes to:
- Decreased appetite and thirst, together with loss of interest in eating and drinking, resulting in diminished food and fluid intake. The loss of interest may begin several months before death or within the few days before the end, varying widely from patient to patient.
- A decline in mental status in many cases contributes to decreased intake of food and fluids.
- As death approaches, many terminally ill patients spend an increasing amount of time asleep, which also limits intake of nourishment and fluids.

Advantages of Dehydration Near the End of Life
There are a number of medical, ethical, and emotional reasons to let nature take its course near the end of life and allow dehydration to occur. It is important to realize that dehydration is not painful. The discomfort that can arise from an associated symptom, such as dry mouth, can be remedied with local treatment (good mouth care, artificial saliva, and ice chips).

Mental Status Change and Lethargy. A major advantage to dehydration near the end of life can be a change in mental status. Drowsiness, lethargy, and a reduced level of consciousness can reduce anxiety and lessen fear of dying. This can be a release for some patients, allowing acceptance and a tranquil departure. Seeing their relative expire peacefully also helps family and friends. The avoidance of psychological suffering as life is ending is desirable, avoiding the devastation to both patient and family.

Natural Processes. Gradual slowing of body systems is part of the normal dying process. Dehydration contributes to this and helps to allow life to end peacefully. Many hospice workers are convinced that patients who are allowed to gently dehydrate toward death produce circulating endorphin-like substances that make the dying process more comfortable.

Decreased Secretions. Dehydration leads to a decreased production of secretions throughout the body, including:

- Decreased pulmonary secretions, with less coughing and congestion; this reduces need for suctioning
- Decreased body fluids, which reduce edema and ascites and can make respiration easier
- Decreased gastrointestinal fluids, with less likelihood of nausea, vomiting, bloating, and regurgitation of stomach contents
- Decreased urine output, with less need for urinal or bedpan, an advantage for the terminally ill bed-bound patient

Artificial Hydration and Nutrition Near the End of Life
Artificial hydration and nutrition of the dying patient with uncomfortable procedures such as nasogastric (NG) or gastrostomy (GT) tubes or intravenous infusions bring their own set of problems:

- The confused patient will constantly manipulate and try to remove any unfamiliar object that is causing discomfort or itch. Even fully conscious patients who are mentally clear and able to understand the reasons for the procedure tolerate NG tubes poorly. If a patient does succeed in pulling out a feeding tube, this could reasonably be interpreted as an indication it is not wanted. To reinsert the tube and tie the arms of a person nearing death is indefensible, but as restraints are now generally discouraged, this is fortunately less likely to happen.

- Itch, irritation, and bleeding of the nasal mucosa and the throat make NG tubes a poor solution.
- Skin irritation from leakage of gastric contents as well as infection at ostomy sites are not uncommon.
- Regurgitation of stomach contents into the esophagus in patients fed by NG or GT tubes with resulting aspiration pneumonia is another hazard of tube feeding.
- Feeding tubes can become blocked and need removal and reinsertion.
- Diarrhea can be caused by the feeding supplement. This is most unpleasant for the patient and caregivers and can mean no improvement in nutritional status.
- A compelling argument for allowing this painless, natural event to occur is that futile, and often uncomfortable, prolongation of dying is avoided. Although it may be medically satisfying to the health professional involved to correct the electrolyte abnormalities, this confers no benefit on the patient in terms of either diagnosis or management of the condition. Keeping this clearly in mind helps to resolve the ethical dilemma that can arise. If a treatment proves not beneficial to the terminal patient or is causing significant discomfort, it is futile and should be stopped.
- If a case arises where the proposed intervention *might* confer some benefit, the health professional should do a risk versus benefit analysis, use clinical judgment, and communicate the recommendations to the patient and family. A trusting relationship with patient and family plus a flexible, frequently adjusted care plan, with agreed upon time limits on doubtful interventions, is essential.

Special Circumstances

Unfinished Business. Artificial hydration near the end of life can be justified to allow for "unfinished business"; if the patient needs time for a relative to arrive, financial affairs to be concluded, or an important event such as the birth of a grandchild to occur, attempts can be made to prolong dying by artificial hydration. I have found in practice that the will to live can be surprisingly powerful, and patients often survive against all odds, with or without tubes or IVs, until after an important event has occurred.

Hypodermoclysis. If the patient feels strongly about being kept hydrated until the end, his or her wishes should be respected, but less uncomfortable and dangerous methods, such as hypodermoclysis, should be considered. Fluid is administered subcutaneously. It is not possible to overload the circulation, and the risk of infection at the site of needle insertion is minimal. The caregivers can look after the equipment and the administration sites, and there is little or no discomfort for the patient.

What Would the Patient Want? If the family wants one course of action, and the patient wants another, the patient's wishes should carry the most weight. If the patient is unable to communicate, ask the family "What would your relative want if he or she could tell me?" The result can be humane, rational treatment for the dying patient.

Late Interference. It is not uncommon for a family member, out of touch with the patient for years, to arrive late on the scene and, in the initial shock and guilt engendered by the patient's condition, to insist that "everything be done." This can occur in the face of the considered decision of the patient and the rest of the family not to use extraordinary measures. If this happens, the health professionals involved need to take time to explain the reasons for the decision to the relative and ensure that the previously decided rational management plan continues.

In the Hospital. The reaction of hospital staff to allow the patient near death to become dehydrated needs to be considered. The acute hospital with its high-technology bias is not a good place for the dying patient. Pain and other symptom control is performed well, and busy staff members are unwilling to take the time needed to discuss important ethical matters with the patient and family. If the patient has to stay in a hospital, hospice workers should be involved in his or her care to ensure a peaceful death with a minimum of suffering and futile interventions.

In a Skilled Nursing Facility. Nursing home staff may have concerns about weight loss and dehydration near the end of life, especially if the physician is not much involved with the patient, family, or facility, or if those involved do not understand the positive, dynamic features of hospice care. Fear of censure from state and federal licensing bodies can also cause irrational and inappropriate interventions to be carried out for dying patients. A good solution here, as in the acute hospital, is to support the patient, caregivers, and nursing home staff by involving the hospice team in the care.

Pressure Ulcers. The issue of dehydration making pre-existing pressure ulcers worse is worth considering. Pressure ulcers that develop near the end of life are a result of many factors, such as immobility and general poor condition relating to the underlying disease. Correcting dehydration does not affect them significantly, and artificial hydration should not be done for this reason alone.

Fear of Lawsuit. Some physicians fear that withholding hydration could place them in legal jeopardy. However, current experience demonstrates that the likelihood of a lawsuit being filed against a physician under these circumstances is very low. If the patient and family perceive the physician to be genuinely caring and involved, the probability of lawsuit becomes extremely small.

Insurance Policy. Another concern is that allowing dehydration near the end of life will invalidate an insurance policy. This is a groundless concern: a considered decision that there is no benefit to hydrating the terminal patient by artificial means is legal; the decision neither kills the patient nor is a form of suicide.

Antibiotics

Withholding antibiotic treatment at the end of life is not killing the patient. Antibiotics either kill the bacteria (bactericidal) or stop them from dividing (bacteristatic). This allows the body's immune system to take over, fight the infection, and complete the cure. Before there were antibiotics, not everyone died from pneumonia, for example. Some people fought off the infection and recovered; others did not. Antibiotics increase the likelihood of recovery from infection. For many centuries, pneumonia at the end of life was called "the old man's friend" because for many patients it conferred a quiet, pain-free, gradual transition to death.

My practice was that if a terminal patient's infection (usually respiratory or urinary tract) was causing pain or irritation of any kind, and my clinical experience told me an antibiotic would help, then I prescribed it. In cases where the terminal patient had an infection that was not causing pain or distress, then I recommended withholding antibiotics. To simply prolong the process of dying, when there is no hope of recovery or functional existence, is ethically indefensible.

Intravenous Therapy, Including Blood Transfusion

Intravenous therapy should be provided if there is a compelling reason and some prospect of improvement or control of unpleasant symptoms. Overloading the circulation, with resulting congestive heart failure and dyspnea, can result from use of intravenous infusions in the dying patient. The need for constant monitoring and even the compulsion to order laboratory tests can cause significant disruption and discomfort to the patient and caregivers. Laboratory values become "abnormal" in the dying patient; body systems wind down as the patient moves closer to death. A vicious cycle of trying to correct abnormal laboratory results with more procedures will confer no benefit on the dying patient. (As always there is an exception to every rule; I try to correct hypercalcemia in my terminally ill patients if it is contributing to nausea.)

Respirators

If there is no hope of patient improvement, respirators should not be used at the end of life. There are other treatments that can relieve breathing difficulty, and an experienced hospice team will be able to help and comfort.

Renal Dialysis

This should be done for the terminal patient only if there is a good reason and some prospect of benefit.

Transfer to the Hospital

Hospitals are the best place for the acutely ill patient and when therapies are needed that can only be given in hospital. Hospitals are not a good place for the patient near the end of life because of the constant noise, people coming and going, lack of privacy, and use of futile treatments and procedures. They are also a home for antibiotic-resistant bacteria. Hospital staffers are not trained in care of the dying patient, and control of unpleasant symptoms is not well done. The general opinion among health professionals involved in end-of-life care is that transfer to a hospital should occur only for a good reason.[5,6]

For example, if one of my terminal patients fractured a hip—a painful condition—I would recommend transfer to a hospital and consultation with an orthopedic surgeon. It might be that the best thing to do to give the patient maximum comfort would be to operate and stabilize the fracture. Doing this can make nursing care easier and the patient's last days more comfortable. On the other hand, if the operation offered no benefit, then splinting and good pain control might be the answer. Common sense, clinical judgment, and a risk/benefit analysis must be weighed carefully in every case.[4]

Withholding or Withdrawing Treatment

When a competent patient makes an informed decision to refuse life-sustaining treatment or have it withdrawn, there is virtual unanimity in state law and in the medical profession that this wish should be respected. Many health professionals and caregivers have more difficulty in accepting withdrawal of existing treatment than withholding it in the first place. It can be reasonable to try a life-prolonging measure like a NG feeding tube for a specified time, then if there is no benefit from it, discontinue it, and give good comfort and supportive care. Ending futile treatments recognizes that they are conferring no benefits and are simply prolonging dying.

What Is "Futile Care"?

"Futile care" is a treatment or procedure that offers no benefit to the individual as a whole. Just because a treatment or procedure exists does not mean it should be used. It can be difficult for the health professional if the family says "Do everything." There needs to be discussion of the risks and benefits of each therapy, and if the practitioner cannot see any benefit for the patient, he or she is not obliged to carry it out.

The following questions are worth considering in this context:

• What benefit will it be to my patient if I do this?
• What are the risks of the procedure?
• Is the procedure uncomfortable or painful?
• What is the likelihood of false-positive or false-negative results?
• What is the potential for the patient recovering functional existence?
• What part does "quality of life" play in deciding what is futile?
• Who decides what is meant by "quality of life"? The physician, the patient, the caregivers?
• Is the intervention simply prolonging dying?

Stopping futile care is not euthanasia; it is compassionate, caring. and in the best interests of the terminal patient.

Euthanasia

The term "euthanasia" comes from two Greek words, *eu* meaning good and *thanatos* being the word for death. The literal meaning is a "good death." In current usage, euthanasia refers to a physician or other health professional deliberately and intentionally using medical means to cause a patient's death. If the health professional acts alone, without the consent of the patient, it is called involuntary euthanasia; it is considered a form of homicide and is illegal in the United States. Voluntary euthanasia is the term used when a health professional ends a patient's life with their consent. Physician-assisted suicide is a form of voluntary euthanasia.

Physician-Assisted Suicide

Physician-assisted suicide (PAS) refers to a practice in which, at the patient's request, the physician provides a lethal dose of medication that the patient intends to use to end his or her life. It is legal only in the state of Oregon at present, but there are moves to legalize it in other states.

The traditional role of the physician has been healer and comforter. The Hippocratic Oath, until recently sworn by all newly qualified physicians, expressly states: "I will use treatment to help the sick according to my ability and judgment, but never with a view to injury and wrongdoing. Neither will I administer a poison to anybody when asked to do so, nor will I suggest such a course."

This clearly prohibits PAS and euthanasia, both of which, until now, were seen as incompatible with being a physician. A segment of the population wishes to have the option of PAS, but this could put pressure on physicians to kill patients. However good the intentions and well meaning the actions, this conflicts with the healer and comforter role, even more now because of the wide array of medications and procedures that work well in palliative care and control of unpleasant symptoms, whether physical, mental, or emotional. The biggest problem is that many physicians are not aware of the available therapies or how best to use them. Also, with the current, fragmented, expensive health-care system, palliative and hospice care is not easily available and/or is too costly for those who could benefit from it. Many people do not know what is involved in this kind of care or how to access it.

The ethical challenge of PAS must be considered. Is it ever acceptable for a physician to kill a patient? There is a wide range of opinions on PAS. Views include those that advocate involuntary euthanasia on people perceived to be of no further value (happening now in the Netherlands) to those who say life must be preserved at all costs, at all times, in all circumstances. There are many shades of opinion between these two extremes.

Ask "Why?"

I have had patients ask me to help them end their life. Whenever this happened, I talked with them and asked why they felt that way. The answers most often given were grounded in hopelessness, depression, and fear. Fear of:

• Uncontrolled pain
• General deterioration
• Progression of the disease
• Becoming too ugly to look at or touch
• Helplessness; loss of independence
• Being ignored; dismissed as of no value
• The unknown

Feeling in control of circumstances matters most to some, especially when it might be the only control they think is left to them: the ability to control the time of their death.

In many cases, the request can be seen as a cry for help. The person cannot see any other way out. Of those in the general population who try to commit suicide and are rescued, most never make a second attempt.

Incidence of Depression in People Requesting Euthanasia

Studies have shown the incidence of clinical depression is over 90%. This can be helped: patients like this respond well to counseling and other support as well as, in some carefully chosen cases, medications. It is more logical to treat the depression, then ask the patient if he or she still wants to be killed or commit suicide.

Other questions worth considering are:

- Has any pressure been put on the individual, either by self or by others, not to be a burden?
- Is there some financial issue or an inheritance involved?
- Is anyone other than the patient making a judgment about quality of life?

Studies that look at physician attitudes to patients' quality of life show that physicians consistently *underestimate* the quality compared with patients' own views. At this vulnerable time the physician's view can significantly influence the patient, especially if he or she is ill and struggling with feelings of hopelessness and depression.

When I received requests for death, I asked the patients to let my hospice team and me help them and their caregivers. Then they could reconsider whether they really wanted to take this final, irrevocable step that would affect not just themselves but also their families, friends and, ultimately, society. When the pain was well controlled, depression addressed, caregivers offered support and comfort, and the many facets of suffering considered, not one of them continued wishing to have life ended. We were treating the reasons for the request. Effectively addressing these issues gave the terminal patient more options, and choosing to be killed was no longer on the list. It also gave the patients time to work through the stages of grieving, interact with their family and friends, and reach acceptance. Other health professionals who work in hospice and palliative care describe similar experiences with their patients.

Jack Kevorkian, MD

A name that occurs in this context is Jack Kevorkian, a pathologist who was nicknamed "Dr. Death" when he was going through hospital wards photographing the fundi of the eyes of dying and dead patients. Born in 1928 in Michigan, he graduated from the University of Michigan medical school in 1956. He advocated medical experimentation on consenting convicts during execution and harvesting their organs for donation to those who needed them. He experimented with transfusing blood from dead bodies into living subjects. (As far as is known, none of the living subjects came to harm.) He became obsessed with dying and death, and in 1987 he advertised himself as a "physician consultant" for "death counseling." Two years later he built his "suicide machine," the Thanatron.

From then until 1999, Dr. Kevorkian was brought to trial and acquitted four times for his involvement in assisted deaths. In 1999 he was convicted of second-degree murder and delivery of a controlled substance for the killing of a patient by lethal injection. He was sentenced to 3 to 7 years in prison. By that time, he had assisted in the death of more than 130 people, either from carbon monoxide inhalation or by using his Thanatron. One disturbing case was that of a 70-year-old man with emphysema and congestive heart failure, where documents were found that suggested the patient changed his mind about committing suicide but that his request to halt the procedure was ignored. Dr. Kevorkian is currently serving time in prison.

Euthanasia in Oregon

In 1997 the Death With Dignity law went into effect in Oregon. Under controlled circumstances, the law allows some terminal patients to request assistance from their physicians in committing suicide. By the end of 2004, 208 individuals in Oregon had ended their life with the help of lethal prescriptions. Since then, about 40 PAS deaths per year have been reported. How many are unreported and how many cases of *involuntary* euthanasia occur are not known, but from interviews a number of physicians admit to ending lives they consider too unpleasant or of no value.

Much legal wrangling has continued over the years about the constitutionality of the right to die and the role physicians should play in the deaths of the patients who request this. In January 2006 the U.S. Supreme Court upheld Oregon's law by a vote of 6 to 3. There are moves in other states to bring in such a law, although opponents will continue to work against it.

Euthanasia in Europe

During the Second World War, under Hitler's Nazi regime in Germany, there was a government-sponsored euthanasia program that eliminated more than 600,000 handicapped and orphaned children and physically and mentally disabled adults. They were either starved to death or killed by lethal injections.

After the fall of the Third Reich, this practice stopped in Germany.

In 2002 the first country in the world to legalize euthanasia was the Netherlands (Holland), where adults 16 years or older can be killed in this way as described below. Teenagers 16 to 18 years old may request and receive euthanasia or assisted suicide. A parent or guardian must have been involved in the decision process but need not agree or approve. Minors from the ages of 12 to 16 years can seek euthanasia with their guardian's consent. The written statement need not be made in conjunction with any particular medical condition. There is no requirement that the suffering be physical or that the patient be terminally ill. The request could have been written years before, based on views that might have changed. The physician could administer euthanasia based on the prior written statement.

The prospect of "euthanasia tourism" exists, because the law does not prohibit physicians from administering euthanasia to nonresidents.

Euthanasia is defined by the Dutch Government Commission on Euthanasia (1985) as "A deliberate termination of an individual's life at that individual's request, by another. Or, in medical practice, the active and deliberate termination of a patient's life, on that patient's request, by a doctor." Physicians will not be prosecuted if they have met the substantive requirements published by the Royal Dutch Medical Association in 1984 (also confirmed by court decisions). These are:

- The patient makes a voluntary request.
- The request must be well considered.
- The wish for death is durable.
- The patient is in unacceptable suffering.
- The physician has consulted a colleague who agrees with the proposed course of action.

"The patient is killed by first an injection to render him or her comatose, followed by a second injection to stop the heart. Official guidelines encourage the doctor to allow the patient to take the lethal dosage, under supervision, if this is practical."—guidelines from the Netherlands.

Recent reports indicate that 1000 or more people each year are administered *involuntary* euthanasia in the Netherlands; that is, they are killed without having requested it.[7] The Dutch have redefined the term "involuntary euthanasia" as "termination of the patient without explicit request."[7,8] For many years, some infants born with conditions such as spina bifida and other disabilities have been killed soon after their birth, some without the parent's request or consent. There are recent proposals to extend the law to allow involuntary killing of mentally incapable and other disabled persons. The physician would be the person to decide on the value of the person's life and whether he or she should be allowed to continue living.[9–11]

The second country to legalize euthanasia was Belgium. The law there is similar to the Dutch legislation, but minors cannot seek assistance to die. In the case of a nonterminal illness, a third medical opinion must be sought.

Swiss law tolerates assisted suicide if the patient commits the act and the helper has no direct interest. However, pressure has been mounting for the practice to be more tightly controlled, partly because of abuses and also the fact that Switzerland has gained a reputation for "death tourism." Again the question must be considered: to effectively manage the reasons for the request and then let the person reconsider, or kill the patient?

Effects of Euthanasia on Physicians

A study[12] reported in May 2006 by the group Physicians for Compassionate Care Education Foundation (PCCEF) found that the psychological effects of "helping patients to die" can be severe for doctors participating in euthanasia and PAS. Data were taken from a number of sources: articles in medical journals, legislative investigations, and the public press. This study is among the first of its kind and says the effects on doctors of the inversion of their traditional medical function as healers can be "substantial": "Doctors describe being profoundly adversely affected, being shocked by the suddenness of the death, being caught up in the patient's drive for assisted suicide, having a sense of powerlessness, and feeling isolated. There is evidence of pressure on and intimidation of doctors by some patients to assist in suicide."

The study quotes a doctor from the Netherlands: "Many physicians who had practiced euthanasia mentioned that they would be most reluctant to do so again." Pieter Admiraal, a leader of Holland's euthanasia movement, is quoted, "You will never get accustomed to killing somebody. We are not trained to kill. With euthanasia, your nightmare comes true."[12]

The PCCEF study corresponds with reports by German authorities during the Second World War that showed negative psychological effects on the doctors and nurses involved in the government-sponsored euthanasia program. They suffered alcoholism and serious mental disorders after prolonged stints working in the killing centers. In a recent session when the British Parliament was debating introducing an euthanasia bill, the following exchange took place:

- Question by Baroness Finlay: "Looking after complex patients can be exhausting. It can be physically and emotionally exhausting. I certainly know of a case where a patient was almost pressured by the doctor, by being offered euthanasia. I wondered if that reflected the doctor's personal distress and whether you have come across cases where the doctor is thinking of euthanasia as the only solution?"

- Response by a physician from the Netherlands: "I was giving consultations in several situations like this when the GP was calling me about a patient with gastrointestinal obstruction. He said, 'The problem is that the patient is refusing euthanasia.' I said, 'What happened?' He said, 'In the past, all these kinds of situations, when people were intractably vomiting, I solved by offering euthanasia. Now this patient does not want it, and I do not know what to do.' That was really striking. Providing euthanasia as a solution to every difficult problem in palliative care would completely change our knowledge and practice and also the possibilities that we have….This is my biggest concern in providing euthanasia and setting a norm of euthanasia in medicine: that it will inhibit the development of our learning from patients, because we will solve everything with euthanasia."[21]

Countertransference in PAS

Countertransference is defined as a phenomenon referring to the attitudes and feelings, only partly conscious, of the analyst toward the patient. Varghese and Kelly[13] have evaluated the involvement of countertransference with assisted suicide. They report that: "The subjective evaluation by a doctor of a patient's 'quality of life' and the role of such an evaluation in making end-of-life decisions of themselves raise significant countertransference issues. Inaccurately putting oneself 'in the patient's shoes' in order to make clinical decisions and evaluations of quality of life leaves the patient vulnerable to the doctor's personal and unrecognized issues concerning illness, death and disability." They state that "fortunately, the ethical code prohibits certain actions on the part of the doctor. In the absence of these prohibitions, the doctor's countertransference feelings about patients could put the public in grave danger." They conclude "Psychopathological factors in the doctor, including reactions to illness, death, and the failure of treatment, can influence the dying patient's end-of-life decision."

It is clear from the above that physician participation in assisted suicide or euthanasia can have a profound harmful psychological effect on the physicians involved. Physicians must take responsibility for causing the patient's death, with a resulting huge burden on conscience and tangled emotions and a large psychological toll on the participating physicians. Many physicians describe feelings of isolation. Published evidence indicates that pressure from patients, and some others, are intimidating doctors to assist in suicides to the point that they feel they have no choice. This shows a woeful ignorance of the methods we have to control unpleasant symptoms, be they physical, psychological, emotional, or financial. Oregon physicians are *decreasingly* present at the time of the assisted suicide.

These significant adverse effects on the doctors participating in assisted suicide and euthanasia, as well as the effects on patients, caregivers, and society, need to be considered when discussing the pros and cons of legalizing these practices and making them freely available.

This situation is not static; it is dynamic. Changes in the law, especially in matters of life and death, must be taken seriously because they can profoundly affect the whole of society.

Useful Resources

www.painfoundation.org/ The American Pain Foundation
www.ampainsoc.org/ The American Pain Society
www.iom.edu/ Institute of Medicine of the National Academies
www.cdc.gov/nchs/ National Center for Health Statistics
www.caringinfo.org/ Caring Connections, a program of the National Hospice and Palliative Care Organization
www.nhpco.org/ National Hospice and Palliative Care Organization
www.npcnow.org/ National Pharmaceutical Council
www.pccef.org/ Physicians for Compassionate Care
www.ninds.nih.gov/ National Institute of Neurological Disorders and Stroke

References

1. Kübler-Ross E. On Death and Dying. New York: Touchstone, 1969.
2. Lynn J. Western Journal of Medicine 1995;163:250–257.

3. Pinellas-Pasco County Medical Examiner Dr. Jon Thogmartin, who led the autopsy team. The official autopsy report was released June 15, 2005, Case #5050439.
4. Schroeder SA. The Legacy of SUPPORT. Annals of Internal Medicine 1999;131:780–782.
5. Lynn J, Schall MW, Milne C, et al. Quality improvements in end of life care: Insights from two collaborations. Joint Committee Journal Quality Improvement 2000;26:254–267.
6. Hendin H. Seduced by Death: Doctors, Patients and the Dutch Cure. New York: W.W. Norton, 1997.
7. Gomez C. Regulating Death: Euthanasia and the Case of the Netherlands. New York: Free Press, 1991.
8. Remmelink J. Medical Decisions About the End of Life. I. Report of the Committee to Study the Medical Practice Concerning Euthanasia. II. The Study for the Committee on Medical Practice Concerning Euthanasia. The Hague, 1991.
9. Sheldon T. Killing or caring? British Medical Journal 2005;330:560.
10. Verhagen E, Sauer PJJ. The Groningen protocol: Euthanasia in severely ill newborns. New England Journal of Medicine 2005;352:959–962.
11. Assisted Suicide: Not for Adults Only? Available at http://www.internationaltaskforce.org/noa.htm
12. Stevens, KR. Emotional and psychological effects of physician-assisted suicide and euthanasia on participating physicians. Issues in Law and Medicine 2006; 21:187.
13. Varghese FT, Kelly B. Countertransference and assisted suicide. Issues in Law and Medicine 2001;16:235–258.

Ethical Considerations of Provider-Patient Challenges

Elin Armeau, PhD, PA-C

The Ethics of Managing the "Whole" Patient

A 70-year-old female had elevated blood pressure, and her dose of medication was increased. She was scheduled to return to the health-care clinic to have her blood pressure monitored on her new medication dosage. She was scheduled for a 15-minute appointment, and the waiting room was full. In the examination room, the provider inquired how the patient was feeling. The patient responded that she had hurt her knee when she was working in the yard the previous day. She stated that she was unable to fill the prior prescription because she did not have money at the time and she was waiting until the following week when her monthly retirement check would arrive.

Additionally, because she will be getting her prescriptions filled, she would like prescriptions for her other medications while she is at the clinic. She has limited transportation available because her husband has also been ill recently. Her anxiety about her husband's health is also an apparent concern to her.

The provider faces a number of ethical considerations how to manage this patient's physical complaints of hypertension and knee pain; her anxiety about her husband's health, her prescription issues, and her transportation issues within the allotted 15-minutes amidst a full waiting room of patients. How does one ethically handle the issue of limited time and resources?

In 1948, the World Health Organization (WHO) stated, "Health is a state of complete physical, mental and social well-being, not merely the absence of disease or infirmity." This definition has not been amended since its origin.[1] The holistic approach to patient care integrates physical, mental, social, and spiritual indicators of health. Within each of these health indicators are daily ethical considerations that practitioners need to address.

Physician-Patient Relationship Models

The physician-patient relationship has evolved from physician-driven paternalism to respect for patient autonomy in the decision-making process. The traditional model of medicine was based on an unequal relationship between physicians and patients. Physicians had a monopoly on medical knowledge, and patients were vulnerable during periods of illness. Certainly, the increasing role of physician assistants and other midlevel providers has dissipated the concept of physician monopoly over medical knowledge and skills. The physician often assumed a role of domination in the decision-making process regarding the patient's care based on his or her judgment what would benefit the patient.[2] In this ethical model, the physician was empowered to override the patient's decision when the physician believed harm would come to the patient who did not follow recommendations.[3,4] This is exemplified by the changes in aggressive life-sustaining therapies.

In contrast to this model of paternalism, the autonomy model focuses on patients' right to choose what treatment they will accept. Autonomy in health care refers to the respect for individuals and their ability to make decisions.[4] The autonomy model is grounded in the concepts of informed consent, the right to refuse treatment, and confidentiality.[3] The physician informs the patient of alternatives and respects the patient's choice. As patients gained access to medical knowledge, their participation in medical decisions gained momentum. The physician must accept that patients may do harm to themselves through refusal to accept beneficial treatment. The decision not to quit smoking or not to adhere to dietary recommendations illustrates the autonomy model. The role of cultural and religious values may affect outcomes and a patient's decision to follow a health-care provider's recommendations for care.

An alternative model, the complementary model, allows for physicians to retain power of decision making based on their medical knowledge and skills. This power can be shared effectively through patient education regarding an illness and management. Issues and choices are explicitly expressed, balancing physicians' advocacy for treatment based on medical knowledge they believe will benefit the patient and/or prevent harm with the patients' right to choice. This team approach is critical to health-care issues that are grounded in lifestyles choices and behaviors and the practice of preventive medicine.

Additionally, financing of health care services directly affects the choices for medical treatment. The administration of insurance plans, limitations of managed health care systems, and prescription costs are a few examples of barriers to health care. Third-party payers, access to Internet resources, and escalating costs of medical technology have progressively influenced the decision-making process over the past two decades.

Managed Care

Historically, the physician held a sovereign status in medical decisions. Under the fee-for-services payment systems, physicians, hospitals, and ancillary services profited from more office visits, longer hospital stays, and utilization of more diagnostic services. However, with the escalation of health-care costs and the growth of third-party payers, the practice of medicine has shifted to limiting consumption of resources. The underlying philosophy of managed care systems is to provide an integrated network of patient care services, financed under a limited prospective budget. Under managed care systems, patients are frequently required to have an assigned primary care provider who serves as a gatekeeper to health-care delivery systems. The primary care provider must balance this gatekeeper role with the role as patient advocate.[5]

In the era of health maintenance organizations (HMOs), preferred provider organizations (PPOs), and managed care systems, the clinical decision-making process is affected by the business of medicine. Managed care and HMOs are aimed at reducing costs while maintaining quality heath care. Limiting the use of resources and increasing efficiency of providers increase profit for these health-care systems.[5] Health-care services, such as diagnostic testing and specialists' services, are limited by costs and reimbursements. In managed care systems, cost considerations create an environment where the patient or the provider is limited in choices of health-care resources. This rationing of health care, based on allocation of resources, generates disparities in health-care practices. Health-care plans vary enormously. Those patients with more comprehensive insurance plans or those who have money to purchase services have ready access to resources, whereas patients without adequate health insurance plans or with limited resources are more vulnerable.[5]

Physical Health

Dilemmas in the U.S. health-care system have consistently focused on three primary issues: cost of care, access to care, and quality of care. Cost of and access to patient care services are driven by politics and economic forces, which are often external to the patient and the provider. Cost incentives of health-care reform have forced providers to practice medicine for the "good of society" but concomitantly create a setting that can potentially limit providers' responsibilities to advocate for individual patients. Health-care policies and processes directly affect the decisions of health-care providers and often limit them or compromise the health-care options for their patients. The ethical challenge is therefore how to maintain quality of health care, given political, cultural, and economic barriers. The sanctity of the patient-provider relationship must be based on trust, not economic considerations.[6]

Capitation of reimbursement to providers coupled with limited referral resources and restricted prescriptive coverage to patients has changed the scope of medical management. These restrictions of resources affect the provision of optimal physical, mental, and social resources for needs of patients.

Clinicians are limited in their choices of diagnostic evaluations and therapeutic modalities by the financial constraints imposed on medical practices as well as by patients' resources to pay for services rendered. Adherence to guidelines under varying health-care systems creates ethical questions when caring for patients who require care that is not covered by health-care plans.[7] For example, a screening colonoscopy is recommended at age 50, but some insurance plans do not cover this procedure unless there are symptoms of disease or a family history of colon cancer. Similarly, high-cost technologies, such as in vitro fertilization, are not equally available within the market-oriented payment system.[8] These types of restrictions of technology are based on cost-benefit analysis in an era of rising costs and limited resources.[9]

Managed care, HMOs, and PPOs emphasize preventive medicine as a mechanism to control long-term costs. However, the practice of preventive medicine is progressively linked to reimbursement rather than to a patient-service orientation. In preventive medicine, the health-care provider must also be aware of the calendar in regard to reimbursement for services. Most insurance carriers require that cancer detection examinations, such as mammograms, cervical PAP smears, and prostate surface antigens, must be scheduled at least 1 year and 1 day after the previous examination. Although this requirement is reasonable based on epidemiological data, in clinical practice it adds another dimension to patient care that is not based on the patient's physical health but rather on economics.

A similar dilemma arises with choices of medications. Again, traditionally, the provider could select and prescribe the optimal therapy to control symptoms and prevent disease. However, in today's health-care market, different insurance companies will provide coverage for some medications and not for others that are in the same class of drug. Often patients will not be able to afford medications that are not covered under their individual insurance or prescription health plans. This is noticed most predominantly for those patients who are retired and those on a very limited fixed income.

Pharmaceutical reimbursement also affect providers' selection of medications for their patients. For example, two patients presented with chronic osteoarthritis of their knees. The arthritis is painful and limits the patients' abilities to enjoy basic activities such as going for a walk at home or climbing up and down stairs. The first patient was prescribed a common nonsteroidal anti-inflammatory drug (NSAID), which was also available over-the-counter but only in a smaller, less effective, dose. Because the medication was available over-the-counter, the insurance would not cover medicine even as prescribed at a higher dose than the nonprescription medicine. This patient would have had to incur the total cost of medication. However, the medication that his insurance would pay for under his health-care policy was an alternative drug for treatment of arthritis that was significantly more costly as it was a newer generation of NSAID. His health-care plan was willing to pay for an expensive prescription medication but not for the inexpensive and more available medication.

The second patient with arthritis had insurance that covered the cheaper NSAID at a low copayment. However, this medication was not effective in pain relief. The practitioner recommended changing to the newer NSAID and had samples available. The challenge component of treatment was that this second patient's insurance would not cover the newer prescription drug and the expense to the patient was excessive. When the samples of medication were no longer available through the physician's office, the patient would be left with an effective drug that he could not afford to continue taking. The provider must decide if offering a treatment with better pain control, followed by the inevitable discontinuation due to cost, is in the patient's best interest.

The decisions for even basic diagnostic and treatment plans are often swayed by the economics of insurance-driven health-care systems rather than optimal patient management. The limited financial or health-care resources of patients progressively necessitate compromises in patient management. Virtue-based medicine, as expressed in the ethics of the Hippocratic oath, is increasingly tempered by the conflicts inherent in advocating for a patient's needs versus societal demands for controlling health-care costs. Society advocates adherence to financial incentives of organized medical practice and is driven by resource allocation.

Traditionally, the physicians weighed the principles of nonmaleficence and beneficence. Nonmalefi-

cence refers to the standard term for "do no harm," and beneficence applies to actions that are intended to benefit the patient.[10] These ethical principles of practice imply that physicians will do everything that might improve the health of their patients. If the bioethical principles of beneficence and nonmaleficence are followed to the fullest extent, the cost of health care and the utilization of health-care resources would continue to soar. Under the model of cost-benefit, the health value of a procedure is tempered by the cost of the procedure to the individual. Often the decision making for patients comes down to the value of their health versus the cost of a medication or a procedure.[9]

Noncompliance and Informed Consent

The decision-making process is grounded in the principle of informed consent. The American Academy of Physician Assistants (AAPA) published guidelines for ethical conduct, which state that in this era of focus on cost containment and resource allocation physician assistants (PAs) should make decisions and advocate for the best care of their patients.[11] Ethically, the PA is obligated to inform the patient of the diagnostic or treatment options that optimize quality of care, regardless of managed care or health insurance plan. However, there is an additional responsibility to inform the patients of financial incentives that limit or conflict with patient care.

Along with health-care economics, physicians and PAs also must address issues of a patient's right to not choose a recommended procedure or treatment. Patients frequently do not have prescriptions filled or follow through with referrals. Historically, physicians dictated the patient's health care. However, since the "Great Society" reforms and the Equal Rights movement of the 1960s, patients have assumed an increasing role in health-care decision making. Rapid access to medical information via the Internet and television has also increased patients' desire to participate in their health-care decisions. Patients respond to the commercialism of medicine and pharmaceutical advertising by making demands for drugs and procedures that may not be necessary or appropriate to their care. Similarly, patients may decline treatment or procedures because they have increased access to information of risks or alternative medicines. Patients have the right to refuse treatments, whether it is based on finances, personal values, or other motivating factors. Refusal is based on patients being aware of the probable benefits and the medical consequences of their decision.[9]

The governing principle is the patient's right to self-determination, based on an informed choice.

Documentation of informed consent and refusal of treatment should specify the procedure, referral, or treatment regimen and state potential benefits and harm. Failure to provide information regarding potential harm relates directly to the ethical concept of nonmaleficence.[12] These outcomes of benefits and harm should be discussed with patients and documented in medical records. Through this action, patients assume the burden of responsibility for resultant health outcomes.

Noncompliant patients also present a challenge to the provider. Noncompliance is often termed nonadherence. Noncompliance involves such patients as a diabetic who does not check his blood sugar as recommended or a patient who does not follow through with a referral appointment or completion of a rehabilitation program.[13] When a practitioner is faced with a patient who is consistently noncompliant in following treatment recommendations, the burden of responsibility for care must be distributed between the patient and the provider. Noncompliance may be grounded in socioeconomic concerns such as finances, transportation, time constraints, or lack of motivation. Regardless of the patient's reason, noncompliance or nonadherence to recommended treatment recommendations should be documented in the medical records.

Mental Health

The economics of health-care practices often present in the form of appointments that are 10 to 15 minutes, allowing for appointments that focus on one patient complaint per office visit. Patients are often scheduled for quick assessments or follow-up appointments such as for checking blood pressure, ear infections, or wound care. However, when patients arrive at the clinic a week or more after they made their appointment, they often present with more serious complaints. Mental health and social health issues such as depression or abuse cannot be addressed ethically in a few minutes. The practitioner must decide to address the simple physical complaint for which the appointment was made and/or the more serious issue. Addressing additional patient complaints often counters the practice guidelines of managed care organizations that employ physicians and PAs. The easy solution of simply making a second appointment is often not in the patient's best interest. This becomes an unfortunate, economically driven dilemma for practitioners and is an ethical challenge in the provision of care. Additionally, potential legal repercussions of not addressing a serious health-care issue augment this conflict.

The AAPA Guidelines for Ethical Conduct of Physician Assistants state that "Physician Assistants

hold as their primary responsibility the health, safety, welfare, and dignity of all human beings." Physical health addresses the mechanics of the profession, including diagnosis and management of disease, illness, and injury. However, this statement also extends that responsibility to include mental and social risk variables that affect illness and wellness.[11]

Prevalence of Mental Illness

Mental disorders affect more than 22% of people over the age of 18 years, or more than 44.3 million people in the United States. Four of the ten leading causes of disability are mental disorders; they are major depression, bipolar disorder, schizophrenia, and obsessive-compulsive disorder.[14] Additionally, Alzheimer's disease, anxiety disorders, attention-deficit hyperactivity disorder, and eating disorders have increasing prevalence rates. There are more than 4 million Americans who have been diagnosed with Alzheimer's disease, and nearly 59% of persons over 85 years of age have Alzheimer's.[15] Recognition of disorders and subsequent referral for evaluation and treatment services fall within the scope of practice of primary care providers. These disorders directly affect a patient's level of understanding and compliance with adherence to preventive recommendations and management of acute and chronic diseases. Additionally, it is estimated that 21% of the population is disabled and has limited ability to complete activities of daily or independent living. Those who are disabled or even perceive themselves as having a disability also experience increased anxiety, pain, sleeplessness, depression, and fewer days of vitality than people without limitations in activities. Attention to these presenting symptoms of mental stressors is as vital to a patient's health as the more apparent symptoms of physical ailments.

Prevalence rates indicate that one out of every five patients meets criteria for diagnosis of a mental health disorder.[16] Therefore, health-care practitioners, employers, managed care organizations, and HMOs should enable access to appropriate services for the delivery of mental health services. Caregivers and family members should be involved in management planning to optimize maintenance of their health and benefit the patient. The National Registry of Certified Group Psychotherapists provides guidelines for patient-focused service indicators regarding access and quality of individual, group, and family psychotherapy services.[17]

The Office of the United Nations High Commissioner for Human Rights states all persons with mental illness have a right to not be discriminated against and the right to receive health and social care as appropriate to need.[18] The language of the principles of human rights is clear. However, when applied to individuals with mental illness, the health insurer or other advocacy agencies do not consistently support the medical recommendations.

The following case of a 35-year-old female who had severe mental retardation exemplifies this conflict. She was diagnosed with endometriosis, presenting with excessively painful menstrual periods with heavy menstrual flow. Because of her physical discomfort, she had associated behavioral components of anger and poor hygiene during her menstrual cycle. Medical intervention and hormone treatments resulted in minimal improvement. Thus, the gynecologist recommended a hysterectomy. This patient was able to express that she wanted her uterus to be removed and understood that it would stop her menstrual cycle as well as prevent pregnancy. Her sister and social caseworker also acknowledged the benefits and risk of a hysterectomy procedure as stated in the informed consent.

Decision-making capacity was assessed on the patient's ability to understand the situation, the proposed treatment, treatment alternatives, and resulting consequences of no treatment.[19] Criteria of decision-making capacity also extended to the patient's ability to communicate her decisions; the durability of this decision over time was assessed through recurrent physician visits and other interactions with other clinicians. The patient, her family, caregivers at the health-care facility, and two physicians supported the hysterectomy procedure. However, Medicaid as her primary insurer would not approve the procedure due to her mental disability and the resultant sterilization.

Although this patient's case represents an extreme on the spectrum of mental disorders, it does clearly exemplify the discrepancies across health care based on mental disabilities and the conflicting application of beneficence.[19] This case of a patient with cognitive impairment illustrates how a clinician may be caught between respecting the patient's choice and competing influences of others, including social welfare agencies and insurers. Guidelines for medical ethics of PAs state that health-care providers should not discriminate against classes or categories of patients in regard to their health-care needs. This principle needs to be universally applied and inclusive of patients with mental disorders.[11]

Practitioners who work with vulnerable populations, including the mentally ill or mentally disabled, should understand the issues of competence, risk/benefit concerns, and surrogates. Level of competence is determined by a patient's ability to communicate choices, understand information that is the basis for choices, and appreciate how these choices are weighed according to one's values.[20] Patients may be competent in some areas of decision making but lack the comprehension to be competent in other issues. If a patient is incapable of making a competent medical decision regarding treatment, a proxy consent is devised, or a surrogate assumes the role of decision maker.[12] The health-care provider's role is to ensure communication of risks and benefits regarding a diagnostic or therapeutic modality to enable the patient or surrogate to reach an informed decision regarding options.

Referrals for Mental Illness

More common mental disorders that the PA will encounter routinely in primary care settings include depression, anxiety, and substance abuse. According to the National Institute of Mental Health, approximately 13.3% of people over age 18 years have an anxiety disorder, and 9.5% have depressive disorders in a given year. These comorbidities are often associated with eating disorders or substance abuse. In 2000, more than 90% of people who died by suicide had a diagnosable mental disorder, commonly depression or substance abuse.[14] Many patients present with complaints of fatigue, headache, palpitation, indigestion, muscle tension, or insomnia. These are common symptoms of depression and anxiety and are often induced by stressful events or changes in patients' lives. Neuroendocrine and catecholamine effects of stress are well delineated and most observable as the "flight or fight" response to an extreme event.[21] However, chronic stress creates breakdowns mentally and physically through this chain of catabolic responses. In medical research, statistical measures of stress are based on culmination of life change units. Life change units include the loss of a loved one, poor relationships, financial difficulties, and new situations. Poor coping responses, such as excesses in overeating, smoking, substance abuse, and lack of exercise, also contribute to decline in health status. Acute and chronic responses to stressful psychosocial events can manifest physically, mentally, and behaviorally.

The temptation for many health-care providers is to focus on the somatic complaints, avoiding exploration or treatment of the underlying causal factors. The fallacy is that the signs of physical illness will continue to manifest until the underlying symptoms of depression and anxiety are managed. This concept is reinforced by limited billing of third-party payers for diagnosis of depression and anxiety in primary care settings. However, referral services and treatment of physical signs and symptoms are included under most health-care plans. Often symptoms of depression or other mental disorder can be overlooked, particularly in a health-care setting where the practitioners have four to five patients scheduled every hour. The cumulative effect of underdiagnosing situational or chronic mental illness results in misperceptions that mental illness is not a serious issue for health insurance companies and perpetuates limited medical treatment. Asking pertinent historical questions and early recognition of symptoms of common mental disorders are keys to the provision of holistic health care and should be incorporated into every individual's health-care plan.

Social Health

Healthy People 2010 primary goals are to (1) increase quality and years of healthy life and (2) eliminate health disparities. Health disparities vary by gender, race, ethnicity, sexual orientation, geographic location, and inequalities in income and education. Demographic variables affect access to health care, environmental exposures, and lifestyle choices. Incidence and prevalence rates of heart disease, obesity, and low birth weight exemplify disparities across socioeconomic levels. In 1900, infectious diseases were the leading causes of death. Today, chronic diseases including heart disease, cancer, stroke, chronic obstructive lung disease, diabetes, kidney disease, and chronic liver disease are leading causes of death. However, across population groups, the impact of sociodemographic variables of income and ethnicity is observed.

Underinsured and uninsured populations utilize fewer health services and have poorer outcomes related to delayed entering of the health-care system. Disability, morbidity, and mortality rates related to chronic illnesses and mental disorders increase in the lower socioeconomic populations.[22] Higher income correlates with improved housing, less occupational and environmental exposures, increased access to medical care, and improved education on health promotion and preventive services.[16]

People ages 25 to 64 years with fewer than 12 years of education have almost double the death rate than persons with more than 13 years of education. Similarly, the infant mortality rate is almost double for mothers with fewer than 12 years of education compared with those who have more than 13 years. Educational levels are linked to income and race, with Hispanics and African Americans being less likely to have 13 or more years of education than other ethnic groups.[16] The heart disease death rate is 40% higher, and the cancer death rate is 30% higher for African Americans than for whites. The leading cause of death for African American men age 25 to 44 years is HIV/AIDS; this death rate is seven times higher than for whites. Hispanics, American Indians, and Alaska Natives have more than twice the incidence and death rate from diabetes than do whites. The infant death rate for African Americans, American Indians, and Alaska Natives is double the rate for whites. Social and environmental variables contribute to disease processes and outcomes and need to be incorporated into primary care and patient care plans.[16]

Ethnicity, education, and income statistics are interrelated and influence access to health care. Certainly, cultural variances including beliefs about the value of medical care and health-seeking behaviors influence early diagnosis and treatment of disease, accounting for some health-care disparities.[22] Barriers of access to health care include transportation, availability of providers, location and proximity of facilities, language barriers, and waiting time for appointments.

Social Isolation

Social isolation has been recurrently linked to increased physical and mental disorders. The importance of social support and socioeconomic variables on disease and on wellness is exemplified by the following case. A 75-year-old widowed female was living alone in a neighborhood that had deteriorated over several decades. Because of the increasing crime rate, her daughter moved her across several states so that she could be closer to family members. The widow presented at the primary care office for a routine examination of her insulin-dependent diabetes mellitus. Since she moved into assisted housing, her income was decreased, and she was having difficulty affording medical supplies to monitor her diabetes. She also felt isolated because she was unable to drive; access to public transportation required walking more than a half-mile to the bus stop. She became dependent on her daughter for transportation to her medical appointments. Because her daughter worked full time and had limited leave time, transporting her mother to medical appointments during the week was difficult. These factors limited the widow's access to podiatry and ophthalmology referral clinics that were recommended in this patient's comprehensive medical care plan for diabetes. Left without transportation in an unfamiliar city, the patient had difficulty attending church, participating in community events, and cultivating new friendships. The result was she felt socially isolated. Her loneliness contributed to inactivity, sleeplessness, poor nutrition, and depression that compounded her signs and symptoms of diabetes.

During an era of managed care and limited time for schedule appointment, the practitioner again may be inclined to address only the physical complaint of diabetes mellitus, avoiding the more time-consuming issues affecting this patient's mental and social welfare. The initial step to improving this patient's quality of life is dependent on the provider's recognition of need for referrals to social services and community transportation resources. Involving the daughter in the health-care plan and seeking referrals sites that are compatible with her work schedule would also improve the access to health care for this patient. Even in an era of restricted office appointments, taking a few minutes to listen quietly to a patient's concerns is sufficient for reassurance that the physician or PA cares about the person's well-being. This provider-patient connection fosters confidence, hope, and encouragement, creating ripples that will improve the well-being of patients. Physician respect for individual patients and their quality of life is a fundamental ethical commitment and should not be outweighed by cost containment practice patterns.

Social Support

Social support networks within communities mediate the effects of disease and reduce the negative effects of stress of a disease. This concept is the foundation of thousands of support groups addressing illnesses including breast cancer, brain injury, cardiac rehabilitation, family violence, eating disorders, and numerous other health and rehabilitation programs. Conversely, lack of social relationships correlates with increased morbidity and mortality rates. Research has indicated that loneliness has a negative effect on the immune system and is a strong predictor of admission to nursing homes for rural elderly.[23] For example, separation and divorce have been associated with increased rates of cancer, infectious disease, pneumonia, heart disease, and psychiatric illness. Social interactions are vital to promotion of health of patients, family, and friends. Social relationships foster a sense of compassion, coherence, and commitment to improving physical, mental, and spiritual health and thus are integral parts of health care.

Family Disease: Domestic Violence

Domestic violence is an individual and societal issue that confronts health-care providers. Incidence and prevalence rates of domestic violence illuminate the need for positive social support systems within families and communities. Almost a third of women report physical or sexual abuse by a husband or boyfriend during their lifetime, and 58% of women over age 30 years have been raped. Domestic violence crosses culture, socioeconomic, sexual orientation, professional, and demographic lines. Among welfare recipients, the majority have experienced domestic abuse and are trapped by the abuse and poverty.

Child and elderly abuse are part of the family disease of violence. Children are more likely to be violent as children and into adulthood if they have experienced violence, witnessed domestic violence, and when violence was the primary mechanism for resolving conflicts within their family. The strongest predictor for a child becoming an abuser later in life is witnessing one's father abusing one's mother, thus perpetuating the abuse across generations. More than 45% of mothers of abused children have been battered, and child abuse is reported in more than a third of the homes where there is adult family violence.[24,25] These are only a few of the staggering statistics of domestic abuse. The health-care provider is often the first point of contact for the recognition and treatment of victims of violence.

Family violence affects children profoundly. Response to violence may be acted out as violent behaviors, substance abuse, mental illness, or striving for unattainable perfectionism. Victims commonly present to health-care providers through primary care and emergency department settings. Recognizing victims and proper referrals for safety and treatment are obligations of practitioners. The American Medical Association defines physical, emotional, psychological, and sexual abuse as behaviors grounded in the abuser's desire to control the victim through physical danger, fear, and degradation.[24,25] Often health-care providers will include sensitive topics of sexual practices and addictions in their patient histories but will omit questions that acknowledge exposure to abuse. Assessment of abuse is important for men and women and should become routinely incorporated into patient interviews. Questions should be asked using a nonjudgmental approach, supportive of the patient's safety.

When abuse is recognized, practitioners have an ethical and legal responsibility to intervene to ensure the safety of their patients. Treating the physical signs of abuse or the interrelated symptoms of depression, suicidal tendencies, or substance abuse is not sufficient. Thorough documentation in medical records is essential and should be precise and professional as medical records may be admissible as testimony in court. The duty to protect the victim is critical and often requires removing the victim from a threatening situation. Health-care providers must have knowledge of community resources that can provide safety, support, and advocacy for the victims. Hospital-based intervention programs often link with these community resources.

Most states have enacted mandatory reporting statues for dependent elders and children. Similar laws regarding nondependent, competent adults vary across states. Failure to report suspected abuse could result in liability for a physician or PA. Regardless of the legal status of the victims, practitioners have a legal duty to protect the victim. They also have a duty to warn third parties of impending or intent to harm if expressed by their patient. This duty to protect victims surpasses the duty of maintaining patient confidentiality. Obtaining advance permission for disclosure of information minimizes breaching patient confidentially.[24,26]

Traditional medical care often does not extend to others affected by the act of violence, including family members and even the perpetrator. The goal of communities is to break the cycle of abuse. Support and safety of victims is the initial step. Treatment plans should include individual counseling, family counseling, support groups, and social services. To break the cycle of abuse, treatment must extend to the abuser and those who witness abuse. Ethical conflicts in treating the perpetrators of abuse should not arise if based on the patient's/perpetrator's need to receive treatment rather than the physician's/PA's like or dislike of the patient.

Family Systems Theory

Family systems theory emphasizes the emotional process that affects the function of each family member. Basic patterns of response to situations are shaped by members' experiences with the nuclear family and are multigenerational. The perpetuation of family violence or addictive behaviors across generations illustrates the emotional processes that are destructive to individuals and families. These processes extend to other relationships and have a societal effect, unless intervention is provided.[27] In accepting the concept of family system diseases, the clinician is thereby empowered to incorporate family members into treatment plans to bring out changes in the home environment, creating security and rebuilding trust among family members. Breaking the cycle of generational responses to family violence or substance abuse requires change. Family systems therapists concur that families repeat destructive interactional routines. Therapists encourage a positive set of structure activities or rituals for role playing and practice behaviors within family therapy sessions. These structured family experiences focus on improving communication and support systems within families.[28] Social support from families, health-care providers, and community organizations are essential for the optimal health of individuals.

Spiritual Health

The medical model of health extends beyond the scope of treating physical ailments and mental illnesses. Social and spiritual well-being are essential components of wellness. The Gallup poll reported that 95% of people in the United States believe in God and that 84% claim that religion is important in their lives. Additionally, about 42% of Americans have sought alternative health care. Just as questions regarding domestic violence and social support systems are often omitted in the patients' histories, spiritual and religious beliefs are frequently ignored. If the premise is accepted that the body, mind, and spirit are interconnected, then spiritual history becomes a vital part of administering holistic health care. Medicine and religion are often combined to help patients cope with infirmity, loneliness, suffering, and death. Spirituality affords hope, meaning, and personal value during medical crises.[29]

Health Belief Systems

Within social structures, social interactions form the guidelines for the development of communication protocols, attitudes, and behaviors. Health belief systems are grounded in social perceptions and acceptance of information, whether confirmed or unconfirmed. Religious commitments are based on individuals identifying with the strongest beliefs within a religious community. Religious beliefs and organizations provide support for patients. Multiple research studies support that being involved in a religious community can aid in disease prevention and in coping with an illness and recovery. Research supports that a religious commitment reduces risks for drug and alcohol abuse, decreases incidence of cardiovascular disease, and lowers rates of suicide and delinquency.[30] Religious commitment, coupled with the social support from belonging to a group, offers a protective factor against physical, emotional, and psychiatric illness.

Three pediatric patients were diagnosed with acute lymphocytic leukemia and admitted to a regional hospital. Their presenting signs and symptoms and stage of disease were equivocal. Two patients had continuous family support 24 hours a day. The family of the third patient lived several hours away from the hospital and had financial limitations that limited their ability to stay at the hospital. Treatment courses were initiated, and the disease of the first two children went into remission, whereas the third child progressively declined and died within a couple weeks. Whether the closeness and prayers of family members affected the morbidity and mortality of these children will remain unproven. However, similar observances have been documented across many clinical settings and diseases. Research findings support those patients who view themselves as spiritual or religious who experience decreased morbidity and mortality rates from cardiovascular disease, substance abuse, and psychiatric illness.[30]

Many community resources and treatment programs often incorporate spiritual principles. The long-term success of many the 12-step recovery programs for addictive behaviors (e.g., anger, eating disorders, gambling, narcotics, and alcohol) is based on patients working to understand their triggers and behaviors that contribute to the cycle of addictive responses. The underlying premise of these programs, which have worked for millions of people worldwide, is that as a result of self-exploration and changes in behaviors an individual will experience a "spiritual awakening." Spirituality is an intrinsic belief offering hope, healing, and guidance. This spiritual awakening then becomes the foundation for coping with life events and long-term relief from the patterns of destructive behaviors.

Spiritual History and Interview

Although a patient's spirituality and religious beliefs should be acknowledged, some practitioners believe that religious activity is out of bounds of medicine. One argument draws parallels between improved outcomes associated with religious affiliation and outcomes associated with marriage. Research evidence supports that marriage is associated with positive health outcomes. However, practitioners do not recommend marriage to patients as a means of decreasing their risk factors. Following this premise, practitioners should not advocate for patients' involvement in spiritual practices. Advocates caution that religion should not be addressed as treatment to improve health nor should illness be linked to moral failure. Even though a complete patient history should incorporate religion or spiritual practices, religion should not be used as an intervention. Religion, prayer, or meditations in clinical practice should be addressed only at the invitation of the patient, not the provider.[31] Similar to medical issues such as mental disorders, risk behaviors, and sexual practices, the practitioners should be open, respectful, and nonjudgmental when conducting a patient interview that is based on moral and religious beliefs. When faced with difficult treatment options, the patient is ultimately the decision maker, and choices will be based on his or her beliefs that give life meaning.

Spirituality in Health Care

If illness can begin in the mind, then so can healing. For many patients, prayer and meditation are utilized as means of affirming contact with a greater consciousness, or God. The basis of these beliefs is that healing changes result from application of spiritual principles. Regardless of personal belief systems, the practitioner should recognize that spirituality and religion are important to many patients.

Contemporary medical ethics supports the principle that medical treatment should reflect the patients' interests, desires, and values. This principle is manifested in informed consents and advance directives that are incorporated into patients' medical treatment plans. Components of a spiritual history should include implications for medical care, including spiritual values, ritualized practices and restrictions, and end-of-life decisions.

Ritualized practices include baptisms, circumcisions, and last rites. Some religions restrict birth control, abortions, or blood products for transfusions. Some religion-supported hospitals limit procedures such as sterilization or elective termination of pregnancy. Spiritual values may influence decisions about the removal of life support, organ donation, and in vitro fertilization. During routine office visits, the PA and the supervising physician(s) should facilitate discussion with patients and patients' families regarding advance directives, living wills, and end-of-life decisions. Documentation in medical records enables practitioners to incorporate patients' choices of health care into treatment plans.

Spiritual Consults

The goal of a spiritual history should be to understand patients' belief system as it influences their health. Practitioners are not obligated to discuss religion, often lack familiarity or experience to offer knowledge, and should avoid imposing their beliefs. Referrals to chaplains, ministries, or counselors are available within medical facilities and communities. Hospital chaplains often serve the patient and their families during times of medical crises. Spiritual or chaplain consults are appropriate during a life-threatening illness or when confronting decisions regarding treatment options. Often these consults are a source of comfort or reassurance for patients.

Selected Patient Care Topics

In October 2002, the WHO established the Ethics and Health Initiative, which addresses global bioethical topics including organ and tissue transplants, stem cell research, genomics, long-term care, and access to health services.[32] Although these topics are addressed internationally, they pose challenges to individual providers and patients.

Genetic Counseling

Genetic testing raises several ethical issues. Genetic testing is used for carrier screening, prenatal diagnostic testing, confirmational diagnosis of symptomatic individuals, and presymptomatic testing for risk of adult-onset disorders such as Huntington's disease, Alzheimer's disease, and some cancers. The potential impact of discrimination or stigmatization due to difference in genetics needs to be weighed with the potential benefit of disease detection.

The Americans With Disabilities Act protects individuals and prohibits discrimination against symptomatic genetic disabilities. However, this act does not address unexpressed genetic disorders nor does it limit request for revealing of pre-employment medical information to employers. The Health Insurance Portability and Accountability Act of 1996 (HIPAA) is the only federal law that addresses genetic discrimination when the illness is not diagnosed. In 2002, HIPAA limited the nonconsensual use of private health information and restricted disclosure of health information to the minimum needed for an intended purpose. Current federal recommendations are also directed against insurance providers' use of genetic information to determine eligibility for health benefits.[33]

As in AIDS testing, pre- and post-testing counseling is also essential to ensure that the patient understands the information and risk of disease based on the results of genetic testing. Awareness of genetic inequalities and risk for developing a life-threatening illness is not always in the patient's best interest. Genetic testing should be voluntary for patients who have the capacity to consent. Determination of disclosure of information to the patient and family members who are at high risk for disease should be discussed in advance and remain confidential. Exceptions to nondisclosure are incidents such as court-ordered disclosure for forensics or paternity testing. Some genetic traits, such as sickle cell disease, are linked to ethnic or racial groups and may precipitate discriminatory practices and eugenics. Decisions for distribution or withholding of resources based on genetic information will become a predominant issue as genetic testing and gene therapy become increasingly accessible to patients. Adhering to principles of informed consent and the principle of nonmaleficence should serve as a guidepost for the clinician.[8]

Reproductive Decision Making

Patients have the right to access to all areas of clinical care regarding reproductive issues. Practitioners must provide unbiased disclosure of information regarding reproductive options, including fertility treatment, family planning, abortion, and sterilization.

About 43% of American women will have an abortion. The decision to terminate a pregnancy is usually based on personal reasons, such as feeling financially insecure, immature, or not responsible enough to bring up a child. About 6% of abortions are due to medical reasons such as prevention of a genetic disorder, and 1% are sought because conception resulted from sexual assault.[34] The decision for elective sterilization includes choosing to remain childless, lacking resources to support more children, or preventing genetic disorders. The reason for the decision belongs to the patient and is often influenced by pressure from peers or family members. The practitioner should provide objective information regarding risks and benefits that will enable the patient to make an informed decision. The PA should differentiate personal ethics from professional ethics when offering professional guidance. Providers should not participate in procedures they consider unethical. Even if providers do not personally consider abortions or sterilizations to be unethical, they should professionally weigh the benefits and risks of the procedures coupled with their dedication to healing. Additionally, the performance of nontherapeutic abortions and elective sterilizations may be limited by institutional philosophies or policies. For example, Catholic hospitals may not provide admitting privileges to physicians who perform these procedures.[5]

The patient's moral or religious biases need to be acknowledged. Artificial insemination and/or birth control are not considered options for many patients due to restrictions of their religions or moral values. Discussions regarding infertility should address medical aspects of care. Additional information on financial burdens, medication support, and emotional support should be provided. If personal values of a PA conflict with disclosure, the patient should be referred to an alternative provider to ensure access to available treatment options.[11]

Organ and Tissue Transplants

Successes in organ and tissue transplants have generated increased demand for organs. More than 45,000 people are awaiting organ transplants. In response to this increasing demand and competition for organs, organ procurement has become a global effort. Questions of free-market enterprise and organ selling are the substance of novels and ethical debates in health care. Defining brain death, living donations, and cloning of fetal tissue and tissue/organ are avenues for organ and tissue procurement. Financial resources and insurance still top the list of accessibility to organs and are often critical to decisions regarding who should receive the transplants.[35] The Human Genome Project also brings into question whether those patients with genetic defects should be given priority above those patients who had behaviors that contributed to disease. Psychosocial variables, such as home environment, support systems, and mental stability of potential recipients, also factor into the decision-making process for organ transplants.

Long-Term Care

Progressive increase in chronic illnesses and long-term disabilities, coupled with societal challenges of an aging population in the United States, have increased the need for long-term care. More than 100 million people have a chronic illness or disability. The list of chronic diseases will continue to proliferate to over 157 million by the year 2020. In 1930, only 5% of the U.S. population was over 65 years of age. When Medicare and Medicaid health-care reforms were initiated to provide health care for the elderly and disabled populations, only 13% of the population was over age 65. However, current population trends indicated that by 2030, 70% of the U.S. population will be over 65 years of age. The population over age 85 is the fastest-growing age group and is expected to increase from 4 million to 9 million by the year 2030.[22] Epidemiological trends suggest continued increase in diseases such as HIV/AIDS, dementia, diabetes, cardiovascular disease, strokes, and chronic obstructive lung disease. These chronic and disabling illnesses, augmented by population trends, necessitate the development of long-term care solutions.

Accessibility, accountability, and efficacy of long-term care are the primary challenges to providers. In 2000, a year of nursing home care cost, on the average, $50,000. This expensive cost of care prohibits placement into long-term care facilities for many patients and their families. More than 28 million people are informal caregivers; two thirds of women age 40 to 69 years anticipate having to provide care for an

elderly relative. Family and friends account for 85% of custodial home care and are unpaid laborers.[22] To qualify for Medicaid coverage of nursing home expenses, families are required to spend down to prescribed poverty levels. The financial and manpower burdens imposed on families are tremendous and increasing annually.

Long waiting periods for availability of beds and restrictions on prior conditions also limit access to health care. Primary health-care providers are constantly confronted with these limitations to patient care. Disclosure of information by providers should delineate choices and outcomes to enable patients and their families to make informed decisions regarding nursing home placement, long-term in-home care, and dependent care. Case management, assisted living, and long-term care facilities should be accessible to patients through health management programs and community resources. Finally, health-care practitioners and counselors should augment discussions with patients and their family members to include life-prolonging measures, living-wills, and referrals to hospice care for patients with terminal illness.

Summary

The statement of values of the PA profession begins with the statement "Physician Assistants hold as their primary responsibility the health, safety, welfare and dignity of all human beings."[11] The Hippocratic oath expresses that it is the duty of physicians to help sick people and to use medical knowledge to benefit health outcomes. Health is dependent on physical, mental, social, and spiritual well-being. Failure to recognize and treat all of these components of health results in a lesser quality of life for patients. Respect and compassion for the quality of life are the fundamental considerations and ethical principles that must preface all provider-patient contacts.

References

1. World Health Organization. WHO definition of health. Retrieved April 15, 2004, from who.int/about/definition/en
2. Ruddick W. Medical ethics. Retrieved April 30, 2004, from nyu.edu/gsas/dept/philo/faculty/ruddick/papers/medethics
3. Brody H. Ethical aspects of the physician-patient relationship. In Wedding D, ed. Behavior and Medicine, 2nd ed. St. Louis: Mosby, 1995; 201-213.
4. Green, B. Medical ethics. Retrieved April 30, 2004, from priory.com.ethics.htm
5. Garrett TM, Baillie HW, Garrett RM. Health Care Ethics: Principles and Problems (4th ed.). Upper Saddle River, NJ: Prentice Hall, 2001.
6. Faria MA Jr. Transformation of medical ethics through time (part II): Medical ethics and organized medicine. Retrieved April 30, 2004, from haciendapub.com/articl35.html

7. Brody H, VandeKieft GK. Managed care. In Sugarman J, ed. Twenty Common Problems: Ethics in Primary Care. New York: McGraw-Hill, 2000; 81-92.

8. Macer DR. Ethical challenges as we approach the end of the Human Genome Project. Retrieved July 14, 2004, from biot.tsukuba.ac.jp/%7Emacer/chgp/chg/68.html

9. Goodman JC, Musgrave GL. National Center for Policy Analysis: Medical ethics. Retrieved April 30, 2004, from ncpa.org/w/w52/html

10. American Academy of Dermatology Association. Position statement on capitation's impact on medical ethics. Retrieved April 30, 2004, from aadassociation.org/Policy/capitation.html

11. American Academy of Physician Assistants. From program to practice: A guide to the physician assistant profession. Alexandria, VA: American Academy of Physician Assistants, 2003.

12. Purtilo R. Ethical Dimensions in the Health Professions, 3rd ed. Philadelphia: W.B. Saunders, 1999.

13. La Puma J. Is medical ethics the same as corporate compliance?. Retrieved April 30, 2004, from managedcaremag.com/archives/9808/9808.ethics.shtml

14. National Institute of Mental Health. The numbers count: Mental disorders in America. Retrieved June 8, 2004, from nimh.nig.gov/publicat/numbers.cfm

15. WrongDiagnosis.com. Statistics about Alzheimer's disease. Retrieved September 24, 2004, from wrongdiagnosis.com/a/alzheimer_disease/stats.htm

16. Healthy People 2010. A systematic approach to health improvement. Retrieved November 11, 2002, from health.gov/healthypeople/document/html

17. American Group Psychotherapy Association. Quality indicators for group psychotherapy programs. Retrieved June 8, 2004, from agpa.org/about/qualind.html

18. Office of United Nations General Assembly. Principles for the protection of persons with mental illness and the improvement of mental health care. Retrieved June 11, 2004, from unhchr.ch/html/menu3/b/68.html

19. Karlawish JH, Casarett D. Competency and decision-making capacity. In Sugarman J, ed. Twenty Common Problems: Ethics in Primary Care. New York: McGraw-Hill, 2000; 225-237.

20. Younger SJ, Gaines AD. The ethics of research with human subjects who are mentally ill. Retrieved September 22, 2004, from Online Ethics Center:file:///C:My%20Documents/mentres.html

21. Griffith CJ. Stress relief: Preventing heart disease. Advance for Physician Assistants 2004:32-35.

22. Bodenheimer TS, Grumbach K. Understanding Health Policy: A Clinical Approach, 3rd ed. New York: McGraw-Hill, 2002.

23. Sanderson H. Shaping our future. Retrieved May 26, 2004, from state.ar.us/dhs/aging/hsjune98.html

24. American Medical Association. Diagnostic and treatment guidelines on domestic violence.

25. National Domestic Violence Hotline. What is domestic violence? Retrieved July 9, 2004, from ndvh.org/dvInfo.html

26. Larkin GL. Suspected abuse and neglect. In Sugarman J, ed. Twenty Common Problems: Ethics in Primary Care. New York: McGraw-Hill, 2000; 161-175.

27. Comella PA. A brief summary of Bowen family systems theory. Retrieved June 8, 2004, from bowentheory.com/abriefsumaryofbowenfamilysystemtheory

28. McDonald L. Applying family system theory to strengthen the family unit. Retrieved June 15, 2004, from weer.wisc.edu/fast/research/FamilySystemTheory.html

29. University of Washington School of Medicine. Spirituality and medicine. Retrieved June 7, 2002, from eduserv.hscer.washington.edu/bioethics/topics/spirit.html

30. Larson DB, Larson SS. Families, relationships, and health. In Wedding D, ed. Behavior and Medicine, 2nd ed. St. Louis: Mosby; 136-148.

31. Sloan RP. Religion, spirituality, and medicine. Retrieved June 7, 2002, from ffrf.org/fttoday/jan_feb00/sloan.html

32. Capron AM, Biller-Andorno N, Bouesseau MC, et al. Ethics and health initiative. Retrieved June 8, 2004, from int/ethics/topics

33. Human Genome Project Information. Genetics privacy and legislation. Retrieved July 14, 2004, from ornl.gov/sci/techresources/Human_Genome/elsi/legislat.shtml

34. Ontario Consultants on Religious Tolerance. Why do women want to have an abortion? Retrieved July 14, 2004, from religioustolerance.org/abo_why.htm

35. Caplan AL, Coelho DH. The ethics of organ transplants. Retrieved June 8, 2004, from hutch.demon.co.uk/prom/organtrans.htm

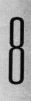

Ethics and State Regulation of PA Practice

Randy D. Danielsen, PhD, PA-C
Ann Davis, PA-C

Evolution of Medical Codes of Ethics

The medical profession has long-adopted bodies of ethical standards that were developed primarily for the benefit of the patient. In the 5th century BC, the Hippocratic oath was considered the beginning, if not the foundation, of a medical code of ethics. It is an oath of ethical professional behavior sworn by new physicians to treat the ill to the best of their ability, to preserve a patient's privacy, and to teach the secrets of medicine to the next generation. In 1803 Thomas Percival published his Code of Medical Ethics, which led to a design of professional conduct for hospital and other charities. This code is considered by some as the most significant contribution to Western medical ethical history after Hippocrates.[1] The American Medical Association (AMA) Code of Medical Ethics was written and published in 1847 and was based on Percival's code. In 1903 the title of the AMA's code was changed to Principles of Medical Ethics and, in 1957, a shorter version was adopted, which contained 10 sections, preceded by a preamble. These were adopted by AMA's House of Delegates in 1980 and, in 2001, the AMA's House of Delegates adopted additional principles.[2]

Ethics in the Physician Assistant Profession

As a member of the health-care profession, the physician assistant (PA) has a responsibility to patients, society, other health professionals, and self. According to Hooker and Cawley, "Physician assistants are expected to behave both legally and morally. They should know and understand the laws governing their practice. Likewise, they should understand the ethical responsibilities of being a health care professional."[3]

Fundamental Principles of the PA Code of Ethics

The PA profession, represented by the American Academy of Physician Assistants (AAPA), has revised its code of ethics numerous times. The fundamental principles underlying the ethical care of patients have not changed; however, the societal framework in which those principles are applied has. Economic pressures of the health-care system, social pressures of church and state, technological advances, and changing patient demographics continually transform the landscape in which PAs practice.

Values
The Statement of Values (Box 8-1) adopted by the AAPA House of Delegates defines the guidelines of ethical conduct for the PA.

Box 8-1	Statement of Values of the Physician Assistant Profession

1. Physician assistants hold as their primary responsibility the health, safety, welfare, and dignity of all human beings.
2. Physician assistants uphold the tenets of patient autonomy, beneficence, nonmaleficence, and justice.
3. Physician assistants recognize and promote the value of diversity.
4. Physician assistants treat equally all persons who seek their care.
5. Physician assistants hold in confidence the information shared in the course of practicing medicine.
6. Physician assistants assess their personal capabilities and limitations, striving always to improve their medical practice.
7. Physician assistants actively seek to expand their knowledge and skills, keeping abreast of advances in medicine.
8. Physician assistants work with other members of the health care team to provide compassionate and effective care of patients.[4]

Adherence to State and Federal Laws
The AAPA also notes the PA's responsibility to adhere to state and federal laws: "Physician assistants are expected to behave both legally and morally. They should know and understand the laws governing their practice. Likewise, they should understand the ethical responsibilities of being a health care professional. Legal requirements and ethical expectations will not always be in agreement. The law describes minimum standards of acceptable behavior, and ethical principles delineate the highest moral standards of behavior."[3]

Adherence to the American Academy of Physician Assistants Policies
It should be noted, according to AAPA bylaws, "If an AAPA member has had his or her physician assistant state license revoked as the result of a final adjudicated disciplinary action for violation of professional practice statutes or regulations, then the individual's AAPA membership shall be automatically revoked. Academy membership is not automatically revoked if the loss of a state license is due to an incident that does not impair the individual's capability to provide medical care, such as a lapse in payment of licensure fees."[5]

AAPA policy states:

"AAPA believes that Academy members have an obligation to disclose what they believe in good faith to be unethical or unprofessional conduct, without reprimand or retaliation.

AAPA will respond to allegations of unethical and unprofessional conduct with the utmost care, diligence, sensitivity, and respect for the rights of all concerned.

AAPA will follow peer-review practices that encompass confidentiality, due notification, fair and equitable process, and an appeal procedure that protect the rights of the members involved.

Upon completion of the peer-review process, the AAPA will report to the appropriate regulatory agencies any suspension or expulsion of membership due to violations of Guidelines for Ethical Conduct for the Physician Assistant Profession.

In keeping with the Guidelines for Ethical Conduct for the Physician Assistant Profession and the principle of self-regulation, AAPA will publish in AAPA News and on the public pages of the AAPA Web site the names of PAs who have lost their membership in the Academy following either a disciplinary process administered by the Judicial Affairs Committee or a final adjudicated disciplinary action by a regulatory agency that result in revocation of licensure for violation of their professional practice statute or regulation."[5]

Adherence to Certification Standards

More recently the National Commission on Certification of Physician Assistants (NCCPA) approved a code of conduct for certified and certifying PAs (Box 8-2). The NCCPA endeavors to assure the public that certified PAs meet professional standards of knowledge and skills. Additionally, NCCPA attempts to ensure that the PAs it certifies are upholding appropriate standards of professionalism and ethics in practice. The NCCPA's Code of Conduct for Certified and Certifying Physician Assistants outlines principles that all certified or certifying PAs are expected to uphold.[6]

Breaches of these principles may be cause for disciplinary review by the NCCPA. Disciplinary actions taken at the conclusion of that review may include formal censures, fines, revocation of certification or eligibility for certification, and/or other actions as deemed appropriate by NCCPA. Some disciplinary actions are reported to state licensing authorities and the National Practitioner Data Bank. This code represents some of the behaviors that may trigger review under NCCPA's Disciplinary Policy.

The NCCPA articulates a code of conduct that focuses on the ethics and professionalism expected from all individuals holding or seeking NCCPA certi-

---

Box 8-2 Code of Conduct for Certified and Certifying PAs

Preamble

The National Commission on Certification of Physician Assistants endeavors to assure the public that certified physician assistants meet professional standards of knowledge and skills. Additionally, NCCPA attempts to ensure that the physician assistants it certifies are upholding appropriate standards of professionalism and ethics in practice. The NCCPA's Code of Conduct for Certified and Certifying Physician Assistants outlines principles that all certified or certifying physician assistants are expected to uphold.

Breaches of these principles may be cause for disciplinary review. Disciplinary actions taken at the conclusion of that review may include formal censures, fines, revocation of certification or eligibility for certification and/or other actions as deemed appropriate by NCCPA. Some disciplinary actions are reported to the state licensing authorities and the National Practitioner Data Bank. This Code of Conduct represents some, though not necessarily all, of the behaviors that may trigger review under NCCPA's Disciplinary Policy.

Principles of Conduct

1. Certified or certifying physician assistants shall protect the integrity of the certification and recertification process.
   a) They shall not engage in cheating or other dishonest behavior that violates exam security (including unauthorized reproducing, distributing, displaying, discussing, sharing or otherwise misusing test questions or any part of test questions) before, during or after an NCCPA examination.
   b) They shall not obtain, attempt to obtain or assist others in obtaining or maintaining eligibility, certification, or recertification through deceptive means, including submitting to the NCCPA any document that contains a misstatement of fact or omits a fact.
   c) They shall not manufacture, modify, reproduce, distribute or use a fraudulent or otherwise unauthorized NCCPA certificate.
   d) They shall not represent themselves in any way as a Physician Assistant-

(box continues on page 178)

Certified (PA-C) designee unless they hold current NCCPA certification.

e) When possessing knowledge or evidence that raises a substantial question of cheating on or misuse of questions from an NCCPA examination, fraudulent use of an NCCPA card, certificate or other document or misrepresentation of NCCPA certification status by a physician assistant or any other individual, they shall promptly inform the NCCPA.

2. Certified or certifying physician assistants shall comply with laws, regulations and standards governing professional practice in the jurisdictions and facilities in which they practice or are licensed to practice.

a) Certified or certifying physician assistants shall respect appropriate professional boundaries in their interactions with patients.

b) Certified or certifying physician assistants shall avoid behavior that would pose a threat or potential threat to the health, well-being or safety of patients apart from reasonable risks taken in the patient's interest during the delivery of health care.

c) Certified or certifying physician assistants shall recognize and understand their professional and personal limitations.

d) Certified or certifying physician assistants shall practice without impairment from substance abuse, cognitive deficiency or mental illness.

e) Certified or certifying physician assistants shall maintain and demonstrate the ability to engage in the practice of medicine within their chosen areas of practice safely and competently. [3]

fication. The code serves as a tool to communicate to other stakeholders the expectations that many PAs are already upholding.

Professional Ethics

Professional ethics pertain to each PA's behavior. The PA's role may be multifaceted and may include such activities as medical practice, consulting, research, teaching, and writing, to mention only a few. PAs and other medical professionals are held to high ethical standards and expectations by their professions and are regulated by individual states to protect vulnerable patients. John Stuart Mill (1806–1873), the philosopher and economist, stated that the "only purpose for which power can rightfully be exercised over any member of a civilized community against his will is to prevent harm to others."[7] It is not surprising that the relationship between law and ethics, especially in medicine, continues to be blurred. As Komesaroff stated in *Archives of Internal Medicine* in 2001: "The reasons why confusion might arise are not difficult to understand: law and ethics share a common language that uses terms like 'rights,' 'responsibility,' 'justice,' and 'innocence,' even if these terms have fundamentally different meanings attached to them; both seek standards for reviewing and controlling personal behaviour; and many ethical problems have unquestionably been brought to light through the medium of litigation and legal judgment."[8]

Regulation of Health Professions

Do No Harm

The goal of preventing harm to others is the basis of health profession regulation. The statement *Primum non nocere* ("First, do no harm") is considered to be a foundation of medical ethics. Many believe that this phrase came from the Hippocratic oath. It does not but seems to have been derived indirectly from Hippocrates' *Epidemics,* in which he wrote, "Declare the past, diagnose the present, foretell the future; practice these acts. As to diseases, make a habit of two things—to help, or at least to do no harm."

State vs. Federal

In the United States, health-care professionals (with the exception of those who are employees of the federal government) are regulated by the states. This is the result of a case decided by the Supreme Court over a century ago. In January 1889, the Supreme Court issued a ruling in the case of *Dent v West Virginia.*[9] The case involved an unnamed "physician" practicing in Newberg, West Virginia, who had been fined $50 for practicing medicine "without a diploma, certificate, or license." The defendant claimed that he was qualified to practice in West Virginia. He had a diploma from the American Medical Eclectic College of Cincinnati, Ohio. The West Virginia Department of Health inspected the diploma and found that it did not meet the specifications of an 1881 West Virginia statute that required graduation from a "reputable medical college" for those wishing to practice medicine in the state.[10]

When the health department refused to accept the physician's training, the physician took the case to court, arguing that if he were prevented from practicing medicine, it would be a great injury to him as it would deprive him of his only means of supporting himself and his family. The jury found the defendant physician guilty of practicing medicine without a license and upheld the fine. The physician appealed to the state supreme court, which upheld the lower court's decision. The case was then appealed to the United States Supreme Court.[10]

Stating the opinion of the majority, Justice Field wrote: "The power of the state to provide for the general welfare of its people authorizes it to prescribe all such regulations as in its judgment will secure or tend to secure them against the consequences of ignorance and incapacity, as well as of deception and fraud." With this ruling, the authority to license and regulate health professionals was given to the states.[11]

State Regulatory Agencies

All states regulate the practice of PAs (Box 8-3). The states issue a license (in some states called certification or registration) and adopt statutes and regulations that govern the supervised practice of PAs and the disciplinary actions that the regulatory agencies may take if a PA violates the laws. In most states the regulatory agency responsible for licensing and regulating PAs is the board of medical examiners. The board appoints an advisory committee of PAs and physicians. Nine states have a regulatory body strictly for PAs. Regardless of which entity has authority, PAs usually share responsibility for regulating and defining PA practice.[11]

Members of regulatory boards are generally appointed by the governor and include voluntary members of the medical profession (physicians), PAs, and the public. The Federation of State Medical Boards describes the responsibility of a state medical board is "to protect consumers of health care through proper licensing and regulation of physicians and, in some jurisdictions, other health care professionals."[11]

Broadly defined, the regulatory agency's ultimate responsibility is the protection of the public from incompetent or unethical practice by PAs. This is accomplished through verifying qualifications, defin-

ing and requiring supervision, delineating scope of practice, and investigating and disciplining PAs who are found to be practicing in violation of PA laws.

Licensure

Although each state is unique, laws for PAs are becoming much more uniform. The criteria for licensure in every state include graduation from an accredited PA program and passage of the Physician Assistant National Certifying Examination (PANCE). Some states make provisions for licensing PAs who are not accredited program graduates but who passed the PANCE when it was available to nonaccredited program graduates before 1985. The PANCE functions as the de facto licensing examination for PAs.

Some state laws add an ethical framework to licensure criteria. Many states require that an applicant for licensure be of "good moral character." Although good moral character generally is not defined, it allows a board, for example, to deny a license to someone who has been convicted of rape, murder, or other serious crimes.

Supervision

PA state laws require and define supervision. In general, supervision is defined as the ability of a physician to exercise direction and control over the work of a PA. Laws require that a supervising physician be available either in person or via telecommunication when a PA is providing care to patients.

Scope of Practice

The definition of PA scope of practice is also becoming uniform. Early state laws included a list of those duties that could be delegated to PAs, e.g., taking the patient history, performing physical examination, and ordering or performing certain laboratory tests. Modern statutes and regulations define PA scope of practice as those activities for which the PA is appropriately trained that are appropriately delegated and supervised by a supervising physician.

Disciplinary Action

In general, disciplinary statutes and regulations for PAs mirror those for physicians. PAs can be disciplined by a board for the same infractions that can trigger discipline for physicians, with the addition of failing to practice with appropriate supervision and holding oneself out as a physician. If a PA is found to be in violation of a law, the board may deny or revoke a license, impose restrictions on a license, levy a fine, issue a public or private letter of reprimand, refer a PA

Box 8-3	Physician Assistant Participation in Professional Regulation*
ALABAMA	Physician Assistant Advisory Committee (Board of Medical Examiners)
ALASKA	PA on State Medical Board
ARIZONA	Arizona Regulatory Board of Physician Assistants
ARKANSAS	Physician Assistant Advisory Committee (Arkansas State Medical Board)
CALIFORNIA	Physician Assistant Committee (Medical Board of California)
CONNECTICUT	PA on Medical Examining Board
DELAWARE	Physician's Assistant Regulatory Council (Board of Medical Practice)
DISTRICT OF COLUMBIA	Physician Assistant Advisory Committee (Board of Medicine)
FLORIDA	Council on Physician Assistants
GEORGIA	Physician Assistant Advisory Committee (Composite State Board of Medical Examiners) PA advisor on CSBME
HAWAII	Physician Assistant Advisory Committee (Board of Medical Examiners)
IDAHO	Physician Assistant Advisory Committee (Board of Medicine)
ILLINOIS	Physician Assistant Committee (Board of Medicine)
INDIANA	Physician Assistant Advisory Committee (Medical Licensing Board)
IOWA	Board of Physician Assistant Examiners
KANSAS	Physician Assistant Council (Board of Healing Arts)
KENTUCKY	Physician Assistant Advisory Committee (Board of Medical Licensure)
LOUISIANA	Physician Assistants Advisory Committee (Board of Medical Examiners)
MAINE	Physician Assistant Advisory Committee (Board of Registration in Medicine)
MARYLAND	Physician Assistant Advisory Committee (Board of Physician Quality Assurance)
MASSACHUSETTS	Board of Registration of Physician Assistants (Department of Consumer Affairs & Business Regulation)
MICHIGAN	Task Force on Physician Assistants PA on Board of Medicine PA on Board of Osteopathic Medicine
MINNESOTA	Physician Assistant Advisory Council (Board of Medical Examiners)
MISSISSIPPI	Physician Assistant Committee (Board of Medical Licensure) PA Committee may be appointed at the discretion of the board; no committee currently appointed
MISSOURI	Advisory Commission for Physician Assistants (Board of Healing Arts)
MONTANA	PA on Board of Medical Examiners PA Advisory Committee (Board of Medical Examiners)

NEBRASKA	Physician Assistant Committee
	(Board of Medical Examiners)
NEVADA	Physician Assistant Advisory Committee
	(Board of Medical Examiners)
NEW HAMPSHIRE	PA on Board of Registration in Medicine
	Physician Assistant Advisory Committee
	(Board of Registration in Medicine)
NEW JERSEY	PA on Board of Medical Examiners
	Physician Assistant Advisory Committee
	(Board of Medical Examiners)
NEW MEXICO	PA on Medical Board
NEW YORK	PAs on State Board of Medicine
	(State Education Department)
	PAs on Board of Professional Medical Conduct
	(State Department of Health)
NORTH CAROLINA	Physician extender on the Board of Medical Examiners
	PA Advisory Committee
	(Board of Medical Examiners)
OHIO	Physician Assistant Policy Committee
	(State Medical Board)
OKLAHOMA	Physician Assistant Committee
	(Board of Medical Supervision and Licensure)
OREGON	Physician Assistant Committee
	(Board of Medical Examiners)
PENNSYLVANIA	One seat on Board of Medicine rotates among PAs, nurse mid-wives, and certified registered nurse practitioners
	One seat on Board of Osteopathic Medicine alternates between a PA and respiratory care practitioner
RHODE ISLAND	Board of Licensure for Physician Assistants
	(Department of Health)
SOUTH CAROLINA	Physician Assistant Committee
	(Board of Medical Examiners)
SOUTH DAKOTA	Physician's Assistant Advisory Committee
	(Board of Medical and Osteopathic Examiners)
TENNESSEE	Committee on Physician Assistants
	(Board of Medical Examiners)
TEXAS	Board of Physician Assistant Examiners
	(connected to Board of Medical Examiners)
UTAH	Physician Assistant Licensing Board
VERMONT	PA on Board of Medical Practice
	PA Committee (inactive)
VIRGINIA	Advisory Committee on Physician's Assistants
	(Board of Medicine)
WASHINGTON	PAs on Medical Quality Assurance Commission
	PA Advisory Committee (inactive)
WEST VIRGINIA	PA on Board of Medicine
WISCONSIN	Council on Physician Assistants
	(Medical Examining Board)
WYOMING	PA on Board of Medicine
	Advisory Committee on Physician Assistants

*Provided by the American Academy of Physician Assistants

CASE STUDIES

Case 8.1
Professional Standards

Joe finished his PA training 2 years earlier and was starting to feel comfortable in his practice with a rural physician. His patients really liked Joe because he was friendly, cared about them, and was always available. Many patients had some difficulty in understanding the role of a PA and were just comfortable in calling him "Doctor Joe". Not wanting to hurt their feelings, he allowed this to continue. In fact, on a number of occasions when patients went to the local hospital emergency room, they listed Joe as their doctor, and even some of the nurses and ancillary personnel started calling Joe "doctor." The local newspaper, anxious to report his good deeds in the community, listed Joe as a physician. Everything was fine until the PA regulatory board contacted Joe after an unhappy patient complained that he thought Joe was not a physician.

Case 8.2
The Issue of Impropriety

Sue, a PA for 15 years, has been a speaker for a national pharmaceutical company for many years, discussing appropriate antibiotic use in various conditions. During her presentations, she states that she prefers the antibiotic promoted by the pharmaceutical company she represents. Just recently, she bought significant market shares in the same pharmaceutical company. The PA state board calls her but finds no credible evidence to support unprofessional conduct.

Case 8.3
Sexual Impropriety

Fred, a newly divorced PA, starts having a sexual relationship with the adult daughter of one of his long-time patients. When the patient indicates disapproval, Fred states that it is not his business because the daughter is an adult. The patient makes a complaint to the regulatory board. An investigation finds no legal violations.

Case 8.4
Ethical Responsibility

Stephanie accepts a new job as a PA with a well-known physician in a suburb of a large town. The physician has practiced in that suburb for over 20 years and is well respected as a competent and caring practitioner. After 6 months on the job, Stephanie notices a significant change in the demeanor of the physician as well as repeated episodes of tardiness to the office. One day, Stephanie thinks she smells alcohol on his breath. When she cautiously asks some of the office and hospital staff if they have noticed any changes, many of them either would not discuss it or had noticed but were unwilling to come forward. When she, appropriately in private, discusses her concerns with the physician, he becomes angry and denies the allegations. Over the next month, Stephanie continues to see evidence of impairment, which, on two occasions, results in inappropriate care to patients. What should the PA do? She is concerned that she may lose her job if she pursues this issue.

Case 8.5
Maintaining Proper Supervision

Jim has been working in a multispecialty clinic for well over 10 years. His long-time physician supervisor leaves the practice, and the clinic selects another physician in the practice to be his legal supervising physician. The physician makes it clear that he does not appreciate PAs and avoids contact with Jim. Jim avoids contact with his supervising physician and elects to interact with other physicians in the clinic. When a patient complaint about medical care reaches the state PA regulatory board, no physician steps forward to support Jim. What ethical issues were breached in this case?

Case 8.6

Ethics in Regulatory Practice

Barbara, a former president of her state PA society, is appointed by the governor to serve as a PA member of the state medical board. The current leadership of the PA society contacts Barbara to enlist her help with a regulatory change to augment PA prescribing authority. Barbara says she will be glad to listen to the proposal but declines to present it to the board. She suggests that the society prepare a presentation for the board and request the board directly that the proposal be included on it's agenda. The society leaders are angry; they do not understand why Barbara refuses to champion their cause.

CASE STUDY DISCUSSION

● **Case 8.1:** Regulatory and/or licensing boards clearly have the authority to discipline PAs when they violate professional standards specified in statute. Most PA practice laws require PAs to explain their role to patients and to wear a name tag or identification indicating their status as a PA. If indeed Joe always wore his name tag or indentification and took every opportunity to explain his role, he likely met the statutory requirements. The ethical question is how far a PA should go to assure that patients understand the PA status. It is important to examine applicable statutes or rules in relation to the potential harm to the public if the PA is in violation. The concern here is that a PA may be impersonating a physician and by doing so may be providing services beyond the scope of a PA. The AAPA notes that: "Physician assistants should not misrepresent directly or indirectly, their skills, training, professional credentials, or identity. Physician assistants should uphold the dignity of the PA profession and accept its ethical values."[12] Ultimately, it is the PA's responsibility and ethical obligation to ensure patients understand who is a PA and what a PA can do.

● **Case 8.2:** Although it appears that no legal violation occurred, is there an ethical problem? The AAPA comments that: "Physician assistants should place service to patients before personal material gain and should avoid undue influence on their clinical judgment. Trust can be undermined by even the appearance of improper influence. Examples of excessive or undue influence on clinical judgment can take several forms. These may include financial incentives, pharmaceutical or other industry gifts, and business arrangements involving referrals. PAs should disclose any actual or potential conflict of interest to their patients."[12]

Certainly, PAs should not avoid the opportunity to participate as speakers on behalf of pharmaceutical or medical equipment companies. However, PAs should avoid even the appearance of impropriety. Is buying significant market shares in a company for which the PA is also a speaker crossing the ethics barrier? Disclosure is very important. If a PA believes that a particular product or drug is superior, it may be ethically proper to say so. Whatever the relationship, the PA should ensure full disclosure to the audience. Joel M. Hill states, "Real or potential conflicts of interest may not indicate that unethical behavior has actually occurred, but should trigger definition of the problem, clarification of internal policy requiring disclosure or other action, and consideration of unintended interpretations by patients or colleagues which may undermine the trust relationship fundamental to quality care."[13]

● **Case 8.3:** Are there any ethical considerations in this case? Once again, the AAPA states: "It is unethical for physician assistants to become sexually involved with patients. It also may be unethical for PAs to become sexually involved with former patients or key third parties. Key third parties are individuals who have influence over the patient. These might include spouses or partners, parents, guardians, or surrogates."[14]

Once again, PAs should avoid even the appearance of impropriety. It may be important for PAs to avoid relationships that have the potential of interfering with patient care. The AAPA goes on to say: "Such relationships generally are unethical because of the PA's position of authority and the inherent imbalance of knowledge, expertise, and status. Issues such as dependence, trust, transference, and inequalities of power may lead to increased vulnerability on the part of the current or former patients or key third parties."[14]

continued

● **Case 8.4:** The AAPA suggests, "PAs should be able to recognize impairment in physician supervisors, PAs, and other health care providers and should seek assistance from appropriate resources to encourage these individuals to obtain treatment."[12] If that fails, "Physician assistants have an ethical responsibility to protect patients and the public by identifying and assisting impaired colleagues....Impaired means being unable to practice medicine with reasonable skill and safety because of physical or mental illness, loss of motor skills, or excessive use or abuse of drugs and alcohol."[12]

What if the impaired practitioner is a PA? The same ethical rules apply. In some states, PAs who have a substance problem and are referred to the regulatory board may not face immediate disciplinary action. Many are allowed to practice while undergoing mutually agreed upon rehabilitation. If they do not meet the conditions of the rehabilitation program or are not successful, they may be subject to disciplinary action at that time.

● **Case 8.5:** The AAPA states "Supervision should include ongoing communication between the physician and the physician assistant regarding patient care. The PA should consult the supervising physician whenever it will safeguard or advance the welfare of the patient. This includes seeking assistance in situations of conflict with a patient or another health care professional." Depending on supervision definition in a particular state, "providing services without required supervision or otherwise attempting tasks beyond the scope of a PA" may be considered unethical conduct.[12]

● **Case 8.6:** When PAs become regulators, their primary responsibility is to uphold the regulatory agency's duty to protect the public. Whereas Barbara's representation of the PA profession is probably not at odds with her role in public protection, it is still not consistent with the terms and covenants of her appointment. PAs would not be happy with a physician member of a regulatory agency who appeared to be primarily interested in addressing concerns of the state medical society. They should expect and honor the same separation of allegiances in their own colleagues.

to a treatment or counseling program, impose probation, or require that the PA complete specific training.

The following case studies illustrate regulatory issues in relation to ethical responsibilities of PA practice. Cases are presented, then followed with discussion of the pertinent ethical and regulatory principles.

Conclusion: Personal Ethics Check

A single chapter on regulatory or professional ethics cannot adequately cover the issues. A PA must develop a sense of personal integrity when it comes to ethics. Kenneth Blanchard and Norman Vincent Peale published a simple ethics check in 1988, which can be valuable in addressing ethical situations.[15] When faced with an ethical decision, PAs should ask themselves the Ethical Check Questions in Box 8-4.

Ultimately, ethical conduct is the responsibility of the individual PA. That conduct includes legal and moral considerations. Unethical behavior of any type is injurious to all involved: the patients, the practice,

| Box 8-4 | The Ethics Check Questions |

1. Is it legal? Will I be violating either civil law or company policy?
2. Is it balanced? Is it fair to all concerned in the short term as well as the long term?
3. Does it promote win-win relationships? How will it make me feel about myself? Will it make me proud? Would I feel good if my decision was published in the newspaper? Would I feel good if my family knew about it?

Blanchard K, Peale NV The Power of Ethical Management. William Morrow & Co., 1988.

the profession, the individual PA, and society. If an issue raises the question in one's mind "Is this ethical?" then certainly it requires introspection and consideration before any action is taken. Even if an unethical act is never revealed, there is a personal price to be paid.

References

1. The Hippocratic Oath. Accessed June 1, 2006, at bbc.co.uk/dna/h2g2/A1103798
2. AMA Code of Ethics. Accessed June 1, 2006, at ama-assn.org/ama/pub/category/8291.html
3. Hooker RS, Cawley JF. Physician Assistants in American Medicine, 2nd ed. New York: Churchill-Livingstone, 1997; 319.
4. Guidelines for Ethical Conduct for the Physician Assistant Profession. Accessed June 1, 2006, at aapa.org/policy/ethical-conduct.html#Heading54
5. Membership Revocation, AAPA. Accessed June 19, 2006, at aapa.org/membership/revocation.html
6. Code of Conduct for Certified and Certifying PAs. Accessed June 1, 2006, at nccpa.net/CER_process_code-ofconduct.aspx 1
7. John Stuart Mill. Accessed June 1, 2006, at http://66.102.7.104/search?q=cache:TYsM9N3Zp2YJ:legalstudies.berkeley.edu/ls107/2006_notes_1_31.doc+%22The+only+purpose+for+which+power+can+rightfully+be+exercised...%22&hl=en&gl=us&ct=clnk&cd=4&client=firefox-a
8. Komesaroff PA. In the public eye: The relationship between law and ethics in medicine. Archives of Internal Medicine 2001;31:413–414.
9. Dent v. West Virginia. 129 U.S. 114 (1889).
10. Younger P, Conner C, Cartwright KK, et al. Physician Assistant Legal Handbook. Aspen Publishers, 1997.
11. What Is a State Medical Board? Federation of State Medical Boards, Dallas: 2004.
12. Guidelines for Ethical Conduct for the Physician Assistant Profession. Accessed June 1, 2006, at aapa.org/policy/ethical-conduct.html#Heading54
13. Can We Serve Two Masters? Conflicts of Interest in Health Care. Accessed June 1, 2006, at parkridgecenter.org/Page646.html
14. Guidelines for Ethical Conduct for the Physician Assistant Profession. Accessed June 1, 2006, at aapa.org/policy/ethical-conduct.html#Heading54
15. Blanchard K, Peale NV. The Power of Ethical Management. New York: William Morrow & Co., 1988.

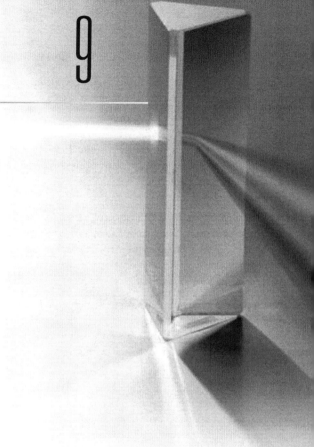

9

Applying for a License and Appearing Before a Regulatory Board

Barry A. Cassidy, PhD, PA-C

Applying for a License to Practice as a PA

In the beginning years of the physician assistant (PA) profession, there were no laws dealing with the practice. Rather, PAs relied on a loose interpretation of the physician's right to delegate tasks under the physician's medical license. As PA practice became more common throughout the country, individual states began passing laws to regulate it. Today all 50 states have legislation regulating PA practice.

The student is given the privilege to learn the art and science of becoming a PA by interacting with patients. In most states students are allowed this privilege through an exemption in the relevant statute that covers PA practice. In Arizona, for instance, the following rules apply: "The board may...grant an exemption from the licensure requirements of this section to...a student enrolled in a physician assistant education program approved by the board in order for that student to work within that program. The student shall register with the board on a form prescribed by the board."[1]

This exemption is given because the law defines the practice of being a PA to be unlawful without a license. To not have this exemption in Arizona would mean the PA student would be guilty of a felony for practicing as a PA without a license. The legislature recognizes that the responsibility for the safety of the patients with whom the student works is delegated to the PA training program. Upon completion of the program, it is easy for the graduate to underestimate the significance of what it means to be given a license to practice as a PA. Being a PA is a very serious matter, and understanding the laws and rules applicable to the practice is essential.

Each state has unique laws that regulate PA practice. Before applying for licensure, it is important to understand the laws of that state. If you do not completely understand the regulations that pertain to PA practice in the state for which you are applying for a license, you are not ready to send in the paperwork. In fact, it is a very good idea to review the laws that regulate PA practice every year to remind yourself of the rules applicable to your practice.

Most states ask applicants to sign a statement that they have read and understood the applicable law. Many states also require that the supervising physicians also acknowledge that they have read the applicable law. Attesting to such a statement deprives an applicant of the claim that they did not know what was expected regarding PA practice.

Answering questions on a state application for licensure is an ethical exercise. Questions are designed to determine if there are issues in one's past or present that might inhibit a jurisdiction from granting a license. At times, there may be general confusion as to what the question is really asking. Remember that the licensing agency is looking to acquire as much information as it can so it can determine whether the PA should practice. Here are some typical questions that might be asked:

PA Program Training Questions

- During your PA training, were you ever required to repeat any segment of your training?
- Have you ever had an action taken against you such as a restriction or limitation, including probation or academic probation, while a participant in this or any other training program?
- Were you ever counseled regarding performance or behavior in your training program?
- Did you ever take a leave of absence, other than for pregnancy, during your PA training program?

Answering these questions truthfully might seem challenging when one contemplates the depth of response to each question that the regulatory board is seeking. For instance, does the board really want to know that a student had to repeat a cardiology physical examination practicum before passing the physical diagnosis course? The bureaucratic answers are yes and no. If the student failed the entire physical diagnosis course and was required to repeat the course, the answer is yes. By acknowledging the failure, the board can determine if additional competency evaluations are necessary before granting a license. If, however, the student successfully completed the course but failed the practicum, requiring a second time, then passed it, it probably is not necessary to report that level of information.

The same is true of answering questions regarding counseling. Part of the molding of a health-care professional involves mentoring. Boards are not interested in the number of times a faculty advisor helps a student refocus. However, they are extremely interested in times when official actions are taken against students for misbehavior, such as cheating, unprofessional conduct, and so on. A landmark study done by Papadakis at the University of California, San Francisco, showed a direct correlation between unprofessional behavior in medical schools and subsequent disciplinary actions taken by the state medical board.[2] Clearly, if an official action was taken that involved a formal academic review committee of the faculty or an official action by the program director or dean, it should be reported. Many states also send a form to the PA training program asking questions similar to those the licensee applicant answered for purposes of verification. If the applicant's response is different than the program's response, difficulties can result. A note of caution is given here. Applicants who have had a disciplinary action taken against them during their training should speak with the program director and ask what their intended statement will be to an inquiry from the state board. It is far better to know what will be sent out in advance than to attempt to minimize a situation that will be misunderstood by the licensing agency.

Questions that ask about disruptions in a training program are designed to elicit the cause of the disruption. Answers such as, "I was in jail for felony assault" are relevant to a regulatory agency. Ultimately, one should answer as truthfully as possible. Oftentimes, the explanation clarifies the issue, and the application is processed routinely. Sometimes, a staff member of the agency will call for clarification. Anything that looks as if information is being hidden does not serve the applicant well. Denial of a license for fraudulent or false information is reported to the National Practitioner Data Bank (NPDB), and such an action can be the basis for denial of licensure in another jurisdiction. When fraud is discovered, an entirely separate course of events occurs that is far more damaging than dealing with an issue appropriately in the beginning.

Dealing with state agencies and filling out licensure applications while meeting deadlines for employment is very stressful. Be courteous to those processing your application. Most regulatory agencies have courteous and respectful staff; when staff members are the recipients of discourteous or demanding attitudes, applications may not be processed expeditiously. It is an unfortunate reality that some medical boards are severely understaffed. As such, staff members do the best they can with what little they have, and kind words go a long way.

Understanding Health-Related Questions

Here are some health-related questions that might appear on an application:

- Do you have a chronic ailment communicable to others?
- Within the last 10 years, have you ever been diagnosed with or treated for bipolar disorder, schizophrenia, paranoia, or any other psychotic disorder?

In its role as a protector of the public, a regulatory board has the legal right to ensure that a practitioner cannot unknowingly harm a patient. For instance, a neurosurgical PA who develops a significant tremor is obviously dangerous in the operating room. A person with uncontrolled bipolar disorder is similarly dangerous to the public. Does this mean that a PA with physical or psychiatric disorders cannot practice medicine? Not necessarily; however, some form of public protection may be indicated. Many states have mechanisms for restricted practices. A neurosurgical PA who has a tremor and can not operate requires public disclosure that the PA's practice is restricted. If it were not public, then other hospital surgical staffs would not know that their patients need protection. A clinician with controlled bipolar disorder is not an imminent threat to the public as long as the person continues an effective therapeutic relationship with a psychiatrist. In situations such as this, boards can enter into a confidential stipulated rehabilitation agreement (SRA). An SRA specifies the agreement for monitoring, such as quarterly reports from the psychiatrist, along with an agreement to stop practicing if the illness becomes uncontrolled. In the event that a clinician becomes unstable, the agreement to not practice is made public.

James B. Stewart highlights the need for public protection and national reporting of incompetent or unethical practitioners in the book *Blind Eye*.[3] Michael Swango was, at first glance, a typical medical student at Southern University Medical School. He was academically advanced and thought to be very bright. However, in his third year of medical school his peers noted peculiar behaviors. He was given the name "Double-O Swango", a parody of James Bond's 007 license to kill. It was noted that patients Swango cared for tended to die. In spite of episodes of unprofessional conduct and not graduating with his medical school class secondary to unethical behaviors, concerns of legal repercussions nevertheless led the way to Swango being given his medical degree.

He was accepted into a neurosurgery residency program at Ohio State University. He completed his first year internship, but during that internship professors, peers, and others expressed grave concerns regarding Swango's behavior. A series of mysterious deaths occurred shortly after nurses reported Swango leaving those patient rooms. It was also alleged that he also attempted to poison fellow residents. Swango was eventually released from his residency program at the university. Nothing, however, was reported to the Ohio Medical Board.

Swango moved back to Quincy, Illinois, and worked as a paramedic. Eventually he was arrested and convicted of poisoning fellow paramedics. His medical licenses in Illinois and Ohio were suspended. He served 2 years of a 5-year term and was released from prison in 1987. On January 18, 1990, Swango went to Virginia and legally changed his name to David Jackson Adams.

During the early 1980s, there was no national clearinghouse for doctors whose licenses were suspended. In spite of the fact that the Federation of State Medical Boards and the American Medical Association did keep lists of doctors who had their licenses suspended, Swango never appeared on their lists. During this same period there was no method for reporting felony convictions involving physicians or PAs. Eventually the National Practitioner Data Bank (NPDB) was created by federal law and went into effect in 1990.

Swango applied for an internal medicine residency program in South Dakota and was accepted into the program. Eventually the program found out about his past and dismissed him. He applied for and was accepted into a psychiatric residency at State University of New York–Stony Brook. A series of unexplained patient deaths occurred at a New York Veterans Administration (VA) hospital. Stony Brook found out about Swango's past and suspended him. Then Swango left the United States and went to Zimbabwe, Africa, to practice as a physician. A series of unexplained deaths led to an investigation. U.S. authorities arrested Swango and eventually he pled guilty to deliberately killing three men in the New York VA hospital and a young woman at Ohio State. It is believed that he may have killed as many as 60 people throughout his career in the United States and Africa.

The case of Michael Swango shows what can happen without a system in place to report illegal practices of health-care practitioners. The creation of the NPDB in 1990 was a step in the right direction. Although the public has no access to its information, it does act as a clearinghouse of important information. NPDB improves the quality of health care by encouraging state licensing boards, hospitals, other health-care entities, and professional societies to identify and discipline those who engage in unprofessional behavior. Further, it restricts the ability of incompetent health-care practitioners to move from state to state without disclosure or discovery of previous medical malpractice payment and adverse action history. Adverse actions involving licensure, clinical privileges, professional society membership, and exclusions from Medicare and Medicaid must be reported.

Similarly, the Healthcare Integrity and Protection Data Bank (HIPDB) was created by U.S. Department of Health and Human Services as a result of the Health Insurance Portability and Accountability Act of 1996 to combat fraud and abuse in health insurance and health-care delivery. Health-care fraud has an enormous financial impact on the quality of health care. Such fraud was estimated in 1997 to have cost between \$30 billion and \$100 billion.[4] The HIPDB augments NPDB reporting and other traditional forms of review and investigation. It provides government agencies and health plans a system of warning regarding fraudulent practices of practitioners or providers.

Content of a PA Law

PA laws and the agencies that regulate them are different in every state (see appendix to this chapter). When a law is made, it represents the voice of the state legislature as to how to best protect the public from unscrupulous or unprofessional practice. Generally, a statute is passed and signed into law. It is impossible to create a law that can be very specific. As such, statutes are a rather "broad brush stroke." They are kept general, recognizing that technology and practice patterns change so that frequent changes do not have to be made. Some states provide for the formulation of rules or administrative codes that better define the interpretation of general statutes or provide substantive policy statements that explain how an agency might proceed in a given situation.

Statutes start with definitions. Whereas this may seem unnecessary, it is quite relevant from a legal standpoint. Consider the Arizona PA Law for the definition of a supervising physician. "'Supervising physician'" means a physician who holds a current unrestricted license, provides a notification of supervision, assumes legal responsibility for the health care tasks performed by the physician assistant and is approved by the board. For purposes of this paragraph, a limited license issued pursuant to section 32-1426, subsection C, before November 2, 1998 is not a restriction."[5]

Based on this definition, one might wonder if a doctor of dental surgery, a chiropractor, a naturopathic physician, or a podiatrist could supervise a PA? However, a "physician" is further defined: "a physician licensed pursuant to chapter 13 or 17 of this title."[6] Chapter 13 and 17 are specific to the allopathic and osteopathic practice of medicine. Therefore, in Arizona, only an MD or DO can legally supervise a PA. Another portion of the definition of a supervising physician addresses a limited license pursuant to section 32-1426, subsection C. Currently, a physician who has any restriction or limitation on his or her license is not eligible to supervise a PA. At one time, there was a large group practice of physicians who were being recruited to move to Arizona; they were given an exemption by the legislature from one of the peculiarities of the licensure requirements. This particular group practice employed many PAs, and without the exemption the physicians would not have been able to supervise PAs.

Other elements of a law may include information such as the structure of the organization, how members are compensated, the powers and duties of the board or subcommittees, how public information is disseminated, qualifications for licensure, withdrawal of applications, renewals of licensure, temporary licensure, cancellation of license, fees for licensure, requirements for change of address, scope of practice, restrictions on practice, prescribing, administering and dispensing drugs, supervising physician responsibilities, employment of PAs, the legal grounds for regulation and discipline, subpoena authority, right to counsel, right to judicial review, injunctions and disciplinary reciprocity.

It is important to pay attention to the definitions of unprofessional conduct. Consider the Arizona PA law and its definitions of unprofessional conduct[7]

21. "Unprofessional conduct" includes the following acts by a physician assistant that occur in this state or elsewhere:

(a) Violation of any federal or state law or rule that applies to the performance of health care tasks as a physician assistant. Conviction in any court of competent jurisdiction is conclusive evidence of a violation.

(b) Claiming to be a physician or knowingly permitting another person to represent that person as a physician.

(c) Performing health care tasks that have not been delegated by the supervising physician.

(d) Habitual intemperance in the use of alcohol or habitual substance abuse.

(e) Signing a blank, undated or predated prescription form.

(f) Gross malpractice, repeated malpractice or any malpractice resulting in the death of a patient.

(g) Representing that a manifestly incurable disease or infirmity can be permanently cured or that a disease, ailment or infirmity can be cured by a secret method, procedure, treatment, medicine or device, if this is not true.

(h) Refusing to divulge to the board on demand the means, method, procedure, modality of treatment or medicine used in the treatment of a disease, injury, ailment or infirmity.

(i) Prescribing or dispensing controlled substances or prescription-only drugs for which the physician assistant is not approved or in excess of the amount authorized pursuant to this chapter.

(j) Any conduct or practice that is or might be harmful or dangerous to the health of a patient or the public.

(k) Violation of a formal order, probation or stipulation issued by the board.

(l) Failing to clearly disclose the person's identity as a physician assistant in the course of the physician assistant's employment.

(m) Failing to use and affix the initials "P.A." or "P.A.-C." after the physician assistant's name or signature on charts, prescriptions or professional correspondence.

(n) Procuring or attempting to procure a physician assistant license by fraud, misrepresentation or knowingly taking advantage of the mistake of another.

(o) Having professional connection with or lending the physician assistant's name to an illegal practitioner of any of the healing arts.

(p) Failing or refusing to maintain adequate records on a patient.

(q) Using controlled substances that have not been prescribed by a physician, physician assistant, dentist or nurse practitioner for use during a prescribed course of treatment.

(r) Prescribing or dispensing controlled substances to members of the physician assistant's immediate family.

(s) Prescribing, dispensing or administering any controlled substance or prescription-only drug for other than accepted therapeutic purposes.

(t) Knowingly making any written or oral false or fraudulent statement in connection with the performance of health care tasks or when applying for privileges or renewing an application for privileges at a health care institution.

(u) Committing of a felony, whether or not involving moral turpitude, or a misdemeanor involving moral turpitude. In either case, conviction by a court of competent jurisdiction or a plea of no contest is conclusive evidence of the commission.

(v) Having a certification or license refused, revoked, suspended, limited or restricted by any other licensing jurisdiction for the inability to safely and skillfully perform health care tasks or for unprofessional conduct as defined by that jurisdiction that directly or indirectly corresponds to any act of unprofessional conduct as prescribed by this paragraph.

(w) Having sanctions including restriction, suspension or removal from practice imposed by an agency of the federal government.

(x) Violating or attempting to violate, directly or indirectly, or assisting in or abetting the violation of or conspiring to violate a provision of this chapter.

(y) Using the term "doctor" or the abbreviation "Dr." on a name tag or in a way that leads the public to believe that the physician assistant is licensed to practice as an allopathic or an osteopathic physician in this state.

(z) Failing to furnish legally requested information to the board or its investigator in a timely manner.

(aa) Failing to allow properly authorized board personnel to examine on demand documents, reports and records of any kind relating to the physician assistant's performance of health care tasks.

(bb) Knowingly making a false or misleading statement on a form required by the board or in written correspondence or attachments furnished to the board.

(cc) Failing to submit to a body fluid examination and other examinations known to detect the presence of alcohol or other drugs pursuant to an agreement with the board or an order of the board.

(dd) Violating a formal order, probation agreement or stipulation issued or entered into by the board or its executive director.

(ee) Except as otherwise required by law, intentionally betraying a professional secret or intentionally violating a privileged communication.

(ff) Allowing the use of the licensee's name in any way to enhance or permit the continuance of the activities of, or maintaining a professional connection with, an illegal practitioner of medicine or the performance of health care tasks by a person who is not licensed pursuant to this chapter.

(gg) False, fraudulent, deceptive or misleading advertising by a physician assistant or the physician assistant's staff or representative.

(hh) Knowingly failing to disclose to a patient on a form that is prescribed by the board and that is dated and signed by the patient or guardian acknowledging that the patient or guardian has read and understands that the licensee has a direct financial interest in a separate diagnostic or treatment agency or in nonroutine goods or services that the patient is being prescribed and if the prescribed treatment, goods or services are available on a competitive basis. This subdivision does not apply to a referral by one physician assistant to another physician

assistant or to a doctor of medicine or a doctor of osteopathy within a group working together.

(ii) Using chelation therapy in the treatment of arteriosclerosis or as any other form of therapy.

(jj) Prescribing, dispensing or administering anabolic or androgenic steroids for other than therapeutic purposes.

(kk) Prescribing, dispensing or furnishing a prescription medication or a prescription-only device as defined in section 32-1901 to a person unless the licensee first conducts a physical examination of that person or has previously established a professional relationship with the person. This subdivision does not apply to:

(i) A physician assistant who provides temporary patient care on behalf of the patient's regular treating licensed health care professional.

(ii) Emergency medical situations as defined in section 41-1831.

(iii) Prescriptions written to prepare a patient for a medical examination.

(ll) Engaging in sexual conduct with a current patient or with a former patient within six months after the last medical consultation unless the patient was the licensee's spouse at the time of the contact or, immediately preceding the professional relationship, was in a dating or engagement relationship with the licensee. For the purposes of this subdivision, "sexual conduct" includes:

(i) Engaging in or soliciting relationships, whether consensual or nonconsensual.

(ii) Making sexual advances, requesting sexual favors or engaging in other verbal conduct or physical contact of a sexual nature with a patient.

(iii) Intentionally viewing a completely or partially disrobed patient in the course of treatment if the viewing is not related to patient diagnosis or treatment under current practice standards.

(mm) Performing health care tasks under a false or assumed name in this state.

To this list of definitions of unprofessional conduct the following requirements and restrictions of the scope of practice[8] and requirements of prescribing, administering and dispensing drugs may be added[9]

32-2531. Health care tasks; scope of practice; restrictions; civil penalty

A. After a supervising physician receives board approval of a notice of supervision, that physician may delegate health care tasks to the physician assistant. The physician assistant may perform these tasks in any setting authorized by the approved supervising physician and the board, pursuant to subsections E and F of this section, including clinics, hospitals, ambulatory surgical centers, patient homes, nursing homes and other health care institutions. These tasks may include:

1. Obtaining patient histories.
2. Performing physical examinations.
3. Ordering and performing diagnostic and therapeutic procedures.
4. Formulating a diagnostic impression.
5. Developing and implementing a treatment plan.
6. Monitoring the effectiveness of therapeutic interventions.
7. Assisting in surgery.
8. Offering counseling and education to meet patient needs.
9. Making appropriate referrals.
10. Prescribing schedule IV or V controlled substances as defined in the federal controlled substances act of 1970 (P.L. 91-513; 84 Stat. 1242; 21 United States code section 802) and prescription-only medications.
11. Prescribing schedule II and III controlled substances as defined in the federal controlled substances act of 1970.
12. Performing minor surgery as defined in section 32-2501.
13. Performing other nonsurgical health care tasks that are normally taught in courses of training approved by the board, that are consistent with the training and experience of the physician assistant and that have been properly delegated by the approved supervising physician.

B. The approved supervising physician shall:

1. Meet the requirements established by the board for supervising a physician assistant and receive written board notification of this compliance.
2. Accept responsibility for all tasks and duties the physician delegates to a physician assistant.
3. Notify the board and the physician assistant in writing if the physician assistant exceeds the scope of the delegated health care tasks.
4. Notify the board if the physician has delegated authority to the physician assistant to prescribe medication. The physician shall also notify the board if the physician makes any changes to this authority.

C. Supervision does not require the personal presence of the physician at the place where health care tasks are performed. The board by order may require the personal presence of a physician when designated health care tasks are performed.

D. A physician assistant shall meet in person with the supervising physician at least once each week to discuss patient management. If the supervising physician is unavailable due to vacation, illness or continuing education programs, a physician assistant may meet with the supervising physician's agent. If the supervising physician is unavailable for any other reason, the fulfillment of this responsibility by the supervising physician's agent is subject to board approval.

E. A physician assistant shall not perform health care tasks in a place which is geographically separated from the supervising physician's primary place for meeting patients without the authorization of the supervising physician and the board.

F. The board may approve the performance of health care tasks by a physician assistant in a place which is geographically separated from the supervising physician's primary place for meeting patients if:

1. Adequate provision for immediate communication between the supervising physician or supervising physician's agent and the physician assistant exists.
2. The physician assistant's performance of health care tasks is adequately supervised and reviewed.
3. A printed announcement which contains the names of the physician assistant and supervising physician and states that the facility employs a physician assistant who is performing health care tasks under the supervision of a licensed physician is posted in the waiting room of the geographically separated site.

G. At all times while a physician assistant is on duty, he shall wear a name tag with the designation "physician assistant" on it.

H. The board by rule may prescribe a civil penalty for a violation of this article relating to charting, wearing tags, identifying prescriptions and posting signs in geographically separated locations. The penalty shall not exceed fifty dollars for each violation. The board shall deposit, pursuant to sections 35-146 and 35-147, all monies it receives from this penalty in the state general fund. A physician assistant and the supervising physician may contest the imposition of this penalty pursuant to board rule. The imposition of a civil penalty is public information, and the board may use this information in any future disciplinary actions.

32-2532. Prescribing, administering and dispensing drugs; limits and requirements; notice

A. Except as provided in subsection F of this section, a physician assistant shall not prescribe, dispense or administer:
  1. A schedule II or schedule III controlled substance as defined in the federal controlled substances act of 1970 (P.L. 91-513; 84 Stat. 1242; 21 United States Code section 802) without delegation by the supervising physician, board approval and drug enforcement administration registration.
  2. A schedule IV or schedule V controlled substance as defined in the federal controlled substances act of 1970 without Drug Enforcement Administration registration and delegation by the supervising physician.
  3. Prescription-only medication without delegation by the supervising physician.
B. All prescription orders issued by a physician assistant shall contain the name, address and telephone number of the supervising physician. A physician assistant shall issue prescription orders for controlled substances under the physician assistant's own Drug Enforcement Administration registration number.
C. Unless certified for fourteen day prescription privileges pursuant to section 32-2504, subsection A, a physician assistant shall not prescribe a schedule II or III controlled substance for a period exceeding seventy-two hours. For each schedule IV or schedule V controlled substance, a physician assistant may not prescribe the controlled substance more than five times in a six month period for each patient.
D. A prescription for a schedule II or III controlled substance is not refillable without the written consent of the supervising physician.
E. Prescription-only drugs shall not be dispensed, prescribed or refillable for a period exceeding one year.
F. Except in an emergency, a physician assistant may dispense schedule II or schedule III controlled substances for a period of use of not to exceed seventy-two hours with board approval or any other controlled substance for a period of use of not to exceed thirty-four days and may administer controlled substances without board approval if it is medically indicated in an emergency dealing with potential loss of life or limb or major acute traumatic pain.
G. Except for samples provided by manufacturers, all drugs dispensed by a physician assistant shall be:
  1. Prepackaged in a unit-of-use package by the supervising physician or a pharmacist acting on a written order of the supervising physician.
  2. Labeled to show the name of the supervising physician and physician assistant.
H. A physician assistant shall not obtain a drug from any source other than the supervising physician or a pharmacist acting on a written order of the supervising physician. A physician assistant may receive manufacturers' samples if allowed to do so by the supervising physician.
I. If a physician assistant is approved by the board to prescribe, administer or dispense schedule II and schedule III controlled substances, the physician assistant shall maintain an up-to-date and complete log of all schedule II and schedule III controlled substances he administers or dispenses.
J. The board shall advise the state board of pharmacy and the United States Drug Enforcement Administration of all physician assistants who are authorized to prescribe or dispense drugs and any modification of their authority.
K. The state board of pharmacy shall notify all pharmacies at least quarterly of physician assistants who are authorized to prescribe or dispense drugs.

What has been listed here is only a small portion of the actual statute and rules that pertain to PA practice in Arizona. Other state statutes are equally complex, but they are definitely something that one must understand.

There are also other portions of law that are applicable to PA practice. For instance, some states require certain practitioners to report when they have settled a malpractice case. Other issues, such as confidentiality of medical records, release of medical records, and retention of medical records, are often in other administrative statutes, separate from the medical or PA practice acts, because the law is applicable to a host of health care professionals. The criminal code also has elements that one needs to know, such as restrictions on controlled substances and the duty to report nonaccidental injuries and treatment of wounds.

Finally, as it relates to the understanding of PA law(s) and an application for licensure, an applicant should make sure that both the applicant and the supervising physician know the rules that regulate PA practice. Once the applicant is licensed, when an issue arises, the supervising physician should not be unaware of their responsibilities under the law.

What to Do When a Complaint Is Filed

Receiving a call from the board that an investigation is being undertaken is unsettling for both the PA and the supervising physician. It is important to develop a plan of response. Most boards are required by law to investigate each complaint they receive. The opening of an investigation does not mean that the PA is automatically guilty of unprofessional conduct. However, the PA must take an inquiry very seriously.

The PA should first notify the supervising physician. (Note that some malpractice carriers pay for legal assistance if a complaint is filed against an insured.) Most letters or subpoenas request that the PA provide pertinent medical records and a response to the allegations that have been made. Particular attention should be paid to the time frames relevant to the reply. The patient's chart should be reviewed immediately. Under no circumstances should anything in the chart be changed or removed. The writing of the response to the letter of inquiry should be taken very seriously. One should not be defensive and stay factual. Others can review the response to ensure that the points are clearly understood. It is important to provide all evidence that supports the licensee's position. The boards receive many complaints that are unjustified, and a concise explanation may often be all that is necessary for the board to make a determination to close the inquiry.

In some cases, the response may also indicate that additional information is necessary in the form of an investigational interview. At this point, one may wish to consider getting legal advice. Administrative law is much different than tort or criminal law. The attorney chosen to represent a PA should have experience representing clients regularly before a medical or PA board. Malpractice carriers and local or state medical societies can provide names of qualified attorneys. Attorneys who have never appeared before a medical or PA board may apply tactics that may work in the criminal arena but fail in the administrative arena. The attorney needs to be very familiar with the PA statutes.

Investigational interviews are fact-finding missions by the board's investigator. If the PA has retained counsel, the attorney should attend. The PA should be well aware of the allegations.

The board will have seen the allegations against the PA and the investigation report. Often, the PA will not have an opportunity to see the investigative report because it contains confidential information not subject to the PA's review. During the hearing the PA may have an opportunity to make an opening statement to the board, or the board members may just begin asking questions. It is important to be well prepared. It is helpful to have notes and records accessible and organized so they are easy to find. During the interview, questions should be answered specifically, and caution should be taken to avoid over-answering or rambling. Because the board members have seen the information in advance, observers may believe the board members have already decided. An administrative hearing is not the same as an evidentiary hearing. Different rules apply to the administrative hearing and the setting is much different. It is extremely valuable for every PA to attend a board meeting to understand what occurs.

If a PA made a mistake and there is no question about it, it is helpful to admit the mistake. For instance, if a PA gives penicillin to a patient who is allergic to penicillin, there is no point trying to make it appear that the event did not occur. Certainly, if there are mitigating circumstances, such as the chart not being available with the reminder that the patient was allergic, it is important to bring those points up because they are relevant. If an honest mistake was made, it is helpful to discuss what has been done in practice to avoid making the same mistake again. This level of honesty can often be the difference between a nondisciplinary action (an advisory letter) versus a disciplinary action such as a letter of reprimand or worse.

If a case is complex, the case may be referred to a formal hearing, which is a full evidentiary hearing. In Arizona, for instance, the case is heard before an administrative law judge, and the PA can subpoena and cross-examine witnesses. The administrative law judge hears the case and then makes recommended findings of facts, conclusions of law, and a recommendation for punishment, if applicable. The case is then referred back to the PA board to review the evidence that has been collected during the hearing and to vote on the recommendations of the administrative law judge.

References

1. ARS 32-2521(B)3(a).
2. Papadakis MA. Unprofessional behavior in medical school is associated with subsequent disciplinary action by a state medical board. Journal of Medical Licensure and Discipline 2004;90:16-23.
3. Stewart J. Blind Eye. New York: Simon & Schuster; 1997.
4. National Practitioner Data Bank/Healthcare Integrity and Protection Data Bank. Accessed December 4, 2004, at npdb-hipdb.com/hipdb.html
5. Title 32, Professions and Occupations, Chapter 25 Physician Assistants ARS 32-2501.
6. Title 32, Professions and Occupations, Chapter 25 Physician Assistants ARS 32-2501(13).

7. ARS 32-2501(21).

8. ARS 32-2531.

9. ARS 32-2532.

10. Summary of AAPA State Regulation of Physician Assistant Practice. Accessed December 7, 2004, at aapa.org/gandp/statelaw.html

APPENDIX

Summary of State Regulation of PA Practice[10]

ALABAMA

Qualifications: Graduation from accredited PA program and NCCPA examination.

Application: By PA for license. PA must be registered to licensed physician prior to practice. Job description must be filed with the board.

Scope of practice: Taking histories, performing physical exams, ordering and/or performing diagnostic and therapeutic procedures, formulating a working diagnosis, developing and implementing a treatment plan, monitoring the effectiveness of therapeutic interventions, assisting at surgery, offering counseling and education, making referrals. PA may not perform any medical service, procedure, function or activity which is not approved by the board.

Prescribing/dispensing: PAs may prescribe non-controlled drugs from board-approved formulary.

Supervision: Oversight and direction but not direct, on-site physician supervision.

Participation in regulation: Four PAs serve on an eight-member Physician Assistant Advisory Committee.

Alabama State Board of Medical Examiners, P.O. Box 946, Montgomery, AL 36101-0946; (334) 242-4116.

www.albme.org

ALASKA

Qualifications: Graduation from accredited PA program and current NCCPA certificate.

Application: By physician and PA; includes plan of collaboration.

Scope of practice: Medical diagnosis and treatment within the scope of practice of the collaborating physician.

Prescribing/dispensing: Prescriptive authority for non-controlled drugs and Schedules III to V drugs (controlled substances). Prescription written and signed by PA must include collaborating physician's name and Drug Enforcement Administration (DEA) number and PA's name and DEA number. PA may order, administer and dispense Schedule II drugs with the approval of the collaborating physician.

Supervision: Periodic assessment by physician and at least monthly telephone or radio review of patient care and records. PAs in remote locations (30 or more road miles from physician's primary office) with less than two years of experience must first work 40 to 160 hours under physician's direct and immediate supervision and periodic assessment must include at least one direct personal contact visit from supervising physician per quarter for at least four hours.

Participation in regulation: One PA serves on medical board.

Alaska Division of Occupational Licensing, 550 West 7th Ave., Suite 1500, Anchorage, AK 99501. www.dced.state.ak.us/occ/pmed.htm

ARIZONA

Qualifications: Graduation from accredited PA program and NCCPA examination within preceding six years.

Application: PA applies for license. Interview, physical examination, mental evaluation, and oral competency examination may be required. PA and supervising physician must submit notification of supervision.

Scope of practice: Histories and physicals; diagnostic and therapeutic procedures; treatment plans; assisting in surgery; patient education and counseling; referrals; minor surgery (not including surgical abortion) and other non-surgical tasks as approved by the board.

Prescribing/dispensing: PA may prescribe non-controlled and controlled drugs. Schedules II and III limited to 72-hour supply or an NCCPA-certified PA or a PA with 45 hours of pharmacology in the preceding three years may prescribe a Schedule II or III for up to 14 days. Schedules IV and V drugs may not be prescribed more than five times in a six-month period for an individual patient. No refills of Schedules II and III drugs. DEA registration required. Except for samples, dispensed drugs must be prepackaged by physician or pharmacist.

Supervision: Physician need not be present on site; weekly meeting required. Board approval needed for PA utilization in separate location.

Participation in regulation: Four PAs serve on ten-member PA regulatory board.

Arizona Regulatory Board of Physician Assistants, 9545 E. Doubletree Ranch Rd., Scottsdale, AZ 85258, (480)551-2700.

www.azpaboard.org

ARKANSAS

Qualifications: Graduation from accredited PA program and NCCPA examination. After July 1, 1999, bachelor's degree required unless PA served as corpsman or was working in an Arkansas federal facility as a PA prior to July 1, 1999 and meets all other qualifications for licensure. PA students enrolled in accredited programs prior to July 1, 1999, not required to have bachelor's degree.

Application: PA applies for license. Physician notifies board of intent to supervise.

Scope of Practice: Duties and responsibilities assigned by supervising physician.

Prescribing/dispensing: PA may prescribe non-controlled and Schedule III-V controlled medications as delegated by supervising physician. PAs authorized to prescribe controlled medications must register with the DEA. All PA prescriptions and orders must identify the supervising physician.

Supervision: Constant physical presence of supervising physician not required as long as PA and supervising physician can be in contact via telecommunication. Supervising physician must be able to reach location where PA is seeing patients within one hour.

Participation in Regulation: Two PAs serve on six-member advisory committee.

Arkansas State Medical Board, 2100 Riverfront Drive, Suite 200, Little Rock, AR 72202-1793; (501)296-1802.
www.armedicalboard.org

CALIFORNIA

Qualifications: Graduation from accredited PA program and NCCPA examination.

Application: By PA for license.

Scope of practice: Medical services delegated in writing, within supervising physician's customary practice and within PA's competence. PA may take histories; perform physical examinations; perform or assist with laboratory, screening, and therapeutic procedures; counsel patients; and assist physician in institutional settings.

Prescribing/dispensing: PA may transmit orally or in writing on patient record or in a drug order an order to a person who may lawfully furnish the medication. Authority limited by delegation from supervising physician. Physician must adopt a practice-specific formulary. "Drug order" means an order for medication which is dispensed to or for a patient issued and signed by a PA and is treated in the same manner as a prescription or order of the supervising physician. PA signing the drug order is deemed a prescriber. Schedule II-V medications administered, provided or for which a drug order is issued require a patient-specific order from a supervising physician. Drug orders for controlled medications require PA's DEA registration number. Medical record of patient receiving prescription medication must be countersigned by a supervising physician within seven days. PA may hand to a patient a properly labeled drug prepackaged by pharmacist, physician, or manufacturer.

Supervision: Physician must be available in person or by electronic communication at all times PA is caring for patients. Written guidelines for supervision must include one or more of the following: same-day examination of patient by physician; countersignature of all medical records within 30 days; protocols for some or all tasks. Supervising physician must review, countersign, and date at least 10% of medical records within 30 days for patients treated by PA for PAs working under protocols.

Participation in regulation: Four PAs serve on nine-member PA regulatory body.

California Physician Assistant Committee, Medical Board of California, 1424 Howe Ave., #35, Sacramento, CA 95825; (916)263-2670.
www.physicianassistant.ca.gov

COLORADO

Qualifications: Graduation from accredited PA program (or equivalent) and NCCPA examination.

Application: By PA for licensure; supervising physician must register with the board.

Scope of practice: PA may perform acts that constitute the practice of medicine, as delegated by the supervising physician. (After July 1, 1990, state-certified Child Health Associates are eligible for licensure as PAs, but practice is restricted to patients under the age of 21 years.)

Prescribing/dispensing: PA may prescribe controlled (Schedules II-V) and non controlled substances. Each prescription must include the name of the supervising physician as well as the PA's name. All drugs dispensed by PAs must be unit doses prepackaged by pharmacist or physician. PA prescribing controlled substances must be registered with DEA.

Supervision: PA must practice with personal and responsible supervision of physician. In acute care hospital PA may practice without physical presence of physician if physician regularly practices in the hospital or if hospital is located in a health professional shortage area; physician must review medical records every two working days. In other settings, physician must be available via telecommunication. New graduate PAs require on-site presence of physician for first 1,000 working hours; for first six months of employment and a minimum of 500 patient encounters charts must be co-signed within seven days. Experienced PAs new to practice require chart review within 14 days for first three months of employment and minimum of 500 patient encounters. All other PAs required to meet with supervising physician at least twice during each 12-month period for performance assessment.

Colorado Board of Medical Examiners, 1560 Broadway St., Suite 1300, Denver, CO 80202; (303)894-7690.
www.dora.state.co.us/Medical

CONNECTICUT

Qualifications: Graduation from accredited PA program, current NCCPA certification, a bachelor's degree and documentation of 60 hours of pharmacology education.

Application: By PA for license; by physician for registration.

Scope of practice: Medical functions delegated by supervising physician in accordance with written protocols.

Prescribing/dispensing: PAs may prescribe non-controlled and Schedule IV and V medications as delegated by supervising physician; dispense drugs in outpatient or non-profit clinics. May order Schedule II and III drugs for inpatients and prescribe Schedule II and III medications for patients in hospitals, emergency departments that are hospital satellites, and after admission evaluation by a physician in long-term care facilities. PAs may renew prescriptions for controlled medications (Schedules II-V) in outpatient settings. Orders for Schedule II and III drugs require supervising physician co-signature within 24 hours.

Supervision: Includes but is not limited to the continuous availability of direct communication between PA and physician either in person or by radio, telephone, or telecommunication; at least weekly personal review of PA's practice; regular chart review; existence of predetermined plan for emergency situations; and designation of an alternate physician in absence of supervisor.

Participation in regulation: One PA serves on medical examining board.

Connecticut Division of Medical Quality Assurance, Dept. of Public Health – PA Licensing, 410 Capitol Ave., MS#12APP, P.O. Box 340308, Hartford, CT 06134-0308; (860)509-7603. www.ct-clic.com/detail.asp?code=1761

DELAWARE

Qualifications: Graduation from accredited PA program and NCCPA examination.

Application: By PA for license.

Scope of practice: Medical acts delegated by supervising physician. PA may take histories, perform physicals, record progress notes in outpatient setting, and relay, transcribe, or execute diagnostic and therapeutic orders. Orders must be countersigned within 24 hours.

Prescribing/Dispensing: PA may prescribe up to a six-month supply of non-controlled drugs and up to a three-month supply of controlled Schedule II-V drugs. PA must have both a state-controlled substance number and a DEA number to prescribe controlled drugs.

Supervision: Physician need not be present as long as is readily accessible by electronic communication and can be present within 30 minutes if necessary. Patients seen by PA receiving controlled drugs should be seen by physician every three months; patients receiving other prescriptions should be seen by physician every six months.

Participation in regulation: Four PAs serve on seven-member PA regulatory council.

Delaware Board of Medical Practice, Cannon Bldg., Suite 203, 861 Silver Lake Blvd., Dover, DE 19904-2467; (302)744-4500 www.state.de.us/license/28

DISTRICT OF COLUMBIA

Qualifications: Graduation from accredited PA program and NCCPA examination.

Application: PA applies for license; job description registration and approval handled separately.

Scope of practice: Acts of medical diagnosis and treatment, prescription, preventive health care, and other functions authorized by the board.

Prescribing/dispensing: PA may prescribe non-controlled substances.

Supervision: Physician must be within 15-mile radius of the city and available in person or by communication device; need not be physically present on premises. Physician must countersign all medical orders and progress notes within 48 hours.

Participation in regulation: One PA serves on three-member PA advisory committee.

District of Columbia Board of Medicine, PA Adv. Comm; 825 North Capitol St. NE, 2nd Floor, Washington, DC 20002; (202)442-4768. www.dchealth.dc.gov

FLORIDA

Qualifications: Graduation from accredited PA program and NCCPA examination. (see NOTE below.)

Application: By PA for license; includes information about supervising physician.

Scope of practice: PA may perform delegated tasks and procedures for which he or she is skilled that are within supervising physician's scope of practice. Some duties may only be performed if the physician is on the premises, such as insertion of chest tubes and monitoring cardiac stress tests. Final diagnoses may not be delegated.

Prescribing/dispensing: Negative formulary exists in Florida. PAs may prescribe drugs not listed on the formulary established by Council on PAs and adopted by medical and osteopathic boards. Formulary must include controlled substances. Prior to prescribing, PA must complete a three-hour course in prescriptive practice, three months of clinical experience in the specialty area of the supervising physician, and 10 hours of CME in the specialty area of practice. The Board issues a prescriber number to the PA.

Supervision: Physical presence or easy availability (by telecommunications) of physician is required. During the initial six months of supervision, medical records must be reviewed and signed by the physician within seven days. After the initial six month period, charts must be cosigned within 30 days.

Participation in regulation: One PA serves on five-member PA Council.

Florida Board of Medical Examiners, 4052 Bald Cypress Way, Bin #C03, Tallahassee, FL 32399; (850) 245-4131.
www.doh.state.fl.us/Mqa/PhysAsst/pa_home.html

Florida Board of Osteopathic Medical Examiners, 4052 Bald Cypress Way, Bin #C06, Tallahassee, FL 32399-3256; (850) 245-4161.
www.doh.state.fl.us/Mqa/osteopath/os_home.html

NOTE: A change in the PA law, allowing certain unlicensed medical school graduates to become PAs in the state of Florida, was repealed in 1991 before it had an opportunity to go into effect. However, a limited number of unlicensed medical school graduates who had been residents of the state for a year and who applied by a certain deadline have been granted temporary certificates and must sit for a state certification examination. Passage of the exam makes these individuals PAs only in Florida.

GEORGIA

Qualifications: Graduation from accredited PA program and NCCPA examination. Personal interview may be required.

Application: By PA for license; by physician for approval to supervise (includes job description and description of locations where PA will practice).

Scope of practice: Delegated medical tasks contained in job description and approved by board.

Prescribing/dispensing: PAs may prescribe Schedules III-V and non-controlled drugs as delegated by physician. Dispensing authorized in public or nonprofit health facilities. PAs who are authorized to prescribe controlled medications must register with the DEA.

Supervision: Supervising physician must be readily available. Board approval required for utilization of PA in satellite clinic where there is a shortage of health care professionals.

Participation in regulation: Four PAs serve on eight-member PA advisory committee. Committee appoints PA to serve as nonvoting medical board member.

Georgia Composite State Board of Medical Examiners, 2 Peachtree St. NW, 36th Floor, Atlanta, GA 30303-3465; (404)656-3913.
www.ganet.org/meb/oa_physasst.html

HAWAII

Qualifications: Graduation from accredited PA program and NCCPA examination; current NCCPA certificate required for biennial renewal.

Application: By PA for license. Must include signed statement from supervising physician(s) who will direct and supervise PA.

Scope of practice: Medical services including histories and physicals, ordering, interpreting or performing diagnostic and therapeutic procedures, formulating a diagnosis, implementing a treatment plan, patient counseling, making referrals and assisting at surgery.

Prescribing/dispensing: PAs may describe Schedule III-V controlled drugs and all legend drugs as delegated by supervising physician. Dispensing activities must comply with federal and state regulations. PA prescribers of controlled medications must register with the DEA. Prescription must include both the PA's DEA number and the physician's DEA number. Medical record of the prescription must be initialed by the physician within seven working days. PAs employed or extended privileges by hospital or extended care facility may write orders for Schedules II-V medications as allowed by facility policy.

Supervision: Physical presence of physician or physician availability via telecommunication. Physician must review PA records within seven working days and must designate a supervising physician in his or her absence.

Participation in regulation: Five PAs serve on advisory committee.

Hawaii Board of Medical Examiners, Dept. of Commerce and Consumer Affairs Division of Professional Licensing, P.O. Box 3469, Honolulu, HI 96801; (808)586-3000.
www.state.hi.us/dcca/pvl/areas_medical.html

IDAHO

Qualifications: Graduation from accredited PA program, baccalaureate degree, and NCCPA examination.

Application: By PA for license. Delegation of Services agreement with supervising physician required for practice. Personal interview of PA, supervising physician, or both may be required.

Scope of practice: PA may take histories, do physical examinations, initiate and interpret laboratory and diagnostic tests, and perform other duties that are included in the supervising physician's scope of practice and are delineated in the Delegation of Services Agreement.

Prescribing/dispensing: PA may apply for approval to prescribe Schedules II-V and non-controlled medications. Application to prescribe must include documentation of all pharmacology course content completed (at least 30 hours). PAs who are authorized to prescribe controlled medications must register with the DEA and Idaho Board of Pharmacy. Dispensing limited to times when pharmacist is not available. PAs in family planning, communicable disease or chronic disease clinics under government contract or grant may also dispense medications.

Supervision: Supervising physician must conduct on-site visit at least monthly. Must be available by phone or in person; hold regularly scheduled conferences; review sampling of charts. Supervising physician must designate an alternate supervising physician in his or her temporary absence.

Participation in regulation: Two PAs serve on PA advisory committee.

Idaho State Board of Medicine, P.O. Box 83720, Boise, ID 83720-0058; (208)327-7000. www.bom.state.id.us

ILLINOIS

Qualifications: Completion of approved program, or verification from NCCPA that applicant has substantially equivalent training and experience. NCCPA examination; current NCCPA certificate required for renewal. No one holding medical degree eligible.

Application: By PA for license. Physician must file notice of supervision.

Scope of practice: Delegated medical duties within the supervising physician's scope of practice, consistent with the PA's education and experience.

Prescribing/dispensing: Physician may delegate prescriptive authority for non-controlled and Schedules III-V medications to PAs. Medication orders issued by PA must be periodically reviewed by supervising physician. Physician must file notice of delegation of prescriptive authority to PA with Department of Professional Regulation. Physician and PA must adopt written guidelines for prescribing. PAs who prescribe controlled medications must register with state-controlled substance authority and DEA.

Supervision: Physician need not be physically present at all times provided consultation available by radio, telephone, or telecommunications. Supervising physician may designate alternate supervising physician in accordance with statute. Physicians within a practice group of the supervising physician may supervise the PA with respect to their patients without being deemed an alternate supervising physician.

Participation in regulation: Three PAs serve on seven-member medical board advisory committee.

Illinois Department of Professional Regulation, 320 West Washington St., Springfield, IL 62786; (217)785-0800. www.ildpr.com/WHO/adjmed.asp

INDIANA

Qualifications: Graduation from accredited PA program and current NCCPA certificate.

Application: By PA for certification by the committee. Must include employment history, statement of supervision from supervising physician, and description of practice setting, including address of supervising physician.

Scope of practice: Medical tasks delegated by supervising physician.

Prescribing/dispensing: No provision.

Supervision: Must be continuous but does not require the physical presence of the physician. Physician shall review all patient encounters within 24 hours.

Participation in regulation: Three PAs serve on a five-member PA committee.

Indiana Health Professions Bureau, Attn: PA Committee, Medical Licensing Board, 402 West Washington St., Suite W066, Indianapolis, IN 46204; (317)234-2060. www.in.gov/hpb/boards/pac

IOWA

Qualifications: Graduation from accredited PA program (or equivalent education and training) and NCCPA examination.

Application: By PA for license. PA must supply information on supervising physician to PA board prior to beginning practice.

Scope of practice: Medical services that are within the supervising physician's scope of practice and for which the PA is qualified by training to perform that are delegated by the supervising physician.

Prescribing/dispensing: PA may prescribe non-controlled and controlled substances (except Schedule II stimulants and depressants). May dispense under certain conditions. PAs who prescribe controlled medications must register with the DEA.

Supervision: Physician need not be physically present, but must be readily available by telecommunication.

Participation in regulation: Three PAs serve on seven-member PA regulatory board.

Iowa Board of Physician Assistant Examiners, Bureau of Professional Licensure, Lucas State Office Building, 321 East 12th St., Des Moines, IA 50319-0075; (515)281-4401.

www.idph.state.ia.us/licensure/board_home.asp?board=pa

KANSAS

Qualifications: Graduation from an accredited PA program (or military experience that meets medical board requirements) and NCCPA examination.

Application: By PA for license, including designation of the responsible physician.

Scope of practice: Delegated acts constituting the practice of medicine and surgery that can be competently performed by the PA, based on his or her education, skill, and experience. Physician required to submit utilization plan.

Prescribing/dispensing: PAs may prescribe Schedule II-V and non-controlled medications as authorized in a written protocol with a supervising physician. PA prescribers of controlled medications must register with the DEA.

Supervision: Physician need not be physically present, but must be immediately available for consultation by telecommunication. Biweekly review of patient records and annual evaluation of PA performance and protocols required. PA may work in different practice location after completing at least 80 hours of on-site supervision with supervising physician, physician periodically sees patients at the same location, and a notice is posted.

Participation in regulation: Three PAs serve on a five member advisory council.

Kansas State Board of Healing Arts, 235 SW Topeka Blvd., Topeka, KS 66603-3068; (785)296-7413.

www.ksbha.org

KENTUCKY

Qualifications: Graduation from board-approved or accredited PA program and NCCPA examination; current NCCPA certificate required for biennial renewal.

Application: By PA for state certification, by physician for approval to supervise (includes job description).

Scope of practice: PA considered to practice medicine or osteopathy with physician supervision. PA may perform duties and responsibilities described in the initial application or supplemental application received by the board. PA may initiate evaluation and treatment in emergency situations without specific approval. PA may not practice in hospitals or other facilities without permissions of facility's governing body.

Prescribing/dispensing: PAs may prescribe non-controlled medications as delegated to do so by supervising physician.

Supervision: Physician need not be physically present provided there is reliable means of direct communication. All records of service must be cosigned by physician in a timely manner. Two years of experience and board approval required for PA to work in satellite setting.

Participation in regulation: Four PAs serve on nine-member PA advisory committee.

Kentucky State Board of Medical Licensure, 310 Whittington Parkway, Suite 1B, Louisville, KY 40222; (502)429-8046.

www.state.ky.us/agencies/kbml

LOUISIANA

Qualifications: Graduation from accredited PA program and current NCCPA certification.

Application: By PA for license; by physician for approval to supervise. Possible interview for initial license if discrepancies exist.

Scope of practice: Medical services within the PA's education, training and experience which are delegated by the supervising physician.

Prescribing/dispensing: PAs may prescribe Schedule III-V and non-controlled medications if delegated by supervising physician to do so and approved by the board. To be approved for prescribing PA must have a minimum of one year of clinical rotations during training and have practiced for a minimum of one year (PAs with less than a full year of clinical rotations may substitute two years of practice). In order to prescribe controlled medications, PA must register with state-controlled drug agency and DEA.

Supervision: Continuous but does not require the physical presence of supervisor at time and place services are rendered. All written entries by PAs shall be cosigned by physician within 24 hours for inpatients, acute care settings, and hospital EDs; 48 hours for nursing home patients and 72 hours in all other cases.

Participation in regulation: Three PAs serve on a five member PA advisory committee.

Louisiana State Board of Medical Examiners, PO Box 30250, New Orleans, LA 70190-0250; (504)568-6820.

www.lsbme.org

MAINE

Qualifications: Graduation from accredited PA program and/or passage of NCCPA exam. Osteopathic PAs: graduation or NCCPA exam plus 3 years' experience.

Application: By PA for license. Supervising physician must submit affidavit stating written plan of supervision is on file in practice setting.

Scope of practice: Delegated medical services within supervising physician's proficiency and scope of practice.

Prescribing/dispensing: PA may prescribe and dispense drugs and medical devices, including non-controlled and Schedules III-V controlled substances. PA and physician may request authorization to prescribe Schedule IIs under specific individual guidelines. Registration with DEA required. PAs supervised by osteopaths can prescribe non-controlled and Schedules III-V controlled drugs.

Supervision: Physician must be available by radio, telephone or telecommunication device. PA and physician establish supervision plan.

Participation in regulation: Two PAs serve on four-member PA advisory committee.

Maine Board of Licensure in Medicine, 137 State House Station, Two Bangor St., Augusta, ME 04333-0137; (207)287-3601.
www.docboard.org/me/me_home.htm

Board of Osteopathic Examiners, 142 State House Station, Two Bangor St., Augusta, ME 04333-0142; (207)287-2480.
www.docboard.org/me-osteo

MARYLAND

Qualifications: Graduation from accredited PA program and NCCPA examination. Applicant who graduates from PA program after Oct. 1, 2003, must have bachelor's degree or equivalent.

Application: By PA for certification; PA and physician apply for approval of delegation agreement.

Scope of Practice: Delegated medical acts within the physician's customary practice, within the PA's training and experience, and consistent with delegation agreement submitted to board.

Prescribing/dispensing: Physician may delegate prescriptive authority including Schedule II-V and non-controlled medications to PA. Must be consistent with delegation agreement. PAs prescribing controlled medications must register with the DEA and state-controlled substance agency. Prescribing PAs must have passed NCCPA exam within previous two years or have completed eight hours of Category I pharmacology CME within previous two years and have bachelor's degree or its equivalent or two years' work experience as a PA or have been previously approved by board to write medication orders.

Supervision: Physician oversight of patient services rendered by PA, including continuous availability to PA in person, through written instructions, or by electronic means.

Participation in regulation: PA serves on medical board.

Maryland Board of Physicians, 4201 Patterson Ave., Baltimore, MD 21215; (410)764-4777 or (800)492-6836.
www.bpqa.state.md.us

MASSACHUSETTS

Qualifications: Graduation from accredited PA program, baccalaureate degree, NCCPA exam.

Application: By PA to PA board for registration. Physician/PA application forms, with list of duties, sent to both boards.

Scope of practice: Medical services delegated by the supervising physician.

Prescribing/dispensing: PA may prescribe non-controlled drugs and controlled substances (Schedules II-V). Prescriptions or orders for Schedule IIs must be reviewed by the physician within 96 hours. PAs who prescribe controlled substances must register with the DEA.

Supervision: Physician need not be physically present when PA renders medical services; patient records must be reviewed in a timely manner.

Participation in regulation: Four PAs and one PA educator serve on the nine-member PA board.

Massachusetts Board of PA Registration, Division of Registration, 239 Causeway St., Ste. 500, Boston, MA 02114; (617)727-4499.
www.state.ma.us/reg/boards/ap/default.htm

MICHIGAN

Qualifications: Graduation from accredited PA program and NCCPA examination.

Application: By PA for license.

Scope of practice: Medical care services delegated by the supervising physician, within the physician's usual scope of practice, and approved by the board.

Prescribing/dispensing: PA may prescribe non-controlled and Schedule III-V medications as delegated by supervising physician. PA may prescribe seven-day supply of Schedule II drugs as discharge medications. Supervising physician's and PA's names must be indicated on prescription. PA prescribers of controlled medications must register with the DEA. PAs may request and distribute complimentary starter doses of medication.

Supervision: Physician must be continuously available for direct communication in person or by radio, telephone, or telecommunication and must regularly review PA performance and patient records, consult, and educate.

Participation in regulation: Five PAs serve on nine-member PA regulatory task force. Task force sends one PA to serve as member of medical board and one PA to serve on osteopathic board.

Michigan Task Force on Physician Assistants, Bureau of Health Professions, P.O. Box 30670, Lansing, MI 48909; (517)335-0918.
www.michigan.gov/mdch

MINNESOTA

Qualifications: Current NCCPA certification. Physician-PA agreement and practice setting description must be in place prior to beginning practice.

Application: By PA for registration; by PA and supervising physician for approval of their practice agreement.

Scope of practice: Delegated patient services within supervising physician's customary practice consistent with PA's training or experience. Specifically allowed are taking histories, doing physical examinations, data interpretation and evaluation to determine treatment, ordering or performing diagnostic and therapeutic procedures, patient counseling, and assisting physician in health care institutions and patient homes.

Prescribing/dispensing: NCCPA-certified PAs may prescribe controlled and non-controlled drugs. PAs authorized to prescribe controlled medications must register with DEA.

Supervision: Constant presence of supervising physician is not required so long as the PA and supervising physician can be in touch via telecommunication.

Participation in regulation: Three PAs serve on seven-member PA advisory council.

Minnesota Board of Medical Practice, 2829 University Ave. South East, Suite 500, Minneapolis, MN 55414-3246; (612)617-2130.
www.bmp.state.mn.us

MISSISSIPPI

Qualifications: Graduation from accredited PA program, current NCCPA certificate, and bachelor's degree until 12/31/04; master's degree in a science or health related field required as of 1/01/05.

Application: By PA for license. Board approval of protocol submitted by PA and supervising physician required prior to PA beginning practice. Interview required.

Scope of practice: Any delegated medical service within the PA's training and skills that forms a component of the physician's scope of practice and is provided with supervision. Board must approve protocol outlining delegated duties.

Prescribing/dispensing: PA may prescribe those non-controlled medications outlined in board-approved protocol.

Supervision: On-site presence of physician required for the first 120 days. Thereafter supervision must be continuous but does not require physical presence of supervising physician. Supervising physician must review and initial 10% of PA charts monthly.

Participation in regulation: Any board-appointed task force or committee must include at least one PA.

Mississippi State Board of Medical Licensure, 1867 Crane Ridge Drive, Suite 200B, Jackson, MS 39216; (601)987-3079.
www.msbml.state.ms.us

MISSOURI

Qualifications: Graduation from accredited PA program and current NCCPA certification. Person employed as PA for three years prior to August 28, 1989, who has passed NCCPA exam and has current certification also eligible.

Application: By PA for license, includes form signed by supervising physician. Personal appearance may be required.

Scope of practice: Histories and physicals; routine office laboratory and screening procedures; routine therapeutic procedures; counseling; assisting at surgery; writing orders; other delegated tasks.

Prescribing/dispensing: Physician assistants shall not prescribe nor dispense any drug, medicine, device or therapy independent of consultation with the supervising physician. PAs may prescribe non-controlled medications pursuant to supervision agreement with supervising physician. Prescriptions shall include name, address, and telephone number of PA and supervising physician. PAs may request, receive and sign for professional samples of non-controlled medications. Dispensing is limited to 72-hour starter dose supply of medication.

Supervision: PA must practice in same facility as supervising physician (certain facilities and clinics exempted). Physician must be immediately available for consultation, assistance and intervention.

Participation in regulation: Two PAs serve on a five-member Advisory Commission for Physician Assistants.

Missouri Board of Healing Arts, State Advisory Commission for Physician Assistants, P.O. Box 4, Jefferson City, MO 65102; (573)751-0098.
http://pr.mo.gov/physician assistants.asp

MONTANA

Qualifications: Graduation from accredited PA program and current NCCPA certificate.

Application: By PA for license; board approval of supervising physician and utilization plan required. Interview may be required.

Scope of practice: Duties delegated by the supervising physician that are within his or her scope of practice and the PA's training and experience.

Prescribing/dispensing: PA may prescribe and dispense drugs, including Schedule II-V controlled substances, as delegated by physician. Schedule II prescriptions may be up to a 34-day supply. PAs who prescribe controlled drugs must register with the DEA.

Supervision: Communication between PA and physician by telephone, radio, or in person as frequently as the board decides is necessary. If practicing in a remote site, PA and supervising physician must work together in direct contact for a minimum of two weeks before PA delivers services in remote site. Supervising physician must visit remote site every 30 days or other interval.

Participation in regulation: One PA sits on the Board of Medical Examiners; one non-voting PA acts as liaison to the Board of Medical Examiners.

Montana State Board of Medical Examiners, P.O. Box 200513, Helena, MT 59620-0513; (406)841-2300.
www.discoveringmontana.com/dli/bsd/license/bsd_boards/med_board/licenses/med/lic_pac.asp

NEBRASKA

Qualifications: Graduation from accredited PA program and NCCPA examination.

Application: By PA for state licensure; by physician for approval to supervise.

Scope of practice: Delegated medical services within the physician's training and within the specialty area(s) for which PA is trained or experienced.

Prescribing/dispensing: PA may prescribe medications as delegated to do so by supervising physician. Delegated authority may include legend drugs and Schedule II-V controlled medications. Schedule II controlled substances limited to prescriptions for pain; limited to 72-hour supply. PAs authorized to prescribe controlled medications must register with the DEA.

Supervision: Physician must be readily available for consultation; telecommunication shall be sufficient. Physician and PA must be together 20% of the time, less if physician shows good cause. Board approval required for PA utilization in secondary site; physician must visit secondary site at least one half-day each month and review 100% of charts.

Participation in regulation: Two PAs serve on five-member PA committee.

Nebraska Health Department, Board of Examiners in Medicine & Surgery. P.O. Box 94986, Lincoln, NE 68509; (402)471-2118.
www.hhs.state.ne.us/crl/msh.htm

NEVADA

Qualifications: Graduation from accredited PA program and current NCCPA certificate.

Application: By PA for license (PA must send in supervision form signed by physician prior to initiating practice).

Scope of practice: Medical services delegated by the supervising physician; within his or her specialty; within the PA's training, experience, and competence; and approved by the board.

Prescribing/dispensing: With board approval, PA may prescribe and dispense controlled and non-controlled drugs and devices as desired by the supervising physician. Registration with pharmacy board and pharmacy law exam required. PAs who prescribe controlled medications must register with the DEA.

Supervision: Supervising physician must be available at all times for consultation, which may be indirect (by telecommunication); physician shall regularly review and initial selected patient records. Board approval required for PA utilization in remote site. Supervising physician shall spend part of a day at least once a month at any location where PA provides medical services to act as consultant to PA and to monitor quality of care.

Participation in regulation: Three PAs serve on PA advisory committee.

Nevada State Board of Medical Examiners, P.O. Box 7238, Reno, NV 89510; (775)688-2559 or (888)890-8210.
www.state.nv.us/medical

Board of Osteopathic Medicine, 2860 E. Flamingo Rd., Suite D, Las Vegas, NV 89121-5270, (702)732-2147
www.osteo.state.nv.us

NEW HAMPSHIRE

Qualifications: Graduation from accredited PA program and current NCCPA certificate.

Application: By PA for license, must include information on supervising physician. Personal interview required.

Scope of practice: Any delegated medical service within the PA's skill and physician's scope of practice.

Prescribing/dispensing: PA may prescribe legend drugs and controlled substances (Schedules II-V); must pass pharmacy law exam. PAs who prescribe controlled medications must register with the DEA.

Supervision: Physician must be available for consultation at all times in person or via radio, telephone or telecommunication; provide regular ongoing evaluation of representative sample of charts. Alternate designated by supervising physician assumes responsibility for PA when supervising physician unavailable.

Participation in regulation: One PA serves on eight-member medical board. Two PAs serve on four-member PA advisory committee.

New Hampshire Board of Medicine, 2 Industrial Park Dr, Suite 8, Concord, NH 03301; (603)271-1203.
www.nh.gov/medicine/pai.html

NEW JERSEY

Qualifications: Graduation from accredited PA program and NCCPA exam.

Application: By PA for license; file notice of employment within 10 days of commencing employment.

Scope of practice: Delegated tasks such as histories and physicals, assisting at surgery, patient education, determining and implementing therapeutic plans.

Supervision: Constant availability through electronic communication; intermittent physical presence; regular review of records; 24-hour countersignature of inpatient medical orders; outpatient chart countersignature in seven days; 48 hours if chart has medication order or prescription.

Prescribing/dispensing: PA may prescribe non-controlled legend drugs as delegated by supervising physician.

Participation in regulation: Three PAs named to five-member PA advisory committee; one PA on medical board.

New Jersey Board of Medical Examiners, PO Box 183, Trenton, NJ 08625-0183; (609)826-7100. For license: PA Advisory Committee, PO Box 45035, Newark, NJ 07101; (973)504-6580.

www.state.nj.us/lps/ca/medical/bme.htm

NEW MEXICO

Qualifications: Graduation from accredited PA program; current NCCPA certificate; bachelor's degree or two years' work experience as certified PA. PAs supervised by osteopathic physicians (DOs): graduation and NCCPA certificate.

Application: By PA for license; by supervising physician for approval. Personal interview with board member or designee and attendance at orientation required. PAs supervised by DOs must attend board meeting when application is discussed.

Scope of practice: Medical services delegated by supervising physician, within PA's skills, and forming a usual component of physician's practice. Written utilization plan must be developed.

Prescribing/dispensing: PA may prescribe, administer, and distribute non-controlled medications and Schedules II-V under direction of supervising physician and within parameters of board-approved formulary and guidelines. PA prescribers of controlled medications must register with the DEA.

Supervision: Must be immediate communication between physician and PA; can be through telecommunication. Physician must review at least ten of the more complicated medical records each month. Physician must visit PA practicing in remote site at least once every two weeks and review at least ten of the more complicated medical records. Quality assurance program must be in place and reviewed at least quarterly.

Participation in regulation: One PA serves on medical board.

New Mexico Medical Board, 491 Old Santa Fe Trail, Lamy Bldg, 2nd Floor, Santa Fe, NM 87501; (505)827-5022 or (800)945-5845.

www.state.nm.us/nmbme

Board of Osteopathic Medical Examiners, 2550 Cerrillos Rd, Santa Fe, NM 87505; (505)476-4695.

www.rld.state.nm.us/b&c/osteo/index.htm

NEW YORK

Qualifications: Graduation from approved PA program and NCCPA examination.

Application: By PA for state registration.

Scope of practice: Medical acts and duties delegated by the supervising physician, within the physician's scope of practice and appropriate to the PA's education, training, and experience.

Prescribing/dispensing: PA may prescribe Schedule III-V and non-controlled medications. PA prescribers of controlled drugs must register with the DEA.

Supervision: Physician not required to be physically present at time and place where PA performs services. Inpatient medical orders must be cosigned within 24 hours.

Participation in regulation: At least two PAs appointed to medical examining board.

New York State Board for Medicine, Office of the Professions, State Education Bldg., 2nd Floor, Albany, NY 12234; (518)474-3817.

www.op.nysed.gov/rpa.htm

NORTH CAROLINA

Qualifications: Graduation from accredited PA program and NCCPA exam.

Application: By PA for license; physician submits statement of supervision.

Scope of practice: Medical acts and tasks delegated by supervising physician and within the PA's training.

Prescribing/dispensing: PA may prescribe non-controlled and controlled drugs in Schedules II-V (Schedules II and III limited to 30-day supply). Pharmacy Board approval required for compounding and dispensing drugs. PA prescribers of controlled medications must register with the DEA.

Supervision: Supervision continuous but physical presence of physician not required at all times. PA must meet with supervising physician monthly for first six months of employment and every six months thereafter to discuss clinical problems and quality improvement measures.

Participation in regulation: Physician extender (PA or NP) serves on medical board. PAs serve in the majority on a 15-member PA Advisory Committee.

North Carolina State Board of Medical Examiners, 1201 Front St., Suite 100, Raleigh, NC 27609-7533; (919)326-1100 or (800)253-9653. www.ncmedboard.org

NORTH DAKOTA

Qualifications: Current NCCPA certification.

Application: By PA for license; includes copy of contract.

Scope of practice: Patient services delegated by supervising physician and approved by board.

Prescribing/dispensing: PAs may prescribe non-controlled drugs and Schedules III-V controlled substances. PA may dispense prepackaged medications (schedules IV and V and non-controlled substances) prepared by pharmacist acting on physician's written order and labeled to show names of PA and physician. Dispensing must be authorized by and within pre-established guidelines of supervising physician. PA prescribers of controlled drugs must register with the DEA.

Supervision: Physician must be continuously available for contact personally or by telephone or radio.

North Dakota State Board of Medical Examiners, 418 E. Broadway, Suite 12, Bismarck, ND 58501; (701)328-6500. www.ndbomex.com

OHIO

Qualifications: Current NCCPA certificate needed for initial registration, change of employment, and renewal.

Application: By PA for certificate of registration (license); by physician for approval.

Scope of practice: Taking histories and performing physical examinations, assisting in surgery, and other tasks approved by the board, in a utilization plan.

Supervision: Physician not required to be physically present but must be available for consultation, and within 60 minutes travel time of PA's location. Medical orders must be cosigned within 24 hours.

Participation in regulation: Three PAs serve on seven-member PA policy committee.

Ohio State Medical Board, 77 S. High St., 17th Floor, Columbus, OH 43215-6127; (614)466-3934. http://med.ohio.gov/PAsubwebindex.htm

OKLAHOMA

Qualifications: Graduation from accredited PA program and passage of examination.

Application: By PA for license. Board must approve PA and physician (includes job description).

Scope of practice: Diagnostic and therapeutic procedures common to the physician's practice.

Prescribing/dispensing: PAs may prescribe non-controlled and Schedules III-V drugs on board-approved formulary. Schedules III-V drugs are limited to 10-day supply or 40 dosage units with one refill, whichever is smaller. PAs who prescribe controlled medications must register with the DEA and the Oklahoma Bureau of Narcotics and Dangerous Drugs.

Supervision: Physician not required to be physically present when, nor specifically consulted before, PA performs delegated task. Board approval required for PA utilization in remote site. In the remote setting, physician shall be present at least half a day each week.

Participation in regulation: Two PAs serve on seven-member PA committee.

Oklahoma State Board of Medical Licensure and Supervision, P.O. Box 18256, Oklahoma City, OK 73154-0256; (405)848-6841. www.osbmls.state.ok.us

OREGON

Qualifications: Graduation from accredited PA program and NCCPA examination.

Application: By PA and physician (includes job description). Interview may be required.

Scope of practice: Medical services delegated by the physician and included in the board-approved job description.

Prescribing/dispensing: PA may prescribe medications, including Schedules II-V controlled substances, as determined by physician and approved by board. PAs prescribing Schedule IIs must have current NCCPA certification. DEA registration required. PA may apply for emergency dispensing authority for medications prepackaged by pharmacist.

Supervision: Physician must always be available for verbal communication. Board approval required for PA utilization at remote site. Supervising physician must provide four hours of on-site supervision every two weeks.

Participation in regulation: Two PAs serve on five-member PA committee.

Oregon Board of Medical Examiners, 1500 SW First Ave., Suite 620, Portland, OR 97201; (503)229-5770 or (877)254-6263. www.bme.state.or.us

PENNSYLVANIA

Qualifications: Graduation from accredited PA program and NCCPA examination; current NCCPA certificate required for renewal. After January 1, 2004, PA must have baccalaureate or higher degree from a college or university and complete not less than 60 clock hours of didactic instruction in pharmacology or other related courses as the board may approve by regulation.

Application: By PA for license; supervising physician must register with board.

Scope of practice: Medical procedures delegated by supervising physician, within normal scope of physician's practice and within the training and expertise of the PA.

Prescribing/dispensing: PAs may prescribe and dispense drugs from formulary that excludes schedules I-II and parenterals except insulin and allergy kits. PAs who prescribe controlled medications must register with the DEA. PAs supervised by osteopathic physicians may not prescribe.

Supervision: Physician's constant physical presence not required as long as contact available through radio, telephone or telecommunication. Board approval required for satellite office. Supervising physician must review and sign medical record of patient cared for by PA within three days. If at a satellite location, supervising physician must visit location at least weekly to provide supervision.

Participation in regulation: One medical board seat reserved for, and rotates among PA, nurse practitioner, respiratory care practitioner, and nurse midwife. One PA or respiratory therapist on osteopathic board.

Pennsylvania State Board of Medicine, P.O. Box 2649, Harrisburg, PA 17105-2649; (717)783-1400.
www.dos.state.pa.us/bpoa/medbd/mainpage.htm
PA State Board of Osteopathic Medicine, same address; (717)783-4858.
www.dos.state.pa.us/bpoa/ostbd/mainpage.htm

RHODE ISLAND

Qualifications: Graduation from accredited PA program and NCCPA examination. No one holding medical degree is eligible.

Application: By PA for license.

Scope of practice: Health care services delegated by supervising physician consistent with the physician's and the PA's expertise.

Prescribing/dispensing: PAs may prescribe legend and Schedule II-V drugs. PA prescribers of controlled medications must register with state drug control office and DEA.

Supervision: Physician not required to be physically present but must be available for easy communication.

Participation in regulation: Two PAs serve on seven-member PA regulatory board.

Rhode Island Board of Licensure for Physician Assistants, Division of Health Services Regulation, Health Professionals, 3 Capitol Hill, Room #104, Providence, RI 02908-5097; (401)222-2827.
www.healthri.org/hsr/professions/phys_assist.htm

SOUTH CAROLINA

Qualifications: Graduation from accredited PA program; current NCCPA certificate required for licensure and license renewal. Must pass examination on state laws governing PA practice.

Application: By PA for license; interview of PA and supervising physician by board member required.

Scope of practice: Medical acts, tasks or functions delegated by supervising physician in written scope of practice guidelines.

Supervision: Supervising physician must be available by telecommunication. Supervising physician must be present at least 75% of the time PA is providing services; PA must have six months clinical experience with supervising physician before off-site supervision authorized; PA may not practice in any location more than 45 miles or 60 minutes from supervising physician without board approval; physician must review and initial charts of patients seen by PA when physician not present within 72 hours (board may authorize exceptions to these provisions).

Prescribing/dispensing: PA may prescribe non-controlled and Schedule V medications as delegated by supervising physician in scope of practice guidelines. PAs who prescribe controlled drugs must register with the DEA.

Participation in regulation: Three PAs serve on an eight-member PA committee.

South Carolina State Board of Medical Examiners, P.O. Box 11289, Columbia, SC 29211-1289; (803)896-4500.
www.llr.state.sc.us/pol/Medical/Default.htm

SOUTH DAKOTA

Qualifications: Graduation from an accredited PA program and NCCPA examination. State residency is also required.

Application: By PA for state license; includes copy of employment contract and personal interview. Physician interviewed in person or by telephone.

Scope of practice: PA in primary care may take histories; do physical examinations; perform routine laboratory tests, diagnostic, and therapeutic procedures; make tentative diagnoses and institute therapy; assist physician in office, hospital, and nursing homes; do x-ray studies; other tasks with board approval. PA in specialty may have similar but not identical responsibilities.

Prescribing/dispensing: PA may prescribe medication including Schedules II-V, limited to 48 hours for schedule II. PAs who prescribe controlled medication must register with the state and the DEA.

Supervision: May be by personal contact or indirect (radio or telephone). If PA utilized in satellite office, physician must provide at least half a day per week of on-site personal supervision.

Participation in regulation: Board has established PA advisory committee with three PA members.

South Dakota State Board of Medical and Osteopathic Examiners, 1323 S. Minnesota Ave., Sioux Falls, SD 57105; (605)336-1965. www.state.sd.us/doh/medical

TENNESSEE

Qualifications: Graduation from accredited PA program and NCCPA examination.

Application: By PA for license; includes name of supervising physician.

Scope of practice: Medical services delegated in writing by supervising physician and form a usual component of the physician's scope of practice.

Prescribing/dispensing: PAs may prescribe non-controlled and Schedules II-V medications. PA prescribers of controlled drugs must register with the DEA.

Supervision: Active and continuous overview, but physician not required to be physically present at all times. Physician shall review 20% of chart notes written by PA every 30 days and must visit remote site once every 30 days.

Participation in regulation: Five PAs serve on five-member PA regulatory committee.

Tennessee Physician Assistant Committee, Department of Health-Related Boards, 3rd Floor, Cordell Hull Bldg., 425 5th Ave. N., Nashville, TN 37247; (615)532-3202 or (800)778-4123. www2.state.tn.us/health/Boards/PA/index.htm

TEXAS

Qualifications: Graduation from accredited PA program and current NCCPA certification.

Application: By PA for license.

Scope of practice: Medical services delegated by the supervising physician within education, training, and experience of PA.

Supervision: Supervision shall be continuous but constant physical presence of physician not required. Establishment of office practice setting separate from that of supervising physician limited to site serving medically underserved, and physician must be on-site to provide medical direction and consultation at least once every 10 business days and randomly review and cosign at least 10% of the charts.

Prescribing/dispensing: PA may carry out or sign a prescription drug order if delegated this task under standing orders. Limited to medically underserved areas, practices with preponderance of medically indigent patients, a physician's primary practice site, hospital, location when physician is present, or an alternate site when specified conditions are met. Authority includes Schedules III-V and non-controlled medications. PAs who prescribe controlled medications must register with the DEA.

Participation in regulation: Three PAs serve on nine-member PA board.

Board of Physician Assistant Examiners, c/o Texas State Board of Medical Examiners, P.O. Box 2018, Austin, TX 78768-2018; (512)305-7022. www.tsbme.state.tx.us

UTAH

Qualifications: Graduation from accredited PA program and NCCPA examination, as well as exam on state laws and rules.

Application: By PA for license; to practice in Utah PA must have a delegation of services agreement with a Utah licensed physician.

Scope of practice: Delegated medical services within supervising physician's scope of practice, within PA's skills, and included on the delegation of services agreement.

Prescribing/dispensing: PA may prescribe schedule II-V and non-scheduled drugs. Any limitations on prescribing may be made in the delegation agreement. Prescriptions for Schedule II and III medications require chart co-signature. PAs who prescribe controlled medications must register with the DEA and hold a state-controlled substance license.

Supervision: Physician must be available for consultation by electronic means if not on site; shall co-sign sufficient number of charts to ensure patient health, safety and welfare.

Participation in regulation: One PA and one PA educator serve on seven-member PA board.

Utah Physician Assistant Licensing Board, P.O. Box 146741, Salt Lake City, UT 84114-6741; (801)530-6628. www.dopl.utah.gov

VERMONT

Qualifications: Graduation from an accredited PA program and NCCPA examination, or completion of board-approved apprenticeship program.

Application: By PA for state certification and by physician (includes employment contract and job description).

Scope of practice: Delegated medical acts within supervising physician's normal scope of practice, consistent with PA education and experience, and approved by board.

Prescribing/dispensing: PA may prescribe those drugs authorized by physician in job description. (May include legend drugs and Schedules II-V medications.) PAs who prescribe controlled medications must register with the DEA.

Supervision: Physician must be available for consultation and review. Board approval required for PA utilization in remote site.

Participation in regulation: One PA serves on medical board.

Vermont Board of Medical Practice, PO Box 70, Burlington, VT 05042-0070; (802)657-4220.

http://www.healthyvermonters.info/bmp/bmp.shtml

VIRGINIA

Qualifications: Graduation from accredited PA program and NCCPA examination; current NCCPA certificate required for renewal.

Application: By PA for license; prior to practice, PA and physician submit description of practice.

Scope of practice: Medical care services delegated by supervising physician, within physician's scope of practice, and approved by the board. Physician must see patient on follow-up visit if condition has not improved and must see patient with continuing illness at least every fourth visit.

Prescribing/dispensing: PAs may prescribe non-controlled drugs and devices and Schedules III-V controlled drugs. PAs who prescribe controlled substances must register with the DEA.

Supervision: Continuous supervision, but supervising physician not required to be present; physician must review PA record of services proportionate to acuity of care and practice setting.

Participation in regulation: Three PAs serve on five-member Advisory Board.

Virginia State Board of Medicine: 6603 W. Broad St., 5th Floor, Richmond, VA 23230-1712; (804) 662-9908.

www.dhp.state.va.us/medicine/default.htm

WASHINGTON

Qualifications: Graduation from accredited PA program and NCCPA examination. PA supervised by osteopathic physician must be a graduate of a board-approved PA program; current NCCPA certification necessary for Rx privileges.

Application: By PA for license. Practice arrangement plan must be filed with the board.

Scope of practice: Medical services delegated by supervising physician and approved by board.

Prescribing/dispensing: PAs may write and sign prescriptions, including controlled substances in Schedule II-V. PAs who prescribe controlled medications must register with the DEA. Osteopathic PAs supervised by osteopathic physicians may prescribe controlled substances in Schedules III-V.

Supervision: Physician not required to be physically present where PA services are rendered. Board approval required for PA utilization in remote site. Osteopathic PAs: chart review within one week.

Participation in regulation: Two PAs serve on medical quality assurance commission.

Washington State Department of Health, Health Professions Quality Assurance, PO Box 47865, Olympia, WA 98504-7865; (360)236-4700.

https://fortress.wa.gov/doh/hpqa1/HPS5/Medical/default.htm

WEST VIRGINIA

Qualifications: Graduation from accredited PA program and NCCPA examination. Bachelor's or master's degree required after 7/1/94.

Application: By PA for license; by supervising physician for approval to supervise (includes job description).

Scope of practice: Medical procedures delegated by supervising physician, within physician's normal scope of practice, included on PA's job description, and approved by the board.

Prescribing/dispensing: PAs with 2 years of experience who have completed board-approved pharmacology course and maintain NCCPA certification may prescribe controlled (Schedules III-V) and non-controlled drugs from formulary. Schedule IIs limited to 72-hour supply. Schedules IV-V limited to 90 dosage units or 30 days. Other drugs not to exceed 6-month supply. Registration with the DEA required. PA may dispense samples and, under certain conditions, legend drugs.

Supervision: Physician's constant physical presence not required provided consultation available by radio, telephone, or telecommunication.

Participation in regulation: One PA serves on medical board.

West Virginia Board of Medicine, 101 Dee Drive, Suite 103, Charleston, WV 25311; (304)558-2921.

www.wvdhhr.org/wvbom

West Virginia State Board of Osteopathy, 334 Penco Road, Weirton, WV 26062; (304)723-4638.

www.wvbdosteo.org

WISCONSIN

Qualifications: Graduation from accredited PA program and current NCCPA certification.

Application: By PA for license.

Scope of practice: Patient services include taking histories; doing physical examinations, routine diagnostic studies, and therapeutic procedures; counseling; monitoring treatment and therapy plans; referrals; and assisting the physician in a hospital or other facility.

Prescribing/dispensing: PA may prescribe Schedule II-V and non-controlled drugs in situations specified in written guidelines developed by supervising physician. Guidelines must be reviewed annually. Supervising physician must sign patient record within 72 hours, review patient record within 72 hours or review by telephone within 48 hours, and sign patient record within one week. PA prescribers of controlled medications must register with the DEA.

Supervision: Physician must be available at all times for consultation either in person or within 15 minutes of contact by telephone, two-way radio, or television. Physician must visit and review on-site any facilities attended by PA at least once a month.

Participation in regulation: Three PAs serve on five-member advisory council.

Wisconsin Medical Examining Board, P.O. Box 8935, Madison, WI 53708-8935; (608)266-2112. http://drl.wi.gov/prof/phya/def.htm

WYOMING

Qualifications: Graduation from accredited PA program and current NCCPA certification.

Application: By PA for license; by physician for approval to supervise.

Scope of practice: Medical services delegated by supervising physician and approved by the board in the specialty area(s) for which physician and PA are trained or experienced.

Prescribing/dispensing: Physicians may delegate prescribing of non-controlled and Schedules II-V medications to PAs; also dispensing of prepackaged medications in rural areas when pharmacy services unavailable. PAs must register with the DEA if they prescribe controlled medications.

Supervision: Physician must be readily available for consultation, in person or by telecommunication.

Participation in regulation: One PA serves on medical board. Two PAs serve on four-member advisory committee.

Wyoming Board of Medical Examiners, 211 W. 19th St., 2nd Floor, Colony Bldg., Cheyenne, WY 82002; (307)778-7053.
http://wyomedboard.state.wy.us

GLOSSARY

A

Absolute An idealistic term used to describe independent reality; all thought is absolutely good or absolutely bad

Abstract A term used to describe that which is real, but without spatial or temporal properties

Altruism Service to others, or the greater good over one's self-interest or benefit

Ambiguity Having multiple meanings

Analysis The process of breaking down a concept to its basic components

Antinomianism Ethical action determined independently of law or rules

Applied ethics Medical (and other) ethical concepts that have application

A priori Independent of experience

Argument Statements that support (or give reason for) a conclusion

Autonomy Freedom to choose or to make decisions

Axiom A statement, proposition, or principle accepted as true

B

Behaviorism A belief that observable action is key to understanding mental phenomena

Belief That which is accepted as true

Beneficence The promotion of the well-being of others

Biomedical ethics The study of ethical issues that arise in the practice of medicine and biomedical research

C

Cardinal virtues Practical wisdom (prudence), courage, temperance, justice

Casuistry An analytical approach to interpreting moral rules

Causality The relationship between events whereby one leads to another (succession)

Causation The relationship between cause and effect

Common good A standard from which all members of a defined community will benefit

Competency Being qualified and having the capacity to handle legal affairs

Confidentiality Maintaining a secret; being entrusted with the confidence of another

Confucianism Chinese school of thought founded by Confucius, which presents moral, ethical, and political teachings

Contextualism The belief that justification of events is judged within their context

Covenant A solemn agreement between two or more parties

Criterion A condition

D

Deconstruction Proof of the error in a philosophical concept or position

Deduction Reasoning from general concepts to specifics; applying theory to specific situations

Definition Meaning of a work, idea, concept, theory, etc.

Deontology Belief in an unchanging moral obligation of rights and duty; a moral duty without regard for consequences

Dignity Moral status attributed to a person

Dissonance Discomfort or distress caused by conflicting beliefs held by an individual

Doctrine A system of beliefs

Dualism Belief that reality has disparate components; the mental and physical have different fundamental natures

E

Egalitarian A social philosophy that advocates human equality

Egoism In any view, the self as central to that view

Empiric Relying on experience; based in experience

Epistemology The study to understand knowledge; what is meant by knowledge; the study of the origin, extent, and nature of knowledge; the study of what people know, its extent and limits

Ethics A set of values; concept(s) of what is right and wrong; rules/concepts to evaluate human actions/behavior; a system of beliefs that guide behavior

Existentialism Human existence explains its characteristics; existence provides the choices that define that existence

F

Fallibilism Belief that absolute certainty about knowledge is impossible

Fatalism Belief that "what will be, will be" regardless of one's deliberations or actions

Fidelity Faithfulness to one's obligations or duties

H

Hedonism The belief that the intrinsic good in life is pleasure; pleasure drives the human and is the highest goal

Heuristics Using rules, guidelines, and processes to problem solve; reducing problems and complexities by rules; a way of reasoning/problem solving

I

Ideology A set of beliefs; a body of thought that provides guidance

Induction Reasoning from specific concepts to generalization; using an observation to form a theory or conclusion

Inference Drawing conclusions from that which best explains; coming to a conclusion based on one's experience/knowledge

Informed consent A legal and professional concept that allows an individual (patient) the freedom to make an informed choice or decision

J

Justice Fair and equal treatment; the right to have what is due

L

Legalism An ethical action in strict conformity to law or rules

Libertarianism Advocating the maximization of individual rights and minimizing the role of the state

M

Macroallocation Distribution of resources on a large scale

Meaning The sense of a verbal or nonverbal construct; that which is signified and understood

Metaethics The branch of ethics dealing with the meaning and justification of ethical terms and norms

Metaphor When a figure of speech that means one thing is used to illustrate another

Morality Cultural or societal rules/principles/concepts that guide/govern/regulate the behavior/actions of the group's members; usually based in some belief system of right or wrong and/or what is good or bad

N

Nihilism View that human existence is without essential value, purpose, and meaning

Nonmaleficence To deliberately not harm

Normativism The doctrine that moral standards or norms determine the rightness or wrongness of actions

P

Paradigm A construct; a framework; a set of rules/theories/concepts, etc.; a pattern; a model

Paradox An apparent truth that leads to a contradiction; a counterintuitive truth; something that seems one way but is another and perhaps an opposite

Paternalism Treating a person like a child to promote his or her well-being but against his or her advice, knowledge, or wishes

Phenomenon An observable event; something that can be observed; that which can be recorded by the senses

Philosophy The study of beliefs/truths/meaning; a doctrine; guidance for living; personal or group beliefs; study of the nature of existence; etc.

Positivism Only scientific knowledge is authentic/real knowledge

Pragmatism Belief that consequences, utility, and practicality define truth

Praxis A concept of putting ideas/thought into action; to put into practice; a cycle of thought-action-reflection-action, etc.

Principle A basic truth, law, or assumption

Professional ethics A code of conduct for a defined group of practitioners who identify themselves as "professionals"

R

Rationalism The belief that reason is the path to truth or the best method of discovery; reason is truth

Reductionism The belief that the complex can be reduced to simple/fundamental phenomena/explanation/theory/meaning

S

Secular ethics Theories of right or wrong based on other than religious doctrine

Situationalism Ethical actions based on and guided by each situation but not directly determined by rules

Solipsism The belief that only one's experience is reality; no one exists but oneself; belief that it is impossible to know another's self

T

Teleology The belief that there is purpose in everything; study of evidence in nature; doctrine of final purpose

Transcendentalism Belief in an ideal spiritual state that "transcends" the physical and empirical and that is perceived by individual intuition

Truth In conformance with reality; reality

U

Utilitarianism Belief/theory that an action is morally right only if it produces more good for people than any alternative action; greatest good for the greatest number

V

Veracity Truthfulness; adherence to the truth

Virtue Moral excellence or righteousness

Voluntariness An act undertaken by one's own free will and without expectation of reward

INDEX

Page numbers followed by "b" denote boxes

Touching, 50
Training. *See* Medical training; PA training
Transference, 116
Transparency model, 55
Transplants, 171–172
Treatment
  life-sustaining, withdrawal of, 30, 147
  PA's role in, 131–132, 134–135
  refusal of, 129–132, 146–147, 164
  spiritual principles included in, 169–170
  withholding of, 30, 147, 154
Triage, 109
Trust
  description of, 46–47, 47b
  empathy and, 44
  end-of-life care and, 148–149
  medical errors and, 53
Truth telling
  description of, 51–53, 128
  end-of-life care and, 148
  informed consent and, 54
Tuskegee Syphilis Study, 32–33

U

Unequal Treatment: Confronting Racial and Ethnic Disparities in Health Care, 112
Unprofessional conduct, 191–194
Utah, 181b, 209
Utilitarianism, 23–24

V

Values
  conflict of, 130–131, 133–134
  key. *See* Key values

purpose of, 131
religious, 131, 134, 137
Vermont, 181b, 209–210
Vices, 39–40
Virginia, 181b, 210
Virtue(s)
  benevolence, 44–45
  compassion, 134
  courage, 42–43
  definition of, 39
  early childhood experiences and, 39
  empathy, 44
  honesty, 39
  humility, 43–44
  integrity, 40–41, 47
  justice. *See* Justice
  necessity of, 40
  prudence, 45–46
  respect, 41–42
  trust, 46–47
  truth telling, 51–53
Virtue ethics, 22, 24
Vulnerability of patient
  description of, 38
  sexual issues, 49–50

W

Washington, 181b, 210
West Virginia, 181b, 210
Wisconsin, 181b, 210–211
Withdrawing of life-sustaining treatment, 30, 147
Withholding of treatment, 30, 147, 154
Wyoming, 181b, 211